# The Prevention and Treatment of Atherosclerosis

# The Prevention and Treatment of Atherosclerosis

Editor

**Anna Kabłak-Ziembicka**

MDPI • Basel • Beijing • Wuhan • Barcelona • Belgrade • Manchester • Tokyo • Cluj • Tianjin

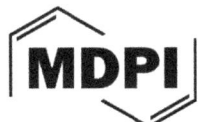

*Editor*
Anna Kabłak-Ziembicka
The John Paul II Hospital
Poland

*Editorial Office*
MDPI
St. Alban-Anlage 66
4052 Basel, Switzerland

This is a reprint of articles from the Special Issue published online in the open access journal *Journal of Clinical Medicine* (ISSN 2077-0383) (available at: https://www.mdpi.com/journal/jcm/special_issues/prevention_and_treatment_of_atherosclerosis).

For citation purposes, cite each article independently as indicated on the article page online and as indicated below:

LastName, A.A.; LastName, B.B.; LastName, C.C. Article Title. *Journal Name* **Year**, *Volume Number*, Page Range.

**ISBN 978-3-0365-3465-7 (Hbk)**
**ISBN 978-3-0365-3466-4 (PDF)**

© 2022 by the authors. Articles in this book are Open Access and distributed under the Creative Commons Attribution (CC BY) license, which allows users to download, copy and build upon published articles, as long as the author and publisher are properly credited, which ensures maximum dissemination and a wider impact of our publications.
The book as a whole is distributed by MDPI under the terms and conditions of the Creative Commons license CC BY-NC-ND.

# Contents

**About the Editor** . . . . . . . . . . . . . . . . . . . . . . . . . . . . . . . . . . . vii

**Anna Kabłak-Ziembicka**
Special Issue "The Prevention and Treatment of Atherosclerosis"
Reprinted from: *J. Clin. Med.* **2022**, *11*, 1023, doi:10.3390/jcm11041023 . . . . . . . . . . . . . . . 1

**Fernando Sabatel-Pérez, Joaquín Sánchez-Prieto, Víctor Manuel Becerra-Muñoz, Juan Horacio Alonso-Briales, Pedro Mata and Luis Rodríguez-Padial**
Improving Familial Hypercholesterolemia Index Case Detection: Sequential Active Screening from Centralized Analytical Data
Reprinted from: *J. Clin. Med.* **2021**, *10*, 749, doi:10.3390/jcm10040749 . . . . . . . . . . . . . . . 5

**Tiago Pereira-da-Silva, Patrícia Napoleão, Marina C. Costa, André F. Gabriel, Mafalda Selas, Filipa Silva, Francisco J. Enguita, Rui Cruz Ferreira and Miguel Mota Carmo**
Cigarette Smoking, miR-27b Downregulation, and Peripheral Artery Disease: Insights into the Mechanisms of Smoking Toxicity
Reprinted from: *J. Clin. Med.* **2021**, *10*, 890, doi:10.3390/jcm10040890 . . . . . . . . . . . . . . . 17

**Ovidiu Mitu, Adrian Crisan, Simon Redwood, Ioan-Elian Cazacu-Davidescu, Ivona Mitu, Irina-Iuliana Costache, Viviana Onofrei, Radu-Stefan Miftode, Alexandru-Dan Costache, Cristian Mihai Stefan Haba and Florin Mitu**
The Relationship between Cardiovascular Risk Scores and Several Markers of Subclinical Atherosclerosis in an Asymptomatic Population
Reprinted from: *J. Clin. Med.* **2021**, *10*, 955, doi:10.3390/jcm10050955 . . . . . . . . . . . . . . . 31

**Keishi Ichikawa, Toru Miyoshi, Kazuhiro Osawa, Takashi Miki and Hiroshi Ito**
Increased Circulating Malondialdehyde-Modified Low-Density Lipoprotein Level Is Associated with High-Risk Plaque in Coronary Computed Tomography Angiography in Patients Receiving Statin Therapy
Reprinted from: *J. Clin. Med.* **2021**, *10*, 1480, doi:10.3390/jcm10071480 . . . . . . . . . . . . . . . 43

**Jakub Baran, Paweł Kleczyński, Łukasz Niewiara, Jakub Podolec, Rafał Badacz, Andrzej Gackowski, Piotr Pieniążek, Jacek Legutko, Krzysztof Żmudka, Tadeusz Przewłocki and Anna Kabłak-Ziembicka**
Importance of Increased Arterial Resistance in Risk Prediction in Patients with Cardiovascular Risk Factors and Degenerative Aortic Stenosis
Reprinted from: *J. Clin. Med.* **2021**, *10*, 2109, doi:10.3390/jcm10102109 . . . . . . . . . . . . . . . 53

**Krzysztof Bryniarski, Pawel Gasior, Jacek Legutko, Dawid Makowicz, Anna Kedziora, Piotr Szolc, Leszek Bryniarski, Pawel Kleczynski and Ik-Kyung Jang**
OCT Findings in MINOCA
Reprinted from: *J. Clin. Med.* **2021**, *10*, 2759, doi:10.3390/jcm10132759 . . . . . . . . . . . . . . . 63

**Dorota Formanowicz, Jacek B. Krawczyk, Bartłomiej Perek, Dawid Lipski and Andrzej Tykarski**
Management of High-Risk Atherosclerotic Patients by Statins May Be Supported by Logistic Model of Intima-Media Thickening
Reprinted from: *J. Clin. Med.* **2021**, *10*, 2876, doi:10.3390/jcm10132876 . . . . . . . . . . . . . . . 73

**Michał Ząbczyk, Joanna Natorska and Anetta Undas**
Fibrin Clot Properties in Atherosclerotic Vascular Disease: From Pathophysiology to Clinical Outcomes
Reprinted from: *J. Clin. Med.* **2021**, *10*, 2999, doi:10.3390/jcm10132999 . . . . . . . . . . . . . . . . **87**

**Anna Kabłak-Ziembicka and Tadeusz Przewłocki**
Clinical Significance of Carotid Intima-Media Complex and Carotid Plaque Assessment by Ultrasound for the Prediction of Adverse Cardiovascular Events in Primary and Secondary Care Patients
Reprinted from: *J. Clin. Med.* **2021**, *10*, 4628, doi:10.3390/jcm10204628 . . . . . . . . . . . . . . . . **103**

**Ewelina A. Dziedzic, William B. Grant, Izabela Sowińska, Marek Dąbrowski and Piotr Jankowski**
Small Differences in Vitamin D Levels between Male Cardiac Patients in Different Stages of Coronary Artery Disease
Reprinted from: *J. Clin. Med.* **2022**, *11*, 779, doi:10.3390/jcm11030779 . . . . . . . . . . . . . . . . **129**

# About the Editor

**Anna Kabłak-Ziembicka** M.D, Ph.D., is Professor for Cardiology and General Medicine at the Department of Interventional Cardiology, Jagiellonian University Medical College and the John Paul II Hospital (Kraków, Poland). She works as a consultant, an academic teacher, and a supervisor of research projects at the Jagiellonian University. She has graduated at the Medical University of Lodz. She has attended the ERASMUS programme at the Medical University of Padua (Italy), and the elective attachments at St. George's Hospital Medical School and the Royal Marsden Hospital (London, U.K.). Postgraduate training includes stays at the Cardiology Department (HerzZentrum, Berlin, Germany), and the Edinburgh Summer School in Clinical Education and the Royal Infirmary Hospital (Edinburgh, U.K.). The PhD thesis on the 'Carotid arteries assessment in patients with coronary artery disease' (2003) was awarded by the Prize of Aurelia Baczko Foundation by the Society for Science Support and Propagation (Warsaw University).She participated in four research grants funded by the Polish Ministry of Science and Higher Education. She contributed to the 'PROG-IMT Study Group' lead by Professor Matthias Lorenz (the Goethe University, Frankfurt) in years 2010-2020.Her research focusses on the relationship between the inflammatory and non-inflammatory biomarkers (such as carotid intima-media thickness, vascular stiffness) and cardiovascular risk factors, atherosclerosis progression, and adverse cardiovascular events; the associations of the serum biomarkers (microRNAs, cytokines) with cardiovascular mortality and morbidity. Further scientific interests include the impact of pharmacological and endovascular interventions in patients with coronary and extra coronary athero-occlusive disease on the outcomes; the management of degenerative aortic valve stenosis, gender-specific alterations of atherosclerosis, and the therapeutic implications of the multi-territorial atherosclerotic occlusive disease.Presently, her scientific portfolio includes 210 scientific original papers and congress presentations published in the international peer-reviewed journals in the field of basic and clinical cardiology and cardiovascular disease indexed in the Journal Citation Reports, and 32 book chapters. Current h-index is 20.

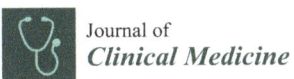

*Editorial*

# Special Issue "The Prevention and Treatment of Atherosclerosis"

Anna Kabłak-Ziembicka [1,2]

1 Department of Interventional Cardiology, Institute of Cardiology, Jagiellonian University Medical College, 31-008 Kraków, Poland; kablakziembicka@op.pl
2 John Paul II Hospital, Prądnicka 80, 31-202 Kraków, Poland

Citation: Kabłak-Ziembicka, A. Special Issue "The Prevention and Treatment of Atherosclerosis". *J. Clin. Med.* 2022, 11, 1023. https://doi.org/10.3390/jcm11041023

Received: 10 February 2022
Accepted: 15 February 2022
Published: 16 February 2022

**Publisher's Note:** MDPI stays neutral with regard to jurisdictional claims in published maps and institutional affiliations.

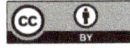

**Copyright:** © 2022 by the author. Licensee MDPI, Basel, Switzerland. This article is an open access article distributed under the terms and conditions of the Creative Commons Attribution (CC BY) license (https://creativecommons.org/licenses/by/4.0/).

This editorial summarizes the 10 scientific papers that contributed to the Special Issue of the *Journal of Clinical Medicine*: 'The Prevention and Treatment of Atherosclerosis'.

Papers published in this Special Issue focused on the biomarkers of cardiovascular diseases and atherosclerosis-associated risk factors and comorbidities.

Arterial properties such as vascular stiffness, carotid intima-media complex thickening (CIMT), and plaque formation are important, as non-traditional cardiovascular risk factors associated with risk of fatal and non-fatal cardiovascular events such as myocardial infarction, stroke, and heart failure episodes. Four papers addressed this clinically relevant problem [1–4].

In a cohort group of 404 patients with cardiovascular risk factors, including 267 patients with moderate-to-severe degenerative aortic valve stenosis, increased values of vascular stiffness (i.e., resistive and pulsatile indices) were associated with 21% to 25% risk increase of heart-failure episodes and major adverse cardiac and cerebral events at 2.5 years follow-up [1].

Formanowicz et al. proposed, based on the self-constructed logistic model of the growth of CIMT, that the optimal patient age for starting the statin treatment is when the CIMT growth curve is at its steepest part on the S-shape curve. Such an approach would allow to prevent CIMT from further thickening, hopefully preventing adverse cardiovascular events [2]. This is in line with the conception of the non-linear CIMT growth, with periods of attenuated and rapid progression described in the review paper of this Special Issue [3]. CIMT, once the measurement approach is unified, is a promising tool to assess the cardiovascular risk in both primary and secondary care patients [3]. Furthermore, markers of subclinical atherosclerosis, including CIMT, pulse wave velocity, aortic and brachial augmentation indexes, and aortic systolic blood pressure, all are associated with four main CV risk scores: SCORE, Framingham, QRISK, and PROCAM in the asymptomatic population [4].

Statin therapy was also addressed in the study by Ichikawa et al., who evaluated the association of serum malondialdehyde low-density lipoprotein (MDA-LDL), an oxidatively modified LDL, with the prevalence of high-risk plaques determined with coronary computed tomography angiography (CTA) in statin-treated patients [5]. The authors of this publication found that a high serum MDA-LDL level is an independent predictor of CTA-verified high-risk plaques, which, despite statin treatment, can lead to cardiovascular events [5].

Similarly, in a very elegant review paper, features of high-risk plaques were addressed in patients with myocardial infarction but non-obstructive coronary artery disease [6]. This condition, despite a lack of stenotic and occlusive lesions in the culprit coronary artery, is associated with a high mortality rate, varying between 2.2% and 3.9% at 12 months follow-up [6]. Due to the high resolution of optical coherence tomography (OCT), OCT displays plaques with high-risk features, such as erosion, thin fibrous cap, ruptured, or large lipid core, as well as enabling to differ between plaque disruption, spontaneous coronary artery dissection, coronary artery spasm, and coronary thromboembolism, which can drive optimal management focused on reducing the morbidity and mortality in that subset of patients [6].

Atherosclerosis is not solely a lipid condition but is also a consequence of local blood coagulation activation that takes place inside atherosclerotic lesions and contributes to their growth. The imbalance between thrombin-mediated fibrin formation and fibrin degradation might enhance atherosclerosis in relation to inflammatory states reflected by increased fibrinogen concentrations, the key determinant of fibrin characteristics [7]. As evidenced, the formation of a dense fibrin structure, which is resistant to lysis, increases patients' risk of atherosclerosis progression and thromboembolic events. Many traditional cardiovascular risk factors, including hyperlipidemia, hypertension, smoking, and diabetes, are associated with altered fibrin clot properties [7]. Active treatment of cardiovascular risk factors increases the fibrin clot permeability and facilitates its lysis [7].

Authors of the next paper searched for the mechanisms of smoking toxicity in patients with peripheral arterial disease (PAD) [8]. Their data suggest that a downregulation of miR-27b mediates the proatherogenic effects of cigarette smoking on the incidence and severity of PAD, which may be attenuated by smoking cessation [8].

Sabatel-Perez et al. presented their strategy for improving familial hypercholesterolemia (FH) detection through the centralized analytical database, which can increase the diagnostic percentage of FH from 5.3% before to 12.2% after the screening strategy was applied [9]. The early detection of FH is important to start and optimize treatment, which greatly reduces the risk of atherosclerotic cardiovascular disease, and perform family-based cascade screening [9].

Finally, the very fashionable topic of vitamin D deficiency, which in the worldwide population may have multiple effects on the cardiovascular system, was explored [10]. The authors found low levels of vitamin D in patients without significant changes within the coronary arteries, and even lower vitamin D levels in patients with single-, double-, or triple-vessel coronary artery disease [10]. Severe (<10 ng/mL) and moderate vitamin D deficiency ($\geq$10 to <20 ng/mL) were observed in 74% of patients with significant coronary artery disease [10].

Overall, these 10 contributions published in this Special Issue further strengthen the relationship between subclinical atherosclerosis, imaging and serum biomarkers, mechanisms of atherosclerosis progression and evolution, and incidence of adverse cardiovascular events.

**Funding:** This research was funded by the Jagiellonian University Medical College, grant number N41/DBS/000752.

**Conflicts of Interest:** The authors declare no conflict of interest.

## References

1. Baran, J.; Kleczyński, P.; Niewiara, Ł.; Podolec, J.; Badacz, R.; Gackowski, A.; Pieniążek, P.; Legutko, J.; Żmudka, K.; Przewłocki, T.; et al. Importance of Increased Arterial Resistance in Risk Prediction in Patients with Cardiovascular Risk Factors and Degenerative Aortic Stenosis. *J. Clin. Med.* **2021**, *10*, 2109. [CrossRef] [PubMed]
2. Formanowicz, D.; Krawczyk, J.B.; Perek, B.; Lipski, D.; Tykarski, A. Management of High-Risk Atherosclerotic Patients by Statins May Be Supported by Logistic Model of Intima-Media Thickening. *J. Clin. Med.* **2021**, *10*, 2876. [CrossRef] [PubMed]
3. Kabłak-Ziembicka, A.; Przewłocki, T. Clinical Significance of Carotid Intima-Media Complex and Carotid Plaque Assessment by Ultrasound for the Prediction of Adverse Cardiovascular Events in Primary and Secondary Care Patients. *J. Clin. Med.* **2021**, *10*, 4628. [CrossRef] [PubMed]
4. Mitu, O.; Crisan, A.; Redwood, S.; Cazacu-Davidescu, I.-E.; Mitu, I.; Costache, I.-I.; Onofrei, V.; Miftode, R.-S.; Costache, A.-D.; Haba, C.M.S.; et al. The Relationship between Cardiovascular Risk Scores and Several Markers of Subclinical Atherosclerosis in an Asymptomatic Population. *J. Clin. Med.* **2021**, *10*, 955. [CrossRef] [PubMed]
5. Ichikawa, K.; Miyoshi, T.; Osawa, K.; Miki, T.; Ito, H. Increased Circulating Malondialdehyde-Modified Low-Density Lipoprotein Level Is Associated with High-Risk Plaque in Coronary Computed Tomography Angiography in Patients Receiving Statin Therapy. *J. Clin. Med.* **2021**, *10*, 1480. [CrossRef] [PubMed]

6. Bryniarski, K.; Gasior, P.; Legutko, J.; Makowicz, D.; Kedziora, A.; Szolc, P.; Bryniarski, L.; Kleczynski, P.; Jang, I.-K. OCT Findings in MINOCA. *J. Clin. Med.* **2021**, *10*, 2759. [CrossRef] [PubMed]
7. Ząbczyk, M.; Natorska, J.; Undas, A. Fibrin Clot Properties in Atherosclerotic Vascular Disease: From Pathophysiology to Clinical Outcomes. *J. Clin. Med.* **2021**, *10*, 2999. [CrossRef] [PubMed]
8. Pereira-da-Silva, T.; Napoleão, P.; Costa, M.C.; Gabriel, A.F.; Selas, M.; Silva, F.; Enguita, F.J.; Ferreira, R.C.; Carmo, M.M. Cigarette Smoking, miR-27b Downregulation, and Peripheral Artery Disease: Insights into the Mechanisms of Smoking Toxicity. *J. Clin. Med.* **2021**, *10*, 890. [CrossRef] [PubMed]
9. Sabatel-Pérez, F.; Sánchez-Prieto, J.; Becerra-Muñoz, V.M.; Alonso-Briales, J.H.; Mata, P.; Rodríguez-Padial, L. Improving Familial Hypercholesterolemia Index Case Detection: Sequential Active Screening from Centralized Analytical Data. *J. Clin. Med.* **2021**, *10*, 749. [CrossRef] [PubMed]
10. Dziedzic, E.A.; Grant, W.B.; Sowińska, I.; Dąbrowski, M.; Jankowski, P. Small Differences in Vitamin D Levels between Male Cardiac Patients in Different Stages of Coronary Artery Disease. *J. Clin. Med.* **2022**, *11*, 779. [CrossRef] [PubMed]

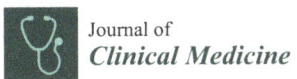 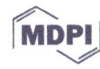

*Article*

# Improving Familial Hypercholesterolemia Index Case Detection: Sequential Active Screening from Centralized Analytical Data

Fernando Sabatel-Pérez [1,2,*], Joaquín Sánchez-Prieto [1], Víctor Manuel Becerra-Muñoz [2], Juan Horacio Alonso-Briales [2], Pedro Mata [3] and Luis Rodríguez-Padial [1]

[1] Department of Cardiology, Complejo Hospitalario Universitario de Toledo, 45004 Toledo, Spain; joaquinsanchezprieto@gmail.com (J.S.-P.); lrpadial@gmail.com (L.R.-P.)
[2] Unidad de Gestión Clínica Área del Corazón, Instituto de Investigación Biomédica de Málaga (IBIMA), Hospital Universitario Virgen de la Victoria de Málaga, Universidad de Málaga (UMA), Centro de Investigación Biomédica en Red de Enfermedades Cardiovasculares (CIBERCV), 29010 Málaga, Spain; vmbecerram@gmail.com (V.M.B.-M.); juanhalonso62@gmail.com (J.H.A.-B.)
[3] Fundación Hipercolesterolemia Familiar, 28010 Madrid, Spain; pmata@colesterolfamiliar.org
* Correspondence: fernandosabatelperez@gmail.com

**Citation:** Sabatel-Pérez, F.; Sánchez-Prieto, J.; Becerra-Muñoz, V.M.; Alonso-Briales, J.H.; Mata, P.; Rodríguez-Padial, L. Improving Familial Hypercholesterolemia Index Case Detection: Sequential Active Screening from Centralized Analytical Data. *J. Clin. Med.* **2021**, *10*, 749. https://doi.org/10.3390/jcm10040749

Academic Editor: Anna Kabłak-Ziembicka

Received: 17 January 2021
Accepted: 9 February 2021
Published: 13 February 2021

**Publisher's Note:** MDPI stays neutral with regard to jurisdictional claims in published maps and institutional affiliations.

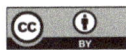

**Copyright:** © 2021 by the authors. Licensee MDPI, Basel, Switzerland. This article is an open access article distributed under the terms and conditions of the Creative Commons Attribution (CC BY) license (https://creativecommons.org/licenses/by/4.0/).

**Abstract:** The majority of familial hypercholesterolemia index cases (FH-IC) remain underdiagnosed and undertreated because there are no well-defined strategies for the universal detection of FH. The aim of this study was to evaluate the diagnostic yield of an active screening for FH-IC based on centralized analytical data. From 2016 to 2019, a clinical screening of FH was performed on 469 subjects with severe hypercholesterolemia (low-density lipoprotein cholesterol ≥220 mg/dL), applying the Dutch Lipid Clinic Network (DLCN) criteria. All patients with a DLCN ≥ 6 were genetically tested, as were 10 patients with a DLCN of 3–5 points to compare the diagnostic yield between the two groups. FH was genetically confirmed in 57 of the 84 patients with DLCN ≥ 6, with a genetic diagnosis rate of 67.9% and an overall prevalence of 12.2% (95% confidence interval: 9.3% to 15.5%). Before inclusion in the study, only 36.8% (n = 21) of the patients with the FH mutation had been clinically diagnosed with FH; after genetic screening, FH detection increased 2.3-fold ($p < 0.001$). The sequential, active screening strategy for FH-IC increases the diagnostic yield for FH with a rational use of the available resources, which may facilitate the implementation of FH universal and family-based cascade screening strategies.

**Keywords:** familial hypercholesterolemia; genetic screening; atherosclerosis prevention; early detection

## 1. Introduction

Familial hypercholesterolemia (FH) is the genetic disorder most frequently associated with premature atherosclerotic cardiovascular disease (ASCVD) [1] due to lifelong elevated levels of low-density lipoprotein cholesterol (LDL-C). Its prevalence in the general population ranges from 1 in every 200 to 300 individuals [2–5]. It has an autosomal dominant transmission pattern whose causative mutations are mainly in the *LDL receptor* gene (*LDL-R*) and, less frequently, mutations in the *apolipoprotein B* (*APOB*) and *proprotein convertase subtilisin/kexin type 9* (*PCSK9*) genes.

Clinical diagnosis of FH is based on clinical and analytical criteria, of which the most widely used and recommended are the Dutch Lipid Clinic Network (DLCN) criteria [6,7], as they have been validated with genetic diagnosis [8,9]. Genetic study is the gold standard for confirming FH, and it is necessary once the clinical diagnosis is probable or definite [10]. FH is markedly related to the development of ASCVD [11,12] with up to 22-fold increased risk compared to the general population [13–15]. Therefore, early detection is essential to both start and optimize treatment, which drastically reduces the risk of ASCVD [16–19], and perform family-based cascade screening. Despite international recommendations in

FH clinical and genetic diagnosis [10], the main problem is the lack of clearly defined screening strategies for the identification of FH index cases in the general population, as well as insufficient genetic test availability [20]. This is why diagnosis is currently performed either after the development of clinical ASCVD or after the fortuitous detection of abnormally high LDL-C levels. Consequently, the majority of patients with FH remain underdiagnosed and undertreated [21].

The aim of this study was to evaluate the genetic diagnostic yield of a sequential, active screening of FH index cases in a population with severe hypercholesterolemia (HCL), based on centralized analytical data, to perform clinical and genetic family-based cascade screening. This screening strategy can contribute to changing how this severe disease is currently detected in Spain.

## 2. Materials and Methods

*2.1. Population Study and Clinical Diagnostic Criteria for Familial Hypercholesterolemia*

We conducted a selective, single-phase, active screening of patients aged ≥18 years with severe HCL, defined as total cholesterol ≥ 290 mg/dL, LDL-C ≥ 220 mg/dL, and triglycerides (TG) ≤ 200 mg/dL, the recommended values at which to start FH screening [7]. Analytical records from both primary and hospital care settings of the whole health area, which are centralized in the Biochemical Laboratory of the Hospital Complex, were reviewed. All samples with the stated profile for the years 2013, 2014, and 2015 were selected. Health professionals not connected with our study had previously requested the biochemical analyses for a variety of reasons. Blood samples were extracted after fasting, and LDL-C levels were calculated using the Friedewald formula [22]. A sample of saliva was taken for genetic testing. The lipid-lowering treatment (LLT) of each patient and their adherence to it was analyzed before inclusion in the study, with LDL-C levels adjusted according to Masana's correction [23], as long as the patient was correctly following the treatment. Maximal lipid-lowering therapy was defined as any LLT that reduces LDL-C levels ≥50% [24].

Demographic and clinical variables, age, classic cardiovascular risk factors, and physical examination were included. We considered ASVCD whenever medical records included a clinical diagnosis of non-thromboembolic stroke, peripheral artery disease (PAD), or ischemic heart disease, both stable and acute coronary syndrome (ACS).

All patients consecutively underwent a medical assessment from December 2016 to March 2019 and were classified following DLCN criteria [25]. These criteria assign a score according to LDL-C levels, family history of HCL in children and/or parents (of the index case), history of premature ASCVD in the index case and/or family members, and the presence of tendon xanthoma or corneal arcus in a person <45 years (Table S1). Consistent with the score obtained, the diagnosis of FH may be possible (3–5 points), probable (6–7 points), or definite (≥8 points). We excluded subjects with a secondary cause of HCL (uncontrolled thyroid condition, HIV on antiretroviral therapy, nephrotic syndrome, end stage chronic kidney disease, uncontrolled diabetes, combined hyperlipidemia, and hepatobiliary diseases), the deceased, subjects with a diagnosis of terminal illness, anyone who refused to participate in the study, and those who were impossible to contact.

This study was approved by the Ethics Committee of the Complejo Hospitalario de Toledo (16 June 2016) and conducted in compliance with the Declaration of Helsinki recommendations for medical research involving human subjects. All of the patients who participated signed informed consent for the purposes contemplated in legislation current at the time the study began.

*2.2. Genetic Testing*

The genetic testing was performed using the Lipid inCode® test (GENinCode, Barcelona, Spain), which is based on next-generation sequencing (NGS). Subsequently, ultrasequencing was used to detect abnormalities in the DNA sequence of the promoter regions that codify and form the exon-intron boundaries of 7 genes: *LDLR, APOB, PCSK9, APOE,*

*STAP1*, *LDLRAP1*, and *LIPA*. The laboratory used the Gendicall 3.0, a bioinformatics tool developed by GENinCode (Gendicall 3.0, GENinCode, Rambla d'Ègara, Terrassa, Spain), to analyze the obtained results. The Lipid inCode® test methodology has previously been used in Spanish studies [26]. Variant annotation was based on the Human Genome Variation Society standard [27] using isoforms from the Reference Sequence (REFSEQ) database, Ensembl 81 source (www.ensembl.org accessed on 10 February 2021). Variant interpretation and pathogenicity classification followed information from the Gendiag.exe database of genetic variants, adhering to the rules published by the American College of Medical Genetics and Genomics (ACMG) [28]. Consistent with ACMG criteria, clinically relevant variants were classified as pathogenic (class I), likely pathogenic (class II), and variants of unknown significance (class III). Since *STAP1* is very unlikely to be a causative FH gene, variants in this gene were not considered [29].

### 2.3. Statistical Analysis

Quantitative variables are presented as a mean ± standard deviation, whereas qualitative variables are given as numbers (%). The Kolmogorov–Smirnov test was used to check the normal distribution of variables. We used standardized effect size measures for baseline characteristics, estimated Cohen's D for quantitative variables, and calculated the odds ratio for qualitative variables, with the respective 95% confidence intervals. Pearson's chi-square test and Fisher's exact test were used to compare the ASCVD percentages between FH mutation and no FH mutation in the DLCN ≥ 6 group, as well as the diagnostic rate before and after the screening. Odds ratios were estimated to assess the probability of a positive genetic result according to the clinical diagnosis of FH.

The statistical significance level was established at $p < 0.05$. All calculations were performed using the IBM SPSS Statistics program, version 25.0 (Chicago, IL, USA).

## 3. Results

### 3.1. Clinical Characteristics of the Studied Population

A total of 752 subjects were evaluated, of which 283 were excluded. Therefore, 469 subjects were included and medically assessed. Of them, 385 subjects (82.1%) received a diagnosis of possible FH, whereas 84 (17.9%) had a diagnosis of probable or definite FH. Genetic tests were performed in all patients with DLCN ≥ 6 as well as 10 patients with DLCN 3–5, selected by means of consecutive sampling to compare the yield of genetic testing between both groups (Figure 1).

Of the 469 subjects, the proportion of men was 40.7%, and the mean age was 53.2 ± 12.8 years. The mean levels of total cholesterol and LDL-C were 331.7 ± 48.3 and 246.8 ± 38.2 mg/dL, respectively. Regarding the treatment, 73.4% of the subjects were on LLT; however, only 23.2% of this treatment was maximal lipid-lowering therapy. Concerning cardiovascular events, 5.5% of the patients had developed ASCVD, which was premature in 42.3% of them. Patients with DLCN ≥ 6, compared with the DLCN 3–5 group, were younger, had higher levels of total cholesterol and LDL-C, and had higher proportions of active or past smoking, LLT, and a family history of premature ASCVD and hypercholesterolemia (Table 1). Finally, the proportion of ASCVD was markedly higher in the DLCN ≥ 6 group, both globally and premature, and these findings were particularly notable in the group with FH mutation who had a global rate of 19.3%, and within this group, events occurred at a premature age in 63.6%. Coronary artery disease was the most frequent ASCVD in DLCN ≥ 6 with FH mutation (Table 2).

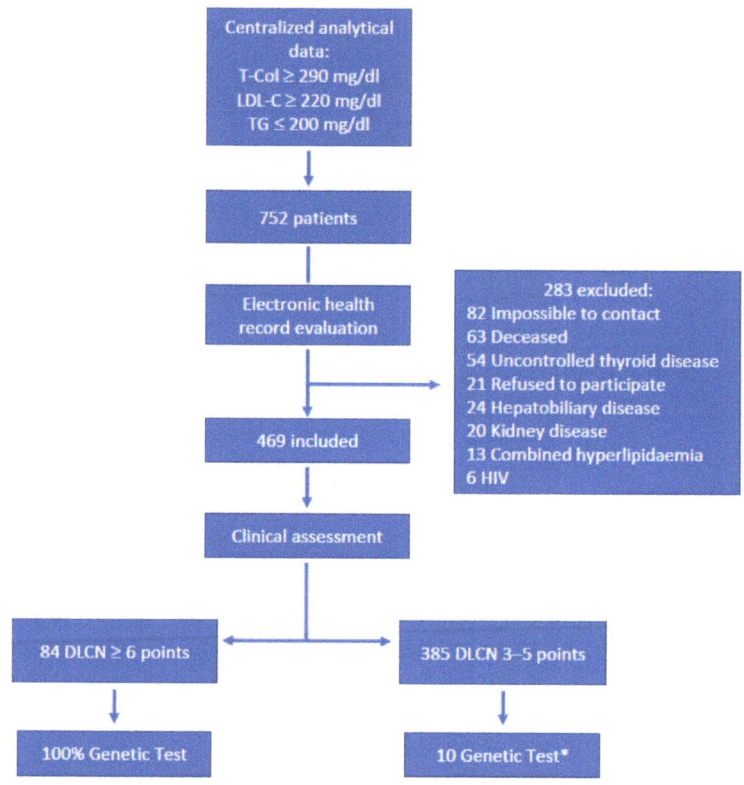

**Figure 1.** Patient selection: Flowchart showing sequential steps during patient selection. * Selected by means of consecutive sampling. T-Col: Total cholesterol. DLCN: Dutch Lipid Clinic Network. HIV: Human immunodeficiency virus. LDL-C: low-density lipoprotein cholesterol. TG: triglycerides.

**Table 1.** Baseline characteristics.

| Variable | Overall (n = 469) | DLCN 3–5 (n = 385) | DLCN ≥ 6 (n = 84) | Standardized Effect Size (95% CI) |
|---|---|---|---|---|
| Male | 191 (40.7) | 162 (42.1) | 29 (34.5) | 0,73 (0.44 to 1.19) |
| Mean age, years | 53.2 ± 12.8 | 54.6 ± 12.3 | 47.1 ± 12.9 | 0.59 (0.36 to 0.82) * |
| Hypertension | 148 (31.6) | 130 (33.8) | 18 (21.4) | 0.54 (0.31 to 0.94) * |
| Diabetes | 47 (10.0) | 43 (11.2) | 4 (4.8) | 0.39 (0.14 to 1.14) |
| Current or past smoking | 233 (49.7) | 181 (47.0) | 52 (61.9) | 1.83 (1.13 to 2.97) * |
| Body Mass Index | 27.7 ± 4.4 | 27.8 ± 4.3 | 27.0 ± 4.7 | 0.19 (−0.04 to 0.43) |
| ASCVD | 26 (5.5) | 13 (3.4) | 13 (15.5) | 5.24 (2.33 to 11.77) * |
| Premature ASCVD | 11 (2.3) | 3 (0.8) | 8 (9.5) | 13.4 (3.48 to 51.68) * |
| Family history of premature ASCVD | 34 (7.2) | 15 (3.9) | 19 (22.6) | 7.21 (3.49 to 14.91) * |
| Family history of HCL | 131 (27.9) | 61 (15.9) | 70 (83.3) | 26.48 (14.02 to 49.99) * |
| Corneal arcus (<45 years) | 7 (6.2) | 0 | 7 (20.6) | - |
| Tendon Xanthoma | 1 (0.2) | 0 | 1 (1.1) | - |

Table 1. Cont.

| Variable | Overall (n = 469) | DLCN 3–5 (n = 385) | DLCN ≥ 6 (n = 84) | Standardized Effect Size (95% CI) |
|---|---|---|---|---|
| Total cholesterol (mg/dL) | 331.7 ± 48.3 | 317.7 ± 21.03 | 396.2 ± 77.5 | −1.62 (−1.97 to −1.27) |
| LDL-C (mg/dL) | 246.8 ± 38.2 | 234.9 ± 15.6 | 301.5 ± 58.5 | −1.74 (−2.08 to −1.41) |
| HDL-C (mg/dL) | 56.2 ± 14.0 | 56.4 ± 13.6 | 55.2 ± 15.9 | 0.89 (−1.47 to 0.33) |
| Triglycerides (mg/dl) | 128.3 ± 36.3 | 129.5 ± 35.8 | 122.8 ± 38.4 | 0.18 (−0.05 to 0.42) |
| TSH (mLU/L) | 2.1 ± 2.12 | 2.1 ± 2.3 | 2.2 ± 1.30 | −0.08 (−0.32 to 0.17) |
| Lipid-lowering treatment | 344 (73.4) | 269 (69.9) | 75 (89.3) | 3.59 (1.74 to 7.42) * |
| Maximal lipid-lowering therapy | 109 (23.2) | 64 (16.6) | 45 (53.6) | 5.79 (3.49 to 9.59) * |

Values are mean ± standard deviation (SD) or n (%). * $p < 0.05$. ASCVD: atherosclerotic cardiovascular disease. CI: Confidence interval. DLCN: Dutch Lipid Clinic Network. HCL: Hypercholesterolemia. HDL-C: high-density lipoprotein cholesterol. LDL-C: low-density lipoprotein cholesterol. TSH: Thyroid stimulating hormone.

Table 2. Atherosclerotic cardiovascular disease rates in DLCN ≥ 6.

| | DLCN ≥ 6 no FH Mutation (n = 27) | DLCN ≥ 6 FH Mutation (n = 57) | p-Value |
|---|---|---|---|
| ASCVD | 2 (7.4) | 11 (19.3) | 0.33 |
| ASCVD without previous FH diagnosis | 2 (100) | 7 (63.6) | 0.47 |
| Premature ASCVD | 1 (50) | 7 (63,6) | 0.43 |
| Premature ASCVD without previous FH diagnosis | 1 (100) | 3 (42.9) | 1 |
| Coronary artery disease | 2 (100) | 7 (63.6) | 0.72 |
| Cerebral vascular disease | 0 | 4 (36.4) | - |
| Peripheral vascular disease | 1 (50) | 1 (9.1) | 0.51 |

Values are n (%). FH: Familial hypercholesterolemia. Other abbreviations as in Table 1.

### 3.2. Genetic FH Diagnosis

Among the 84 subjects with DLCN ≥ 6, clinical FH diagnosis was confirmed with genetic testing in 57 (12.2% of the 469 included, 67.9% of those genetically studied). Differentiating by FH clinical diagnosis, 33 (58.9%) of the 56 patients with probable FH and 24 (85.7%) of the 28 patients with a definite FH (≥8 points) were genetically confirmed. The rate of genetic confirmation among patients with a clinical diagnosis of possible FH was 20%. The odds ratio for detection mutations in the DLCN ≥ 6 group compared to the DLCN 3–5 group was 8.44 (95% CI (1.68 to 42.49); $p = 0.005$; Figure 2, Table 3).

Before their inclusion in the study, only 21 out of the 57 patients (36.8%) with genetic diagnosis had been clinically diagnosed with FH. Following the study strategy used in this research, the real detection rate in the cohort increased from 5.3% to at least 12.2% (2.3-fold increase; $p < 0.001$); it was also possible to reclassify four patients with no FH mutation who had been clinically diagnosed with FH before the present study (Figure 3).

Table 3. Genetic testing results.

| | All | FH Mutation | No FH Mutation | Odds Ratio (95% CI) | p-Value * |
|---|---|---|---|---|---|
| Previous FH diagnosis | 26 | 21 (80.8) | 5 (19.2) | 2,94 (0.99–8.73) | 0.08 |
| Possible FH | 10 | 2 (20) | 8 (80) | 1 (Reference) | - |
| Probable FH | 56 | 33 (58.9) | 23 (41.1) | 5.74 (1.12–29.54) | 0.037 |
| Definite FH | 28 | 24 (85.7) | 4 (14.3) | 24.0 (3.68–156.7) | 0.001 |
| DLCN ≥ 6 | 84 | 57 (67.9) | 27 (32.1) | 8.44 (1.68–42.49) | 0.005 |

Values are n (%). * $p < 0.05$. ** Percentages according to no FH mutation of the respective DLCN group. Abbreviations as in Tables 1 and 2.

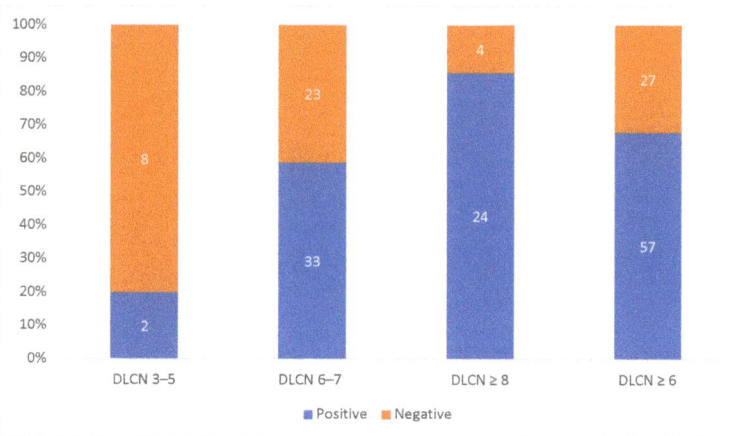

**Figure 2.** The positive and negative rates in the genetic study. Bar graph presenting the percentages of genetic diagnosis according to DLCN criteria. DLCN: Dutch Lipid Clinic Network.

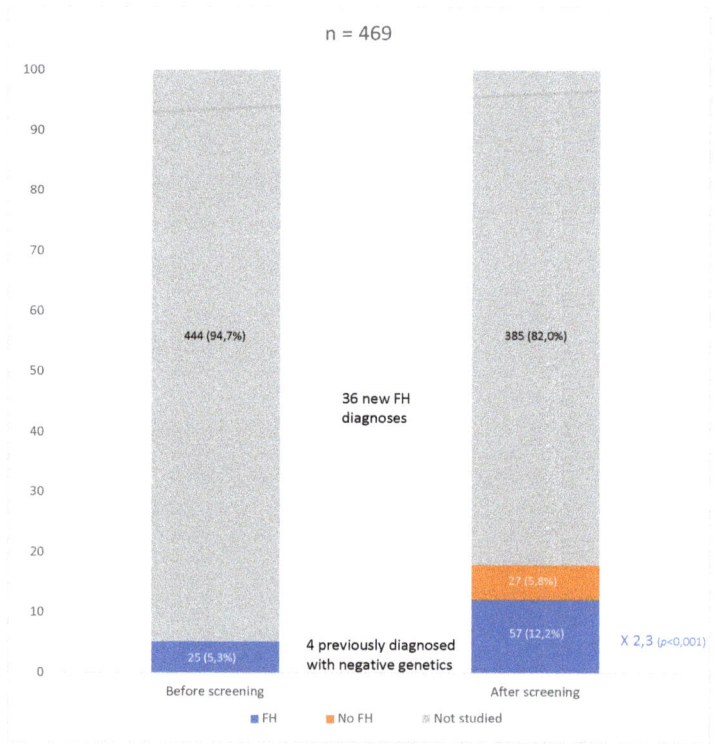

**Figure 3.** Diagnostic percentage of familial hypercholesterolemia, before and after screening, Bar graph where we can appreciate the percentage of diagnosis of familial hypercholesterolemia (FH) in the DLCN $\geq$ 6 group before carrying out the screening strategy (25 patients, 5.3%; although 4, 0.9%, had negative genetics and 21, 4.4%, were positive) and after the strategy (57, 12.2%, genetically confirmed with 2.3-fold increase in FH diagnosis, $p < 0.001$). The 10 patients with DLCN 3–5 and genetic study were counted as not studied. DLCN: Dutch Lipid Clinic Network.

The most frequent mutation was in the *LDLR* gene (92.9%), followed by *APOB* (5.3%) and *APOE* (1.8%). In our study, a mutation of the *LDLR* or *APOB* genes explained 98.2% of the total mutations (Tables S2 and S3).

## 4. Discussion

This study showed a high diagnostic yield with a universal, sequential active screening of FH index cases. The prevalence of FH within the studied cohort of patients with severe HCL was 12.2%, with a genetically confirmed FH rate in the DLCN $\geq 6$ group of 67.9%. We estimate that the strategy proposed in this study will contribute to modifying how FH index case screening is conducted because in our health setting, where only 36.8% of the patients with FH mutation had been previously diagnosed, the FH detection increased 2.3 times.

Our screening strategy presents several advantages that might justify the higher detection rates obtained. It focuses on patients with a higher probability of having FH by clinical diagnosis (DLCN $\geq 6$), since this is the group that is really considered FH [10] and, therefore, are candidates for advanced lipid-lowering therapies in accordance with the recommendations of Spanish guidelines [7,30]. Additionally, it allows optimization of diagnostic yield in accordance with the available resources. This is why, unlike cascade screening, potential index cases with DLCN 3–5 were not genetically tested, except for 10 patients, to estimate the diagnostic yield of our study (20%), in a similar way as previously described [31–33].

The first step in the search for patients was to detect those who had high LDL-C levels using widely available tools such as the computerized, centralized analytical data of the population in the health area obtained from both primary and hospital care. The exclusive use of LDL-C levels for the FH screening may be debatable, as not all patients with genetic mutations express the HCL phenotype [10]. Nevertheless, it is the most useful tool for initial screening because it is the most characteristic and frequent phenotype abnormality, particularly among the young [34], it is easily recognizable by any clinician, and it is the indicator that best predicts a later positive diagnosis of FH [9,35]. The advantage of this study was supplementing the initial analytical screening with a direct medical assessment, which increased diagnostic accuracy with a concise check of the items included in the DLCN criteria. In fact, 83.3% of the genetically tested patients had a family member with a history of hypercholesterolemia that would score points on the DLCN, data that might easily be omitted from digital medical records.

Recent studies have evaluated the genetic yield of FH with NGS. Reeskamp et al. [36] reported an overall prevalence of genetically confirmed FH of 14.9% within a cohort of 1528 patients with clinical FH diagnosis at a national referral center for genetic diagnosis. The FH detection rate in subjects with DLCN $\geq 6$, once stratified by higher LDL-C levels and stricter diagnostic FH criteria, was more than 50%. The higher prevalence in this study may be related to including subjects with DLCN 3–5 for genetic testing. Our better diagnosis yield in the DLCN $\geq 6$ group could be because our cohort exhibited higher mean LDL-C levels, fewer missing patient data for DLCN calculation, and restricted access to genetic testing. In Wang et al. [37], among 313 patients with severe HCL (LDL-C $\geq$ 190 mg/dL), 65.5% of them with DLCN $\geq 6$, a FH causative mutation was identified in 148 (47.3%). The detection rate increased up to 88% in those with LDL-C $\geq$ 310 mg/dL. Trinder et al. [38] found a pathogenic FH variant in 275 of 626 patients (43.9%) with previous clinical FH diagnosis who were referred for NGS. Of their cohort, 456 patients (72.8%) had a probable or definite clinical FH diagnosis. The percentage of genetic confirmation in patients with DLCN 6–7 and DLCN $\geq 8$ was 37.4% and 74.3%, respectively. We reported a lower prevalence of genetically confirmed FH compared to these two studies. However, only 17.9% of our cohort had DLCN $\geq 6$, and subjects with possible FH were not genetically tested (except for 10). Despite this, in our study, the LDL-C level was the most weighted item of the DLCN criteria, and the greatest diagnosis rate was in DLCN $\geq 8$, as in Wang et al., where the higher the LDL-C level, the higher the diagnostic yield. Our higher percentage of genetic diagnosis in both the DLCN 6–7 and DLCN $\geq$ 8 groups, compared to Trinder et al., could be explained because the same professional who applied the DLCN criteria also obtained the samples for genetic analysis. Consequently, there might have been stricter patient classification.

Other screening strategies for FH have previously been studied, both among general and selected populations. Khera et al. [15] studied a population with severe HCL without ASCVD and obtained a 2% prevalence of FH. The difference in the results may be explained because the definition of severe HCL was LDL-C $\geq$ 190 mg/dL, with the consequent loss of specificity compared to our cut-off point of LDL-C $\geq$ 220 mg/dL. In addition, this study did not include patients with ASCVD, and there was no direct medical assessment. Benn et al. [2] reported a prevalence of 5% of FH in subjects with LDL-C $\geq$ 220 mg/dL, conducted using a large cohort of the general Danish population. The best diagnostic yield was obtained in patients with LDL-C $\geq$ 230 mg/dL (13%). Nevertheless, the percentage of genetic diagnosis of FH in DLCN 6–7 and $\geq$8 points was 6% and 24%, respectively, whereas our study showed 58.9% and 85.7%, respectively. This result may be due to only having analyzed four genetic variations and not performing a direct medical assessment of the patients, therefore omitting important data. However, our study represents a selected population sample, which might explain the difference in FH prevalence compared to the two previous studies. Abul-Husn et al. [39] described a similar situation in their randomized cohort of patients whose digital medical records they analyzed to perform a retrospective diagnosis of FH according to DLCN criteria. Of their cohort, 10% had the severe HCL phenotype, with 2.5% prevalence of FH and 12.8% of genetic diagnosis in the group with LDL-C $\geq$ 250 mg/dL. Finally, in Amor-Salamanca et al., the prevalence of genetically confirmed FH was 9% in those cases $\leq$65 years admitted for ACS and with LDL-C $\geq$ 160 mg/dL [28]. Nonetheless, index cases were detected after the development of clinical ASCVD; therefore, following such a strategy does not allow the identification of asymptomatic FH patients.

As previously stated, this study confirms that the diagnosis of index cases continues to be random [1,25] and clearly improvable [20]. Given the prognostic significance of early detection and treatment both for FH index cases and relatives, we consider it necessary to apply screening strategies at the general population level. The screening strategy presented, which focuses on the search for patients with a higher probability of having FH, increases diagnostic accuracy and allows subsequent family-based cascade screening, in addition to an efficient and rational use of healthcare resources [40].

One of the notable limitations of our study is that it was not conducted among the general population, but rather in a severe HCL population. The objective of this study was to establish a realistic scenario, which is why we focused on subjects with a higher probability of having FH. Self-selection bias may exist in patients with previous ASCVD as well as family history of hypercholesterolemia and/or premature ASCVD. In addition, selection bias may have existed with the patient selection strategy and may have influenced the final result due to the deliberate exclusion of patients with an apparent secondary cause of hypercholesterolemia who could have FH. It is also possible that this strategy may have allowed subjects with FH and not such abnormally high LDL-C to go unnoticed, as well as those with a clinical possible FH diagnosis, although it was estimated that this represents a small number of the adult population [10], the majority of whom can be identified in a family-based cascade screening. Likewise, due to financial restrictions, it was not possible to conduct genetic testing of all the medically assessed patients, although we indicate that a large number of tests was performed. Finally, it was not possible to analyze some data from the medical records of relatives of index cases, such as the presence of tendon xanthoma, nor data related to non-resident relatives in the health area studied.

## 5. Conclusions

In conclusion, after applying a strategy of active, sequential screening of index cases, the prevalence of FH in the severe HCL cohort of patients was 12.2%, with a high percentage of genetically confirmed FH among the target population (67.9%). It is essential to accurately select patients who should undergo genetic testing based on centralized analytical data for a subsequent medical assessment, which can reliably stratify the patients who have suspected FH. Our data support the applicability of an active screening strategy at the general population level, with a rational use of the available resources, which would facilitate the early detection and treatment of FH index cases and the application of family-based cascade screening.

**Supplementary Materials:** The following are available online at https://www.mdpi.com/2077-0383/10/4/749/s1, Table S1: Dutch Lipid Clinic Network criteria, Table S2. Causative mutations in DLCN ≥ 6 group, Table S3: Genetic variants in DLCN ≥ 6 group.

**Author Contributions:** Conceptualization: F.S.-P., J.S.-P., P.M. and L.R.-P.; Methodology: F.S.-P., P.M. and L.R.-P; Investigation: F.S.-P. and J.S.-P.; Formal analysis: F.S.-P., V.M.B.-M. and J.H.A.-B.; Writing—original draft: F.S.-P.; Writing—review & editing: F.S.-P., J.S.-P., V.M.B.-M., J.H.A.-B., P.M. and L.R.-P.; Supervision: J.S.-P., P.M. and L.R.-P.; Funding acquisition: L.R.-P.; Project administration: L.R.-P. All authors have read and agreed to the published version of the manuscript.

**Funding:** This research received funding support for genetic testing from Sanofi-Aventis España SA and Amgen España SA, as well as support for statistical analysis and translation from the Chair of Advanced Therapies in Cardiovascular Pathologies, University of Málaga.

**Institutional Review Board Statement:** The study was conducted according to the guidelines of the Declaration of Helsinki, and approved by the Ethics Committee of the Complejo Hospitalario de Toledo (16 June 2016).

**Informed Consent Statement:** Informed consent was obtained from all subjects involved in the study.

**Data Availability Statement:** Data is contained within the article and supplementary Materials.

**Acknowledgments:** The authors would like to thank Mario Gutiérrez Bedmar, professor in the Department of Preventive Medicine and Public Health at Malaga University, Spain, for his invaluable help.

**Conflicts of Interest:** The authors declare no conflict of interest.

# References

1. Watts, G.F.; Gidding, S.S.; Mata, P.; Pang, J.; Sullivan, D.R.; Yamashita, S.; Raal, F.J.; Santos, R.D.; Ray, K.K. Familial hypercholesterolaemia: Evolving knowledge for designing adaptive models of care. *Nat. Rev. Cardiol.* **2020**. [CrossRef] [PubMed]
2. Benn, M.; Watts, G.F.; Tybjærg-Hansen, A.; Nordestgaard, B.G. Mutations causative of familial hypercholesterolaemia: Screening of 98 098 individuals from the Copenhagen General Population Study estimated a prevalence of 1 in 217. *Eur. Heart J.* **2016**, *37*, 1384–1394. [CrossRef]
3. Beheshti, S.O.; Madsen, C.M.; Varbo, A.; Nordestgaard, B.G. Worldwide Prevalence of Familial Hypercholesterolemia: Meta-Analyses of 11 Million Subjects. *J. Am. Coll. Cardiol.* **2020**, *75*, 2553–2566. [CrossRef]
4. Hu, P.; Dharmayat, K.I.; Stevens, C.A.T.; Sharabiani, M.T.A.; Jones, R.S.; Watts, G.F.; Genest, J.; Ray, K.K.; Vallejo-Vaz, A.J. Prevalence of Familial Hypercholesterolemia Among the General Population and Patients With Atherosclerotic Cardiovascular Disease. *Circulation* **2020**, *141*, 1742–1759. [CrossRef]
5. Akioyamen, L.E.; Genest, J.; Shan, S.D.; Reel, R.L.; Albaum, J.M.; Chu, A.; Tu, J.V. Estimating the prevalence of heterozygous familial hypercholesterolaemia: A systematic review and meta-analysis. *BMJ Open* **2017**, *7*, e016461. [CrossRef] [PubMed]
6. Mach, F.; Baigent, C.; Catapano, A.L.; Koskinas, K.C.; Casula, M.; Badimon, L.; Chapman, M.J.; De Backer, G.G.; Delgado, V.; Ference, B.A.; et al. 2019 ESC/EAS Guidelines for the management of dyslipidaemias: Lipid modification to reduce cardiovascular risk: The Task Force for the management of dyslipidaemias of the European Society of Cardiology (ESC) and European Atherosclerosis Society (EAS). *Eur. Heart J.* **2019**, *41*, 111–188. [CrossRef]
7. Alonso, R.; Perez de Isla, L.; Muñiz-Grijalvo, O.; Mata, P. Barriers to Early Diagnosis and Treatment of Familial Hypercholesterolemia: Current Perspectives on Improving Patient Care. *Vasc. Health Risk Manag.* **2020**, *16*, 11–25. [CrossRef] [PubMed]
8. Damgaard, D.; Larsen, M.L.; Nissen, P.H.; Jensen, J.M.; Jensen, H.K.; Soerensen, V.R.; Jensen, L.G.; Faergeman, O. The relationship of molecular genetic to clinical diagnosis of familial hypercholesterolemia in a Danish population. *Atherosclerosis* **2005**, *180*, 155–160. [CrossRef] [PubMed]
9. Civeira, F.; Ros, E.; Jarauta, E.; Plana, N.; Zambon, D.; Puzo, J.; Martinez de Esteban, J.P.; Ferrando, J.; Zabala, S.; Almagro, F.; et al. Comparison of Genetic Versus Clinical Diagnosis in Familial Hypercholesterolemia. *Am. J. Cardiol.* **2008**, *102*, 1187–1193. [CrossRef] [PubMed]

10. Sturm, A.C.; Knowles, J.W.; Gidding, S.S.; Ahmad, Z.S.; Ahmed, C.D.; Ballantyne, C.M.; Baum, S.J.; Bourbon, M.; Carrié, A.; Cuchel, M.; et al. Clinical Genetic Testing for Familial Hypercholesterolemia. *J. Am. Coll. Cardiol.* **2018**, *72*, 662–680. [CrossRef]
11. Nanchen, D.; Gencer, B.; Muller, O.; Auer, R.; Aghlmandi, S.; Heg, D.; Klingenberg, R.; Räber, L.; Carballo, D.; Carballo, S.; et al. Prognosis of Patients with Familial Hypercholesterolemia after Acute Coronary Syndromes. *Circulation* **2016**, *134*, 698–709. [CrossRef]
12. Pérez De Isla, L.; Alonso, R.; Mata, N.; Fernández-Pérez, C.; Muñiz, O.; Díaz-Díaz, J.L.; Saltijeral, A.; Fuentes-Jiménez, F.; De Andrés, R.; Zambón, D.; et al. Predicting cardiovascular events in familial hypercholesterolemia: The SAFEHEART registry (Spanish Familial Hypercholesterolemia Cohort Study). *Circulation* **2017**, *135*, 2133–2144. [CrossRef]
13. De Isla, L.P.; Alonso, R.; Mata, N.; Saltijeral, A.; Muñiz, O.; Rubio-Marin, P.; Diaz-Diaz, J.L.; Fuentes, F.; De Andrs, R.; Zambn, D.; et al. Coronary heart disease, peripheral arterial disease, and stroke in familial hypercholesterolaemia: Insights from the SAFEHEART registry (Spanish familial hypercholesterolaemia cohort study). *Arterioscler. Thromb. Vasc. Biol.* **2016**, *36*, 2004–2010. [CrossRef] [PubMed]
14. Perak, A.M.; Ning, H.; de Ferranti, S.D.; Gooding, H.C.; Wilkins, J.T.; Lloyd-Jones, D.M. Long-Term Risk of Atherosclerotic Cardiovascular Disease in US Adults With the Familial Hypercholesterolemia Phenotype. *Circulation* **2016**, *134*, 9–19. [CrossRef]
15. Khera, A.V.; Won, H.H.; Peloso, G.M.; Lawson, K.S.; Bartz, T.M.; Deng, X.; van Leeuwen, E.M.; Natarajan, P.; Emdin, C.A.; Bick, A.G.; et al. Diagnostic Yield and Clinical Utility of Sequencing Familial Hypercholesterolemia Genes in Patients with Severe Hypercholesterolemia. *J. Am. Coll. Cardiol.* **2016**, *67*, 2578–2589. [CrossRef]
16. Versmissen, J.; Oosterveer, D.M.; Yazdanpanah, M.; Defesche, J.C.; Basart, D.C.G.; Liem, A.H.; Heeringa, J.; Witteman, J.C.; Lansberg, P.J.; Kastelein, J.J.P.; et al. Efficacy of statins in familial hypercholesterolaemia: A long term cohort study. *BMJ* **2008**, *337*, a2423. [CrossRef] [PubMed]
17. Besseling, J.; Hovingh, G.K.; Huijgen, R.; Kastelein, J.J.P.; Hutten, B.A. Statins in Familial Hypercholesterolemia: Consequences for Coronary Artery Disease and All-Cause Mortality. *J. Am. Coll. Cardiol.* **2016**, *68*, 252–260. [CrossRef] [PubMed]
18. Kastelein, J.J.P.; Ginsberg, H.N.; Langslet, G.; Hovingh, G.K.; Ceska, R.; Dufour, R.; Blom, D.; Civeira, F.; Krempf, M.; Lorenzato, C.; et al. ODYSSEY FH I and FH II: 78 week results with alirocumab treatment in 735 patients with heterozygous familial hypercholesterolaemia. *Eur. Heart J.* **2015**, *36*, 2996–3003. [CrossRef] [PubMed]
19. Raal, F.J.; Stein, E.A.; Dufour, R.; Turner, T.; Civeira, F.; Burgess, L.; Langslet, G.; Scott, R.; Olsson, A.G.; Sullivan, D.; et al. PCSK9 inhibition with evolocumab (AMG 145) in heterozygous familial hypercholesterolaemia (RUTHERFORD-2): A randomised, double-blind, placebo-controlled trial. *Lancet* **2015**, *385*, 331–340. [CrossRef]
20. Wilemon, K.A.; Patel, J.; Aguilar-Salinas, C.; Ahmed, C.D.; Alkhnifsawi, M.; Almahmeed, W.; Alonso, R.; Al-Rasadi, K.; Badimon, L.; Bernal, L.M.; et al. Reducing the Clinical and Public Health Burden of Familial Hypercholesterolemia: A Global Call to Action. *JAMA Cardiol.* **2020**, *5*, 217–229. [CrossRef]
21. Nordestgaard, B.G.; Chapman, M.J.; Humphries, S.E.; Ginsberg, H.N.; Masana, L.; Descamps, O.S.; Wiklund, O.; Hegele, R.A.; Raal, F.J.; Defesche, J.C.; et al. Familial hypercholesterolaemia is underdiagnosed and undertreated in the general population: Guidance for clinicians to prevent coronary heart disease. *Eur. Heart J.* **2013**, *34*, 3478–3490. [CrossRef]
22. Friedewald, W.T.; Levy, R.I.; Fredrickson, D.S. Estimation of the concentration of low-density lipoprotein cholesterol in plasma, without use of the preparative ultracentrifuge. *Clin. Chem.* **1972**, *18*, 499–502. [CrossRef] [PubMed]
23. Masana, L.; Ibarretxe, D.; Plana, N. Maximum Low-density Lipoprotein Cholesterol Lowering Capacity Achievable With Drug Combinations. When 50 Plus 20 Equals 60. *Rev. Española Cardiol. Engl. Ed.* **2016**, *69*, 342–343. [CrossRef]
24. Escobar, C.; Anguita, M.; Arrarte, V.; Barrios, V.; Cequier, Á.; Cosín-Sales, J.; Egocheaga, I.; López de Sa, E.; Masana, L.; Pallarés, V.; et al. Recommendations to improve lipid control. Consensus document of the Spanish Society of Cardiology. *Rev. Esp. Cardiol.* **2020**, *73*, 161–167. [CrossRef]
25. Mata, P.; Alonso, R.; Ruiz, A.; Gonzalez-Juanatey, J.R.; Badimón, L.; Díaz-Díaz, J.L.; Muñoz, M.T.; Muñiz, O.; Galve, E.; Irigoyen, L.; et al. Diagnóstico y tratamiento de la hipercolesterolemia familiar en España: Documento de consenso. *Aten Primaria* **2015**, *47*, 56–65. [CrossRef]
26. Amor-Salamanca, A.; Castillo, S.; Gonzalez-Vioque, E.; Dominguez, F.; Quintana, L.; Lluís-Ganella, C.; Escudier, J.M.; Ortega, J.; Lara-Pezzi, E.; Alonso-Pulpon, L.; et al. Genetically Confirmed Familial Hypercholesterolemia in Patients with Acute Coronary Syndrome. *J. Am. Coll. Cardiol.* **2017**, *70*, 1732–1740. [CrossRef]
27. Den Dunnen, J.T.; Dalgleish, R.; Maglott, D.R.; Hart, R.K.; Greenblatt, M.S.; Mcgowan-Jordan, J.; Roux, A.F.; Smith, T.; Antonarakis, S.E.; Taschner, P.E.M. HGVS Recommendations for the Description of Sequence Variants: 2016 Update. *Hum. Mutat.* **2016**, *37*, 564–569. [CrossRef] [PubMed]
28. Richards, S.; Aziz, N.; Bale, S.; Bick, D.; Das, S.; Gastier-Foster, J.; Grody, W.W.; Hegde, M.; Lyon, E.; Spector, E.; et al. Standards and guidelines for the interpretation of sequence variants: A joint consensus recommendation of the American College of Medical Genetics and Genomics and the Association for Molecular Pathology. *Genet. Med.* **2015**, *17*, 405–424. [CrossRef]
29. Loaiza, N.; Hartgers, M.L.; Reeskamp, L.F.; Balder, J.-W.; Rimbert, A.; Bazioti, V.; Wolters, J.C.; Winkelmeijer, M.; Jansen, H.P.G.; Dallinga-Thie, G.M.; et al. Taking One Step Back in Familial Hypercholesterolemia. *Arterioscler. Thromb. Vasc. Biol.* **2020**, *40*, 973–985. [CrossRef] [PubMed]
30. Ascaso, J.F.; Civeira, F.; Guijarro, C.; López Miranda, J.; Masana, L.; Mostaza, J.M.; Pedro-Botet, J.; Pintó, X.; Valdivielso, P. Indications of PCSK9 inhibitors in clinical practice. Recommendations of the Spanish Sociey of Arteriosclerosis (SEA), 2019. *Clin. Investig. Arterioscler.* **2019**, *31*, 128–139. [CrossRef]

31. Graham, C.A.; McIlhatton, B.P.; Kirk, C.W.; Beattie, E.D.; Lyttle, K.; Hart, P.; Neely, R.D.G.; Young, I.S.; Nicholls, D.P. Genetic screening protocol for familial hypercholesterolemia which includes splicing defects gives an improved mutation detection rate. *Atherosclerosis* **2005**, *182*, 331–340. [CrossRef]
32. Taylor, A.; Wang, D.; Patel, K.; Whittall, R.; Wood, G.; Farrer, M.; Neely, R.; Fairgrieve, S.; Nair, D.; Barbir, M.; et al. Mutation detection rate and spectrum in familial hypercholesterolaemia patients in the UK pilot cascade project. *Clin. Genet.* **2010**, *77*, 572–580. [CrossRef]
33. Palacios, L.; Grandoso, L.; Cuevas, N.; Olano-Martín, E.; Martinez, A.; Tejedor, D.; Stef, M. Molecular characterization of familial hypercholesterolemia in Spain. *Atherosclerosis* **2012**, *221*, 137–142. [CrossRef]
34. Wald, D.S.; Bestwick, J.P.; Wald, N.J. Child-parent screening for familial hypercholesterolaemia: Screening strategy based on a meta-analysis. *BMJ* **2007**, *335*, 599. [CrossRef] [PubMed]
35. Kirke, A.B.; Barbour, R.A.; Burrows, S.; Bell, D.A.; Vickery, A.W.; Emery, J.; Watts, G.F. Systematic Detection of Familial Hypercholesterolaemia in Primary Health Care: A Community Based Prospective Study of Three Methods. *Hearth Lung Circ.* **2015**, *24*, 250–256. [CrossRef] [PubMed]
36. Reeskamp, L.F.; Tromp, T.R.; Defesche, J.C.; Grefhorst, A.; Stroes, E.S.G.; Hovingh, G.K.; Zuurbier, L. Next-generation sequencing to confirm clinical familial hypercholesterolemia. *Eur. J. Prev. Cardiol.* **2020**. [CrossRef]
37. Wang, J.; Dron, J.S.; Ban, M.R.; Robinson, J.F.; McIntyre, A.D.; Alazzam, M.; Zhao, P.J.; Dilliott, A.A.; Cao, H.; Huff, M.W.; et al. Polygenic Versus Monogenic Causes of Hypercholesterolemia Ascertained Clinically. *Arterioscler. Thromb. Vasc. Biol.* **2016**, *36*, 2439–2445. [CrossRef]
38. Trinder, M.; Li, X.; DeCastro, M.L.; Cermakova, L.; Sadananda, S.; Jackson, L.M.; Azizi, H.; Mancini, G.B.J.; Francis, G.A.; Frohlich, J.; et al. Risk of Premature Atherosclerotic Disease in Patients With Monogenic Versus Polygenic Familial Hypercholesterolemia. *J. Am. Coll. Cardiol.* **2019**, *74*, 512–522. [CrossRef]
39. Abul-Husn, N.S.; Manickam, K.; Jones, L.K.; Wright, E.A.; Hartzel, D.N.; Gonzaga-Jauregui, C.; O'Dushlaine, C.; Leader, J.B.; Kirchner, H.L.; Lindbuchler, D.M.; et al. Genetic identification of familial hypercholesterolemia within a single U.S. Health care system. *Science* **2016**, *354*, aaf7000. [CrossRef] [PubMed]
40. Lazaro, P.; Perez de Isla, L.; Watts, G.F.; Alonso, R.; Norman, R.; Muniz, O.; Fuentes, F.; Mata, N.; Lopez-Miranda, J.; Gonzalez-Juanatey, J.R.; et al. Cost-effectiveness of a cascade screening program for the early detection of familial hypercholesterolemia. *J. Clin. Lipidol.* **2017**, *11*, 260–271. [CrossRef]

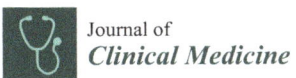 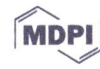

Article

# Cigarette Smoking, miR-27b Downregulation, and Peripheral Artery Disease: Insights into the Mechanisms of Smoking Toxicity

Tiago Pereira-da-Silva [1,2,*], Patrícia Napoleão [3], Marina C. Costa [3,4], André F. Gabriel [3,4], Mafalda Selas [1], Filipa Silva [1], Francisco J. Enguita [3,4], Rui Cruz Ferreira [1] and Miguel Mota Carmo [5]

1. Department of Cardiology, Hospital de Santa Marta, Centro Hospitalar Universitário de Lisboa Central, 1169-024 Lisbon, Portugal; mafalda.selas@gmail.com (M.S.); felipafernandes@gmail.com (F.S.); cruzferreira@netcabo.pt (R.C.F.)
2. NOVA Doctoral School, NOVA Medical School | Faculdade de Ciências Médicas, Universidade NOVA de Lisboa, 1169-056 Lisbon, Portugal
3. Instituto de Medicina Molecular João Lobo Antunes, Faculdade de Medicina, Universidade de Lisboa, 1649-028 Lisbon, Portugal; napoleao.patricia@gmail.com (P.N.); marinacosta@medicina.ulisboa.pt (M.C.C.); andre.gabriel@medicina.ulisboa.pt (A.F.G.); fenguita@medicina.ulisboa.pt (F.J.E)
4. Cardiomics Unit, Centro Cardiovascular da Universidade de Lisboa, Faculdade de Medicina, Universidade de Lisboa, 1649-028 Lisbon, Portugal
5. Chronic Diseases Research Center (CEDOC), NOVA Medical School, Faculdade de Ciências Médicas, Universidade NOVA de Lisboa, 1150-082 Lisbon, Portugal; mabmc@sapo.pt
* Correspondence: tiagopsilva@sapo.pt; Tel.: +351-919908505

**Abstract:** Cigarette smoking is a risk factor for the development of peripheral artery disease (PAD), although the proatherosclerotic mediators of cigarette smoking are not entirely known. We explored whether circulating microRNAs (miRNAs) are dysregulated in cigarette smokers and associated with the presence of PAD. Ninety-four participants were recruited, including 58 individuals without and 36 with PAD, 51 never smokers, 28 prior smokers, and 15 active smokers. The relative expression of six circulating miRNAs with distinct biological roles (miR-21, miR-27b, miR-29a, miR-126, miR-146, and miR-218) was assessed. Cigarette smoking was associated with the presence of PAD in multivariate analysis. Active smokers, but not prior smokers, presented miR-27b downregulation and higher leukocyte, neutrophil, and lymphocyte counts; miR-27b expression levels were independently associated with active smoking. Considering the metabolic and/or inflammatory abnormalities induced by cigarette smoking, miR-27b was independently associated with the presence of PAD and downregulated in patients with more extensive PAD. In conclusion, the atheroprotective miR-27b was downregulated in active smokers, but not in prior smokers, and miR-27b expression was independently associated with the presence of PAD. These unreported data suggest that the proatherogenic properties of cigarette smoking are mediated by a downregulation of miR-27b, which may be attenuated by smoking cessation.

**Keywords:** atherosclerosis; cigarette smoking; miR-27b; peripheral artery disease

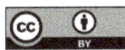

## 1. Introduction

Cigarette smoking is a major health hazard, being accountable for substantial cardiovascular morbidity and mortality worldwide due to its proatherogenic effects [1]. Cigarette smoking increases the risk of atherosclerosis development by several fold and is a more influential risk factor for peripheral artery disease (PAD) than for atherosclerosis of other territories, including coronary arteries [2]. Some of the mechanisms associated with cigarette-smoking-induced atherogenesis include the activation of inflammation, dysregulation of the lipid metabolism, increase in oxidative stress, and endothelial dysfunction [1,2]. Nevertheless, the pathophysiology associated with the initiation and progression of atherosclerosis secondary to cigarette smoking is not entirely known [1,2].

MicroRNAs (miRNAs) are small noncoding RNA molecules that regulate the genetic expression at the post-transcriptional level [3]. Cigarette smoking is associated with an altered expression of circulating miRNAs, including an upregulation of pro-inflammatory miRNAs [4,5]. On the other hand, specific miRNAs participate in different steps of atherogenesis, and a dysregulated expression of circulating miRNAs was described in patients with stable atherosclerosis of different territories [3,6]. However, to the best of our knowledge, coexistent associations among cigarette smoking, miRNA dysregulation, and the presence of atherosclerosis in humans have not been reported. The identification of miRNA dysregulation in association with both cigarette smoking and atherosclerosis could provide insights into the pathophysiology of cigarette-smoking toxicity. In fact, miRNAs may mediate the causal relationship between cigarette smoking and atherosclerosis development, especially PAD, which is particularly influenced by cigarette smoking [2].

Of the diversity of miRNAs associated with atherosclerosis regulation, miR-27b, miR-21, miR-29a, miR-126, miR-146, and miR-218 participate in distinct pathways and/or have distinct mechanisms of action, as described in experimental models, and were also reported to be dysregulated in patients with stable atherosclerosis [3,6–9]. Of note, miR-27b is a pleiotropic miRNA, and its expression is associated not only with atherosclerotic disease but also with non-atherosclerotic cardiovascular processes, such as cardiomyocyte hypertrophy and non-cardiovascular diseases, including cancer, non-alcoholic fatty liver disease, and viral infections [10–18]. Specifically, regarding atherosclerosis, miR-27b regulates lipid metabolism, development of lipid-induced atherosclerotic lesions, vascular inflammation, endothelial function, and angiogenesis [19–26]. Overall, the reported effects of miR-27b in experimental models are atheroprotective [19–26]. Among the relevant roles of the remaining miRNAs in the development and expression of atherosclerosis, miR-21 regulates vascular smooth cell and endothelial cell functions, miR-29a regulates fibrosis and extracellular matrix composition, miR-126 regulates endothelial function in response to shear stress, miR-146 regulates endothelial function in response to inflammatory cytokines, and miR-218 regulates endothelial cell migration [3,7,8].

We explored whether circulating miRNAs are simultaneously dysregulated in cigarette smokers and associated with the presence of PAD.

## 2. Materials and Methods

The study protocol was approved by the ethics committees of the involved institutions (Centro Hospitalar Universitário de Lisboa Central, Nr. 245/2015, in 2015, and the NOVA Medical School | Faculdade de Ciências Médicas, Universidade NOVA de Lisboa, Nr. 000176, in 2015). The investigation conformed to the principles outlined in the Helsinki Declaration. All the participants signed informed consent forms.

### 2.1. Recruitment of Participants

Two groups of participants from our center were recruited, with and without PAD. PAD was defined as a significant ($\geq$50%) stenosis on Doppler ultrasound at rest [27,28] or the combination of chronic claudication and an ankle-brachial index equal to or less than 0.9 [28,29]. Doppler ultrasound was performed for the characterization of PAD, according to a standardized protocol, using the GE Logiq S7 Expert Ultrasound System, and measurements were performed while following published guidelines [28,29].

We excluded patients with critical limb ischemia (with ischemic rest pain), those with acute ischemic events within 12 months in any arterial territory, those with lower-extremity bypass surgery performed within 12 months, those with any prior percutaneous arterial treatment, those with heart failure, hemodynamically significant valvular heart disease, hematological disorders, active infection (based on symptoms and/or signs, including fever, and leukocyte count, white blood cell differential, and C-reactive protein levels), history of malignancy, chronic kidney disease (stage 4 or 5), or severe hepatic dysfunction, those under 18 years of age, and those unable or unwilling to consent to study participation.

*2.2. Data Collection*

Data were collected prospectively after patient inclusion. A standardized record including clinical, demographic, laboratory, echocardiographic, and Doppler ultrasound data was obtained from each participant. Participants were classified according to cigarette-smoking status as never smokers, prior smokers (if cessation occurred at least six months before), or active smokers (in cases of daily cigarette smoking, irrespective of the number of cigarettes) [30].

*2.3. Candidate miRNAs*

Six candidate miRNAs (miR-21, miR-27b, miR-29a, miR-126, miR-146, and miR-218) were selected based on the following criteria: miRNAs are associated with the regulation of atherosclerosis development and expression in experimental models [3,7,8]; each of the miRNAs regulates distinct pathways of atherosclerotic disease and/or has distinct mechanisms of action [3,7,8]; miRNAs were reported to be dysregulated in patients with stable atherosclerosis [6,9].

*2.4. Quantification of Expression Levels of Candidate miRNAs*

Peripheral blood was collected early in the morning under fasting conditions. Serum was separated by centrifugation (500× $g$ for 10 min) within 15 min of sampling. Aliquots were stored at −80 °C, and samples were thawed only once.

Total RNA was extracted from serum samples using the miRCURY™ RNA Isolation Kit (Qiagen, Hilden, Germany). Complementary DNA was synthesized from total RNA using the Universal complementary DNA (cDNA) synthesis kit from the miRCURY™ LNA miRNA system (Qiagen, Hilden, Germany). miRNA amplification was performed using quantitative reverse-transcription polymerase chain reaction (using the miRCURY™ LNA SYBR Green PCR Kit and LNA™ PCR primers, Qiagen, Hilden, Germany), and the melting curve was determined according to the following conditions: 95 °C for 10 min, followed by 45 cycles of 95 °C for 10 s and 60 °C for 60 s. All reactions were performed in triplicate. The amplification data were assessed using DataAssist™ Software v3.01. Cycle threshold (Ct) values greater than 40 were considered undetermined [31–34]. The relative expression levels of the six candidate miRNAs were calculated using the delta Ct (ΔCt) method, normalizing for the UniSp6 RNA spike-in control [34–37]. Higher ΔCt miRs represent lower circulating levels of the candidate miRNAs [34–37]. Where appropriate, the fold-change in the miRNA expression levels was expressed using the Livak method ($2^{-\Delta\Delta Ct}$) [38].

*2.5. Statistical Analysis*

Discrete variables are presented as frequencies (percentages); continuous variables are presented as the mean (standard deviation) in normally distributed data or median (interquartile range (IQR)) in variables without a normal distribution (Shapiro–Wilk test). Categorical variables were analyzed using the chi-square or Fisher's exact tests. Continuous variables were analyzed using Student's *t*-test or the Mann–Whitney test when normality was not verified. Comparisons between multiple groups were performed using an analysis of variance (ANOVA) in normally distributed data and the Kruskal–Wallis test in variables without a normal distribution; the Bonferroni post-hoc correction was used for multiple pairwise comparisons. Pearson's correlation was used to test correlations between continuous variables. Three distinct multivariable logistic regression models were successively tested: (1) using classical cardiovascular risk factors as the independent variables and PAD as the dependent variable; (2) using metabolic and inflammatory data and miRNA expression levels as the independent variables and active smoking as the dependent variable; and (3) using miRNAs and other laboratory parameters dysregulated in cigarette smokers as the independent variables and PAD as the dependent variable. Variables with a *p*-value of <0.10 in univariate analyses were tested in the multivariable models. A correction for collinearity was performed as appropriate. The level of significance was set at α = 0.05. Analyses were conducted using SPSS software, version 26.0 (IBM Corp, Armonk, NY, USA).

## 3. Results

### 3.1. Characteristics of Participants According to the Presence of PAD and Cigarette-Smoking Status

A total of 94 participants were recruited, including 58 without and 36 with PAD (Table 1). Patients with PAD presented a higher prevalence of classical cardiovascular risk factors (including cigarette smoking), concomitant coronary and carotid artery disease, and use of antiplatelet and statin therapy, as well as higher creatinine levels, compared to patients without PAD. The ΔCt miR-27b and ΔCt miR-146 values were significantly higher in patients with PAD (Table 1), corresponding to a 17.0- and 3.4-fold downregulation of miR-27b and miR-146 [38], respectively, in patients with PAD.

Of the 94 participants, 51 were never smokers, 28 were prior smokers, and 15 were active smokers (Table 2). The mean pack-year was 53 (22) in prior smokers and 45 (21) in active smokers, with a median time from cigarette-smoking cessation of 10 (7–11) years in prior smokers. The prevalence of PAD and the proportion of bilateral PAD (among patients with PAD) increased from never smokers to prior smokers and to active smokers. Moreover, the leukocyte, neutrophil, and lymphocyte counts were higher in active smokers compared with other groups. MiR-27b was the only dysregulated miRNA according to cigarette-smoking status; the ΔCt miR-27b values were significantly higher in active smokers compared with prior smokers ($p = 0.004$; corresponding to a downregulation of miR-27b in active smokers), and there was a trend for higher ΔCt miR-27b values in active smokers compared with never smokers ($p = 0.053$; corresponding to a trend for downregulation of miR-27b in active smokers), with no significant differences between never smokers and prior smokers.

Active smokers presented significantly higher ΔCt miR-27b values (22.00 (4.35)) compared with non-active smokers, including never smokers and prior smokers (18.66 (4.33)), corresponding to a 10.0-fold downregulation of miR-27b expression levels in active smokers [38] (Figure 1).

### 3.2. Cigarette Smoking Was Independently Associated with the Presence of PAD

Considering all the risk factors for the development of cardiovascular disease that differed according to the presence of PAD in the univariate analysis, the age, cigarette-smoking status, and creatinine levels were independently associated with the presence of PAD in the multivariate logistic regression analysis (Table 3).

### 3.3. MiR-27b Was Dysregulated in Active Smokers Independently of Other Metabolic and Inflammatory Parameters

Considering the metabolic and inflammatory parameters and the miRNAs dysregulated in active smokers in the univariate analysis, the leukocyte count and ΔCt miR-27b were independently associated with active smoking in the multivariate logistic regression analysis (Table 4).

### 3.4. MiR-27b Was Independently Associated with the Presence of PAD

Considering all the metabolic and inflammatory parameters and the miRNA (miR-27b) dysregulated in active smokers in the univariate analysis, only ΔCt miR-27b was independently associated with the presence of PAD ($\beta = 1.13$, 95% confidence interval: 1.01–1.28, $p = 0.037$). Moreover, ΔCt miR-27b was significantly higher in bilateral PAD (24.0 (17.2–25.7)) compared with unilateral PAD (20.3 (15.1–23.2), $p = 0.041$ vs. bilateral PAD) and with absent PAD (18.3 (14.8–21.6), $p = 0.004$ vs. bilateral PAD). Such results corresponded to a 4.0- and 52.0-fold reduction in miR-27b in bilateral PAD compared with unilateral and absent PAD, respectively [38].

Table 1. Characteristics of participants without and with peripheral artery disease.

| Characteristics of Participants | Without Peripheral Artery Disease | With Peripheral Artery Disease | p-Value |
|---|---|---|---|
| n | 58 | 36 | |
| **Clinical characteristics** | | | |
| Age, years | 61 (53–70) | 68 (60–73) | 0.009 |
| Male, n (%) | 51 (88) | 33 (92) | 0.419 |
| Hypertension, n (%) | 42 (72) | 36 (100) | <0.001 |
| Dyslipidemia, n (%) | 48 (83) | 35 (97) | 0.031 |
| Diabetes mellitus, n (%) | 15 (26) | 17 (47) | 0.029 |
| Cigarette-smoking status, n (%) | | | 0.001 |
| Never smoker | 39 (67) | 12 (33) | |
| Prior smoker | 15 (26) | 13 (36) | |
| Active smoker | 4 (7) | 11 (31) | |
| LVEF > 50%, n (%) | 58 (100) | 36 (100) | – |
| Antiplatelet therapy, n (%) | 37 (64) | 35 (97) | <0.001 |
| Statin therapy, n (%) | 42 (72) | 32 (91) | 0.023 |
| Coronary artery disease, n (%) | 32 (55) | 36 (100) | <0.001 |
| Carotid artery disease, n (%) | 12 (55) | 18 (50) | 0.003 |
| **Peripheral artery disease** | | | |
| Bilateral disease, n (%) | 0 (0) | 25 (69) | <0.001 |
| Prior bypass surgery, n (%) | 0 (0) | 8 (22) | <0.001 |
| **Laboratory parameters** | | | |
| Hemoglobin, g/dL | 13.8 (1.5) | 13.6 (1.6) | 0.586 |
| Leukocyte count, $10^9$/L | 7.0 (1.9) | 7.7 (1.7) | 0.081 |
| Neutrophil count, $10^9$/L | 4.0 (1.7) | 4.5 (1.4) | 0.192 |
| Lymphocyte count, $10^9$/L | 1.9 (1.6–2.3) | 2.2 (1.6–2.7) | 0.100 |
| Neutrophil/lymphocyte ratio | 2.2 (1.0) | 2.2 (1.0) | 0.943 |
| Platelet count, $10^9$/L | 223 (58) | 227 (44) | 0.749 |
| Fasting glycemia, mg/dL | 92 (83–104) | 90 (82–121) | 0.978 |
| Percentage of glycosylated hemoglobin | 5.7 (5.4–6.2) | 5.9 (5.5–7.4) | 0.295 |
| Creatinine, mg/dL | 0.85 (0.77–0.97) | 0.94 (0.80–1.34) | 0.036 |
| Total cholesterol, mg/dL | 164 (130–206) | 166 (147–205) | 0.781 |
| LDL-cholesterol, mg/dL | 92 (72–130) | 109 (83–135) | 0.250 |
| HDL-cholesterol, mg/dL | 43 (34–51) | 36 (31–43) | 0.062 |
| Triglycerides, mg/dL | 115 (71–163) | 117 (88–178) | 0.429 |
| C-reactive protein, mg/L | 4.0 (1.9) | 3.6 (1.5) | 0.529 |
| **miRNAs** [1] | | | |
| miR-21 | 14.89 (4.51) | 15.99 (4.65) | 0.282 |
| miR-27b | 18.23 (14.58–21.59) | 22.32 (16.50–24.13) | 0.032 |
| miR-29a | 20.42 (3.57) | 21.80 (3.12) | 0.152 |
| miR-126 | 16.89 (14.89–22.46) | 19.69 (16.28–24.06) | 0.060 |
| miR-146 | 18.70 (3.40) | 20.48 (4.23) | 0.048 |
| miR-218 | 22.69 (22.48–23.33) | 14.49 (−8.6–23.50) | 0.186 |

Categorical variables are expressed as the frequency (percentage), and continuous variables are expressed as the mean (standard deviation) or median (interquartile range). HDL—high-density lipoprotein; LDL—low-density lipoprotein; LVEF—left-ventricular ejection fraction; miRNA—microRNA. [1] Delta cycle threshold (ΔCt) values are presented for each miRNA (higher ΔCt values correspond to lower miRNA expression levels).

**Table 2.** Characteristics of participants according to cigarette-smoking status.

| Characteristics of Participants | Never Smokers | Prior Smokers | Active Smokers | $p$-Value |
|---|---|---|---|---|
| $n$ | 51 | 28 | 15 | |
| **Clinical characteristics** | | | | |
| Age, years | 65 (56–73) | 67 (58–71) | 59 (53–68) | 0.415 |
| Male, $n$ (%) | 43 (84) | 28 (100) | 13 (87) | 0.090 |
| Hypertension, $n$ (%) | 36 (71) | 28 (100) | 14 (93) | 0.002 |
| Dyslipidemia, $n$ (%) | 43 (84) | 26 (93) | 14 (93) | 0.424 |
| Diabetes mellitus, $n$ (%) | 17 (33) | 10 (36) | 5 (33) | 0.975 |
| LVEF > 50%, $n$ (%) | 51 (100) | 28 (100) | 15 (100) | – |
| Antiplatelet therapy, $n$ (%) | 36 (71) | 24 (86) | 12 (80) | 0.298 |
| Statin therapy, $n$ (%) | 37 (73) | 24 (86) | 13 (93) | 0.156 |
| Coronary artery disease, $n$ (%) | 31 (61) | 24 (86) | 13 (86) | 0.024 |
| Carotid artery disease, $n$ (%) | 14 (51) | 10 (36) | 6 (40) | 0.576 |
| **Peripheral artery disease** | | | | |
| Number of patients | 12 (24) | 13 (46) | 11 (73) | 0.001 |
| Bilateral disease, $n$ (%) | 8 (16) | 11 (39) | 6 (40) | 0.002 |
| Prior bypass surgery, $n$ (%) | 2 (4) | 5 (18) | 1 (7) | 0.101 |
| **Laboratory parameters** | | | | |
| Hemoglobin, g/dL | 13.4 (1.5) | 14.1 (1.4) | 14.1 (1.4) | 0.063 |
| Leukocyte count, $10^9$/L | 6.6 (1.5) | 7.3 (1.8) | 9.2 (1.8) | <0.001 [1,2] |
| Neutrophil count, $10^9$/L | 3.8 (3.0–4.4) | 3.9 (3.2–5.3) | 4.6 (3.7–5.8) | <0.001 [1,2] |
| Lymphocyte count, $10^9$/L | 1.8 (1.5–2.2) | 2.1 (1.6–2.4) | 2.3 (1.8–3.5) | 0.027 [1] |
| Neutrophil/lymphocyte ratio | 2.0 (1.5–3.0) | 2.2 (1.7–2.7) | 2.3 (1.9–2.8) | 0.568 |
| Platelet count, $10^9$/L | 219 (51) | 218 (54) | 255 (51) | 0.058 |
| Fasting glycemia, mg/dL | 92 (83–116) | 91 (85–112) | 89 (72–117) | 0.565 |
| Percentage of glycosylated hemoglobin | 5.7 (5.3–7.1) | 5.8 (5.4–6.2) | 5.9 (5.6–6.1) | 0.787 |
| Creatinine, mg/dL | 0.86 (0.78–1.08) | 0.86 (0.76–1.00) | 1.01 (0.75–1.71) | 0.447 |
| Total cholesterol, mg/dL | 178 (51) | 154 (43) | 172 (48) | 0.060 |
| LDL-cholesterol, mg/dL | 108 (41) | 89 (38) | 116 (32) | 0.059 |
| HDL-cholesterol, mg/dL | 42 (34–51) | 41 (29–46) | 35 (31–42) | 0.236 |
| Triglycerides, mg/dL | 116 (79–156) | 104 (73–178) | 158 (112–243) | 0.139 |
| C-reactive protein, mg/L | 3.5 (1.6) | 3.7 (1.8) | 4.0 (1.9) | 0.339 |
| **miRNAs [3]** | | | | |
| miR-21 | 15.44 (4.40) | 14.55 (4.62) | 16.42 (5.09) | 0.454 |
| miR-27b | 19.29 (4.42) | 17.44 (3.98) | 22.00 (4.35) | 0.014 [2] |
| miR-29a | 21.01 (3.04) | 19.74 (3.86) | 23.19 (3.12) | 0.059 |
| miR-126 | 17.42 (15.20–23.98) | 16.10 (14.89–19.48) | 22.40 (17.65–24.15) | 0.075 |
| miR-146 | 20.03 (15.74–22.21) | 17.79 (16.26–20.12) | 21.69 (18.23–23.58) | 0.150 |
| miR-218 | 22.31 (15.67–23.02) | 22.31 (15.67–23.02) | 8.45 (−8.46–21.50) | 0.120 |

Categorical variables are expressed as the frequency (percentage), and continuous variables are expressed as the mean (standard deviation) or median (interquartile range). HDL—high-density lipoprotein; LDL—low-density lipoprotein; LVEF—left-ventricular ejection fraction; miRNA—microRNA. [1] $p < 0.05$, active smokers vs. never smokers; [2] $p < 0.05$, active smokers vs. prior smokers; [3] delta cycle threshold ($\Delta$Ct) values are presented for each miRNA (higher $\Delta$Ct values correspond to lower expression levels of candidate miRNAs).

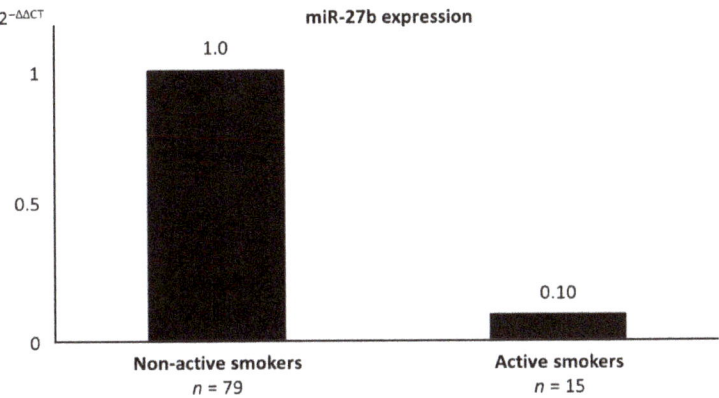

**Figure 1.** Relative expression of miR-27b according to the cigarette-smoking status. The relative expression of miR-27b ($2^{-\Delta\Delta Ct}$) is presented for non-active smokers, including never smokers and prior smokers, and for active smokers.

**Table 3.** Predictors of peripheral artery disease in multivariate logistic regression analysis.

| Independent Predictors | β | 95% CI | p-Value |
|---|---|---|---|
| Age, years | 1.11 | 1.04–1.18 | 0.002 |
| Cigarette smoking | 4.11 | 1.89–8.95 | 0.031 |
| Creatinine, mg/dL | 6.29 | 1.12–33.49 | <0.001 |

95% CI—95% confidence interval.

**Table 4.** Parameters dysregulated in active smokers in multivariate logistic regression analysis.

| Independent Predictors | β | 95% CI | p-Value |
|---|---|---|---|
| Leukocyte count | 2.33 | 1.37–3.94 | 0.002 |
| ΔCt miR-27b | 1.33 | 1.02–1.72 | 0.034 |

95% CI—95% confidence interval, ΔCt—delta cycle threshold.

## 4. Discussion

In this prospective study, three main findings stood out: cigarette smoking was associated with the presence of PAD, cigarette smoking was associated with miR-27b downregulation, and miR-27b downregulation was associated with the presence and severity of PAD. These results suggest that miR-27b mediates the proatherogenic effects of cigarette smoking.

Cigarette smoking is a recognized causal risk factor for PAD development [1,2]. On the other hand, the expression of circulating miRNAs is influenced by exogenous factors, such as cigarette smoking [4]. In this study, the atheroprotective miR-27b was downregulated in active smokers compared with non-active smokers (including never smokers and prior smokers), independently of other metabolic and inflammatory parameters. These results suggest a detrimental effect of active cigarette smoking on miR-27b expression, similar to the reported effect of cigarette smoking on other atheroprotective miRNAs [39]. MiR-27b was significantly downregulated in active smokers compared with prior smokers but not with never smokers, although there was a trend towards miR-27b downregulation in active smokers compared with never smokers. The latter may be explained by the limited sample size used in this study. Based on an extensive post-hoc analysis, the absence of differences in miR-27b expression levels between active smokers and never smokers is difficult to explain, and we did not find additional factors that could contribute to such results. Nevertheless, the numerical differences between active smokers and never smokers were close to the margin of statistical significance and are consistent with a culprit effect of active smoking in downregulating miR-27b compared with prior smokers and, likely, never smokers as well. There were no significant differences in miR-27b expression levels between prior smokers and never smokers. Such results may be explained by a sensitivity of miR-27b expression levels to active smoking without a legacy effect [39,40]. Specifically, smoking cessation was reported to completely revert the dysregulation of some miRNAs observed in active smokers [39,40], and this may also be the case of miR-27b. These data reinforce the atheroprotective effects of smoking cessation. Published data addressing the effect of smoking on miR-27a/b expression are limited [39–41]. Of two studies addressing miR-27a, one reported an upregulation and the other reported no dysregulation in active smokers [39,40]. Nevertheless, miR-27a and miR-27b may differ in their mechanisms of action and expression levels in specific diseases, and the aforementioned results concerning miR-27a expression in active smokers may not be applicable to miR-27b [42–44]. Specifically, for miR-27b, a nonsignificant downregulation was reported in human oral keratinocytes in association with cigarette smoke exposure [41]. In our study, the downregulation of circulating miR-27b in active smokers was significant after adjusting for other metabolic and inflammatory parameters.

The dysregulation of some circulating miRNAs is known to be associated with the development of atherosclerosis, and miR-27b was reported to be atheroprotective on the basis of experimental studies [19–26]. This possibly explains the association between the reduced miR-27b expression and the higher prevalence and severity of PAD observed in this study. Complementary atheroprotective mechanisms of miR-27b were previously reported [19–26]. Xie W. et al. [19] elegantly showed that miR-27 reduces vascular lipid accumulation, partially mediated by the suppression of expression of scavenger receptors associated with lipid uptake in vascular macrophages. Interestingly, systemic treatment with miR-27 decreased aortic plaque size and lipid content in mice [19]. Consistently, in another study, miR-27b was identified as a crucial regulatory hub in lipid metabolism in human and mouse liver and was shown to downregulate the expression of key genes involved in lipid metabolism, including Angptl3 and Gpam, which mitigates the accumulation of lipids in circulation [20]. Regarding inflammation, miR-27b downregulates lipoprotein lipase gene expression and thereby reduces vascular inflammatory response, which limits atherogenesis [19]. Moreover, miR-27b restrains the activity of NF-κB and the production of several pro-inflammatory factors, including interleukin (IL)-1β, IL-6, and tumor necrosis factor alpha [21], inhibits interleukin-17-induced monocyte chemoattractant protein-1 [22] and targets Bcl-2-associated athanogene 2 in macrophages [21]. This contributes to a decreased monocyte-macrophage activation [23]. Considering the key role of vascular inflammation, particularly the monocyte-macrophage activation, in the development and expression of atherosclerosis, the aforementioned molecular mechanisms are consistent with the atheroprotective effects of miR-27b [45,46]. On the other hand, as miR-27b represses repulsive semaphorins, especially semaphorin 6A, it facilitates the formation of tight endothelial monolayers and stable vessels in response to shear stress [24]. In addition, miR-27b was identified as a proangiogenic miRNA [25], regulating angiogenesis through the angiogenic inhibitor semaphorin 6A and Notch ligand Dll4 [23,26]. Regarding studies addressing miR-27b expression in patients with PAD, data is conflicting. Signorelli et al. [11] reported an upregulation of miR-27b in patients with PAD compared with controls. On the other hand, Stather et al. [10] reported a downregulation of miR-27b in patients with PAD, and our findings are consistent with their results. Contrary to the study by Signorelli et al. [11], Stather et al. [10] confirmed the presence of PAD using imaging methods, used one derivation and two validation sample sets, reported the diagnostic accuracy of miR-27b for detecting PAD, and presented a pathway enrichment analysis. There is a known biological variation in miRNAs measurements, occasionally with conflicting expression levels among different studies focused on the same disease [47]. The miR-27b downregulation observed in our study reinforces the results of the study by Stather et al. [10], where a very robust methodology was used.

The downregulation of miR-27b in active smokers and the independent association between miR-27b and the presence of PAD in this study suggest that miR-27b is downregulated due to active cigarette smoking and that such dysregulation contributes to PAD (Figure 2). The results are, therefore, consistent with miR-27b acting as a mediator of cigarette-smoking toxicity, specifically in PAD development.

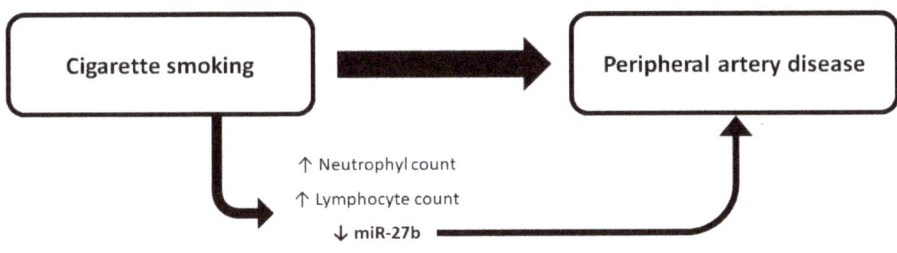

**Figure 2.** Putative role of miR-27b in the toxicity induced by cigarette smoking. Cigarette smoking was associated with the presence of peripheral artery disease and with miR-27b downregulation; downregulation of the atheroprotective miR-27b was associated with the presence and severity of peripheral artery disease; miR-27b may mediate the atherogenesis induced by cigarette smoking. The suspension points represent metabolic and inflammatory parameters potentially dysregulated in association with cigarette smoking, in addition to neutrophil count, lymphocyte count, and miR-27b expression.

In this study, miR-146 was also downregulated in patients with PAD. MiR-146 is induced in endothelial cells in response to pro-inflammatory cytokines and acts as a negative feedback regulator of inflammatory signaling in endothelial cells by dampening the activation of pro-inflammatory transcriptional programs, including the NF-κB, AP-1, and MAPK/EGR pathways, and by promoting eNOS expression [3,7,48]. Moreover, miR-146a was reported to decrease endothelial inflammation by inhibiting NAPDH Oxidase 4 expression in a diabetic atherothrombosis model [49]. The anti-inflammatory effects of miR-146 contribute to counteracting atherogenesis [3,7,48,49] and may explain the association between miR-146 downregulation and the presence of PAD observed in our study. The remaining miRNAs (miR-21, miR-29a, miR-126, and miR-218) were not dysregulated in association with PAD, despite their involvement in biological pathways associated with atherosclerosis regulation, as reported in experimental studies [48,50–60]. A comprehensive review of their biological roles is out of the scope of this study, but some of the main targets are herein addressed. MiR-21 has both atheroprotective and proatherogenic effects [50]. It enhances vascular smooth muscle cell migration and proliferation by targeting TSP-1 and c-Sk [50,51]. On the other hand, miR-21 inhibits both endothelial cell apoptosis, through PTEN [52], and endothelial cell proliferation, through RhoB [53]. In addition, miR-21 promotes inflammatory activation of endothelial cells by targeting PPARα, which induces the expression of adhesion molecules and cytokines [54]. MiR-29a acts in distinct pathways, as it represses transcripts of several components of the extracellular matrix; of note, miR-29a downregulates the expression of ELN, COL1A1, and COL3A1, resulting in a reduction of the elastin and collagen content in the atherosclerotic plaque [55,56]. In fact, antagonizing the antifibrotic effect of miR-29a leads to a reduced size of atherosclerotic lesions, enhanced fibrous cap thickness, and reduced necrotic zones [55]. MiR-126 promotes endothelial proliferation and limits atherosclerosis by suppressing Dlk1 [57]. Interestingly, miR-126 is a mechanosensitive miRNA that is downregulated through the transcription factor klf2a in response to disturbed flow and shear stress [58]. Finally, miR-218 regulates Slit/Robo signaling through the repression of Robo1, Robo2, and glucuronyl C5-epimerase and thereby regulates endothelial cell migration and vascular patterning [59,60]. As supported by the aforementioned experimental data, further clinical studies are warranted to confirm the role of these miRNAs as biomarkers of atherosclerosis.

There are strengths of this study that should be acknowledged. As far as we know, we describe for the first time coexistent associations among cigarette-smoking status, dysregulation of circulating miR-27b, and PAD. The results were consistent with the aforementioned biological roles of miR-27b in experimental studies [19–26]. Moreover, the miR-27b downregulation in more severe, bilateral PAD further added to the consistency of the results. Importantly, the multivariable analyses carried out in this study, adjusting for confounders, contributed to the accuracy of our findings.

Our study has some limitations. The results indicate associations among cigarette smoking, miR-27b dysregulation, and PAD development, but not a causal effect. Nevertheless, the adjustment for confounders in the multivariable analyses and the consistency of the results with the aforementioned experimental data [19–26] suggest that miR-27b is very likely a mediator in such a pathophysiology chain. Of note, this is a single-center study that included only European participants, which may limit the applicability of results to other clinical settings. Populations with different ethnicities may express distinct microRNA profiles, either in healthy individuals or in specific disease subsets [61,62]. Therefore, further multicentric studies recruiting participants from distinct geographical areas are warranted for external validation of our findings.

## 5. Conclusions

Cigarette smoking was associated with the presence of PAD. Active smokers, but not prior smokers, presented a downregulation of miR-27b, and such dysregulation was associated with the presence and severity of PAD. These unreported data suggest that miR-27b mediates the proatherogenic effects of cigarette smoking and that cigarette smoking cessation may be associated with an attenuation of miR-27b dysregulation. Our results provide insights into the pathophysiology of cigarette-smoking toxicity and associated PAD.

**Author Contributions:** Conceptualization, T.P.-d.-S., P.N. and M.M.C.; methodology, P.N., M.C.C. and A.F.G.; validation, P.N., M.C.C., A.F.G. and F.J.E.; formal analysis, T.P.-d.-S. and P.N.; investigation, T.P.-d.-S., P.N., M.C.C., A.F.G., M.S. and F.S.; resources, M.S. and F.S.; data curation, T.P.-d.-S., M.S. and F.S.; writing—original draft preparation, T.P.-d.-S. and P.N.; writing—review and editing, T.P.-d.-S., P.N., M.C.C., A.F.G., M.S., F.S., F.J.E., R.C.F. and M.M.C.; visualization, T.P.-d.-S.; supervision, P.N., R.C.F. and M.M.C.; project administration, P.N. and M.M.C. All authors have read and agreed to the published version of the manuscript.

**Funding:** This research received no external funding.

**Institutional Review Board Statement:** The study was conducted according to the guidelines of the Declaration of Helsinki, and approved by the ethics committees of the involved institutions (Centro Hospitalar Universitário de Lisboa Central, Nr. 245/2015, on 1 October 2015, and NOVA Medical School | Faculdade de Ciências Médicas, Universidade NOVA de Lisboa, Nr. 000176, on 11 November 2015).

**Informed Consent Statement:** Informed consent was obtained from all subjects involved in the study.

**Data Availability Statement:** The data presented in this study are available on request from the corresponding author. The data are not publicly available due to personal data protection.

**Acknowledgments:** This study is part of the PhD thesis program of one of the authors (T.P.-d.-S.), supervised (M.M.C.) and co-supervised (P.N.) by the other two, conducted at the NOVA Medical School | Faculdade de Ciências Médicas, Universidade NOVA de Lisboa, Lisbon, Portugal. The authors are grateful to Joana Castro, from Medinres—Medical Information and Research, for her advice with respect to the statistical analysis.

**Conflicts of Interest:** The authors declare no conflict of interest.

## References

1. Siasos, G.; Tsigkou, V.; Kokkou, E.; Oikonomou, E.; Vavuranakis, M.; Vlachopoulos, C.; Verveniotis, A.; Limperi, M.; Genimata, V.; Papavassiliou, A.G.; et al. Smoking and Atherosclerosis: Mechanisms of Disease and New Therapeutic Approaches. *Curr. Med. Chem.* **2014**, *21*, 3936–3948. [CrossRef]
2. Lu, J.T.; Creager, M.A. The relationship of cigarette smoking to peripheral arterial disease. *Rev. Cardiovasc. Med.* **2004**, *5*, 189–193.
3. Feinberg, M.W.; Moore, K.J. MicroRNA Regulation of Atherosclerosis. *Circ. Res.* **2016**, *118*, 703–720. [CrossRef] [PubMed]
4. Willinger, C.M.; Rong, J.; Tanriverdi, K.; Courchesne, P.L.; Huan, T.; Wasserman, G.A.; Lin, H.; Dupuis, J.; Joehanes, R.; Jones, M.R.; et al. MicroRNA Signature of Cigarette Smoking and Evidence for a Putative Causal Role of MicroRNAs in Smoking-Related Inflammation and Target Organ Damage. *Circ. Cardiovasc. Genet.* **2017**, *10*. [CrossRef]
5. Kaur, G.; Begum, R.; Thota, S.; Batra, S. A systematic review of smoking-related epigenetic alterations. *Arch. Toxicol.* **2019**, *93*, 2715–2740. [CrossRef]
6. Pereira-da-Silva, T.; Coutinho Cruz, M.; Carrusca, C.; Cruz Ferreira, R.; Napoleão, P.; Mota Carmo, M. Circulating mi-croRNA profiles in different arterial territories of stable atherosclerotic disease: A systematic review. *Am. J. Cardiovasc. Dis.* **2018**, *8*, 1–13.
7. Andreou, I.; Sun, X.; Stone, P.H.; Edelman, E.R.; Feinberg, M.W. miRNAs in atherosclerotic plaque initiation, progression, and rupture. *Trends Mol. Med.* **2015**, *21*, 307–318. [CrossRef]
8. Chen, L.-J.; Lim, S.H.; Yeh, Y.-T.; Lien, S.-C.; Chiu, J.-J. Roles of microRNAs in atherosclerosis and restenosis. *J. Biomed. Sci.* **2012**, *19*, 79. [CrossRef]
9. Navickas, R.; Gal, D.; Laucevičius, A.; Taparauskaitė, A.; Zdanytė, M.; Holvoet, P. Identifying circulating microRNAs as biomarkers of cardiovascular disease: A systematic review. *Cardiovasc. Res.* **2016**, *111*, 322–337. [CrossRef]
10. Stather, P.W.; Sylvius, N.; Wild, J.B.; Choke, E.; Sayers, R.D.; Bown, M.J. Differential MicroRNA Expression Profiles in Peripheral Arterial Disease. *Circ. Cardiovasc. Genet.* **2013**, *6*, 490–497. [CrossRef]
11. Signorelli, S.S.; Volsi, G.L.; Pitruzzella, A.; Fiore, V.; Mangiafico, M.; Vanella, L.; Parenti, R.; Rizzo, M.; Volti, G.L. Circulating miR-130a, miR-27b, and miR-210 in Patients With Peripheral Artery Disease and Their Potential Relationship With Oxidative Stress. *Angiology* **2016**, *67*, 945–950. [CrossRef]
12. Wang, J.; Song, Y.; Zhang, Y.; Xiao, H.; Sun, Q.; Hou, N.; Guo, S.; Wang, Y.; Fan, K.; Zhan, D.; et al. Cardiomyocyte overexpression of miR-27b induces cardiac hypertrophy and dysfunction in mice. *Cell Res.* **2011**, *22*, 516–527. [CrossRef]
13. Liu, B.; Chen, W.; Cao, G.; Dong, Z.; Xu, J.; Luo, T.; Zhang, S. MicroRNA-27b inhibits cell proliferation in oral squamous cell carcinoma by targeting FZD7 and Wnt signaling pathway. *Arch. Oral Biol.* **2017**, *83*, 92–96. [CrossRef]
14. Murata, Y.; Yamashiro, T.; Kessoku, T.; Jahan, I.; Usuda, H.; Tanaka, T.; Okamoto, T.; Nakajima, A.; Wada, K. Up-Regulated MicroRNA-27b Promotes Adipocyte Differentiation via Induction of Acyl-CoA Thioesterase 2 Expression. *BioMed Res. Int.* **2019**, *2019*, 1–9. [CrossRef]
15. Cazalla, D.; Steitz, J.A. Down-Regulation of a Host microRNA by a Viral Noncoding RNA. *Cold Spring Harb. Symp. Quant. Biol.* **2010**, *75*, 321–324. [CrossRef] [PubMed]
16. Guo, Y.E.; Riley, K.J.; Iwasaki, A.; Steitz, J.A. Alternative Capture of Noncoding RNAs or Protein-Coding Genes by Herpesviruses to Alter Host T Cell Function. *Mol. Cell* **2014**, *54*, 67–79. [CrossRef]
17. Marcinowski, L.; Tanguy, M.; Krmpotic, A.; Rädle, B.; Lisnić, V.J.; Tuddenham, L.; Chane-Woon-Ming, B.; Ruzsics, Z.; Erhard, F.; Benkartek, C.; et al. Degradation of Cellular miR-27 by a Novel, Highly Abundant Viral Transcript Is Important for Efficient Virus Replication in Vivo. *PLoS Pathog.* **2012**, *8*, e1002510. [CrossRef]
18. Machitani, M.; Sakurai, F.; Wakabayashi, K.; Nakatani, K.; Tachibana, M.; Mizuguchi, H. MicroRNA miR-27 Inhibits Adenovirus Infection by Suppressing the Expression of SNAP25 and TXN2. *J. Virol.* **2017**, *91*, e00159–e00217. [CrossRef]
19. Xie, W.; Li, L.; Zhang, M.; Cheng, H.-P.; Gong, D.; Lv, Y.-C.; Yao, F.; He, P.-P.; Ouyang, X.-P.; Lan, G.; et al. MicroRNA-27 Prevents Atherosclerosis by Suppressing Lipoprotein Lipase-Induced Lipid Accumulation and Inflammatory Response in Apolipoprotein E Knockout Mice. *PLoS ONE* **2016**, *11*, e0157085. [CrossRef]
20. Vickers, K.C.; Shoucri, B.M.; Levin, M.G.; Wu, H.; Pearson, D.S.; Osei-Hwedieh, D.; Collins, F.S.; Remaley, A.T.; Sethupathy, P. MicroRNA-27b is a regulatory hub in lipid metabolism and is altered in dyslipidemia. *Hepatology* **2013**, *57*, 533–542. [CrossRef] [PubMed]
21. Liang, S.; Song, Z.; Wu, Y.; Gao, Y.; Gao, M.; Liu, F.; Wang, F.; Zhang, Y. MicroRNA-27b Modulates Inflammatory Response and Apoptosis during Mycobacterium tuberculosis Infection. *J. Immunol.* **2018**, *200*, 3506–3518. [CrossRef]
22. Huang, K.; Shen, Y.; Wei, X.; Zhang, F.; Liu, Y.; Ma, L. Inhibitory effect of microRNA-27b on interleukin 17 (IL-17)-induced monocyte chemoattractant protein-1 (MCP1) expression. *Genet. Mol. Res.* **2016**, *15*. [CrossRef]
23. Veliceasa, D.; Biyashev, D.; Qin, G.; Misener, S.; Mackie, A.R.; Kishore, R.; Volpert, O.V. Therapeutic manipulation of angiogenesis with miR-27b. *Vasc. Cell* **2015**, *7*, 6. [CrossRef]
24. Boon, R.A.; Hergenreider, E.; Dimmeler, S. Atheroprotective mechanisms of shear stress-regulated microRNAs. *Thromb. Haemost.* **2012**, *108*, 616–620. [CrossRef]
25. Kuehbacher, A.; Urbich, C.; Zeiher, A.M.; Dimmeler, S. Role of Dicer and Drosha for Endothelial MicroRNA Expression and Angiogenesis. *Circ. Res.* **2007**, *101*, 59–68. [CrossRef]
26. Urbich, C.; Kaluza, D.; Frömel, T.; Knau, A.; Bennewitz, K.; Boon, R.A.; Bonauer, A.; Doebele, C.; Boeckel, J.-N.; Hergenreider, E.; et al. MicroRNA-27a/b controls endothelial cell repulsion and angiogenesis by targeting semaphorin 6A. *Blood* **2012**, *119*, 1607–1616. [CrossRef]

27. Hwang, J.Y. Doppler ultrasonography of the lower extremity arteries: Anatomy and scanning guidelines. *Ultrasonography* **2017**, *36*, 111–119. [CrossRef]
28. Aboyans, V.; Ricco, J.-B.; Bartelink, M.-L.E.; Björck, M.; Brodmann, M.; Cohnert, T.; Collet, J.-P.; Czerny, M.; De Carlo, M.; Debus, S.; et al. Editor's Choice—2017 ESC Guidelines on the Diagnosis and Treatment of Peripheral Arterial Diseases, in collaboration with the European Society for Vascular Surgery (ESVS). *Eur. J. Vasc. Endovasc. Surg.* **2018**, *55*, 305–368. [CrossRef]
29. Collins, R.; Burch, J.; Cranny, G.; Aguiar-Ibáñez, R.; Craig, D.; Wright, K.; Berry, E.; Gough, M.; Kleijnen, J.; Westwood, M. Duplex ultrasonography, magnetic resonance angiography, and computed tomography angiography for diagnosis and assessment of symptomatic, lower limb peripheral arterial disease: Systematic review. *BMJ* **2007**, *334*, 1257. [CrossRef]
30. Hackshaw, A.; Morris, J.K.; Boniface, S.; Tang, J.-L.; Milenković, D. Low cigarette consumption and risk of coronary heart disease and stroke: Meta-analysis of 141 cohort studies in 55 study reports. *BMJ* **2018**, *360*, 5855. [CrossRef] [PubMed]
31. Deo, A.; Carlsson, J.; Lindlöf, A. How to Choose A Normalization Strategy for Mirna Quantitative Real-Time (QPCR) Arrays. *J. Bioinform. Comput. Biol.* **2011**, *9*, 795–812. [CrossRef] [PubMed]
32. Wolfinger, R.D.; Beedanagari, S.; Boitier, E.; Chen, T.; Couttet, P.; Ellinger-Ziegelbauer, H.; Guillemain, G.; Mariet, C.; Mouritzen, P.; O'Lone, R.; et al. Two approaches for estimating the lower limit of quantitation (LLOQ) of microRNA levels assayed as exploratory biomarkers by RT-qPCR. *BMC Biotechnol.* **2018**, *18*, 6. [CrossRef]
33. Zhang, X.; Shao, S.; Geng, H.; Yu, Y.; Wang, C.; Liu, Z.; Yu, C.; Jiang, X.; Deng, Y.; Gao, L.; et al. Expression Profiles of Six Circulating MicroRNAs Critical to Atherosclerosis in Patients With Subclinical Hypothyroidism: A Clinical Study. *J. Clin. Endocrinol. Metab.* **2014**, *99*, 766–774. [CrossRef] [PubMed]
34. Kumar, D.; Narang, R.; Sreenivas, V.; Rastogi, V.; Bhatia, J.; Saluja, D.; Srivastava, K. Circulatory miR-133b and miR-21 as Novel Biomarkers in Early Prediction and Diagnosis of Coronary Artery Disease. *Genes* **2020**, *11*, 164. [CrossRef]
35. Vegter, E.L.; Ovchinnikova, E.S.; Van Veldhuisen, D.J.; Jaarsma, T.; Berezikov, E.; Van Der Meer, P.; Voors, A.A. Low circulating microRNA levels in heart failure patients are associated with atherosclerotic disease and cardiovascular-related rehospitalizations. *Clin. Res. Cardiol.* **2017**, *106*, 598–609. [CrossRef]
36. Stather, P.W.; Sylvius, N.; Sidloff, D.A.; Dattani, N.; Verissimo, A.; Wild, J.B.; Butt, H.Z.; Choke, E.; Sayers, R.D.; Bown, M.J. Identification of microRNAs associated with abdominal aortic aneurysms and peripheral arterial disease. *BJS* **2015**, *102*, 755–766. [CrossRef]
37. Huang, Y.-Q.; Ying-Ling, Z.; Chen, J.-Y.; Zhou, Y.-L.; Cai, A.-P.; Huang, C.; Feng, Y.-Q. The Association of Circulating MiR-29b and Interleukin-6 with Subclinical Atherosclerosis. *Cell. Physiol. Biochem.* **2017**, *44*, 1537–1544. [CrossRef]
38. Livak, K.J.; Schmittgen, T.D. Analysis of relative gene expression data using real-time quantitative PCR and the $2^{-\Delta\Delta CT}$ Method. *Methods* **2001**, *25*, 402–408. [CrossRef]
39. Takahashi, K.; Yokota, S.-I.; Tatsumi, N.; Fukami, T.; Yokoi, T.; Nakajima, M. Cigarette smoking substantially alters plasma microRNA profiles in healthy subjects. *Toxicol. Appl. Pharmacol.* **2013**, *272*, 154–160. [CrossRef]
40. Suzuki, K.; Yamada, H.; Nagura, A.; Ohashi, K.; Ishikawa, H.; Yamazaki, M.; Ando, Y.; Ichino, N.; Osakabe, K.; Sugimoto, K.; et al. Association of cigarette smoking with serum microRNA expression among middle-aged Japanese adults. *Fujita Med J.* **2013**, *2*, 1–5. [CrossRef]
41. Bhat, M.Y.; Advani, J.; Rajagopalan, P.; Patel, K.; Nanjappa, V.; Solanki, H.S.; Patil, A.H.; Bhat, F.A.; Mathur, P.P.; Nair, B.; et al. Cigarette smoke and chewing tobacco alter expression of different sets of miRNAs in oral keratinocytes. *Sci. Rep.* **2018**, *8*, 1–13. [CrossRef]
42. Fazeli, S.; Motovali-Bashi, M.; Peymani, M.; Hashemi, M.-S.; Etemadifar, M.; Nasr-Esfahani, M.H.; Ghaedi, K. A compound downregulation of SRRM2 and miR-27a-3p with upregulation of miR-27b-3p in PBMCs of Parkinson's patients is associated with the early stage onset of disease. *PLoS ONE* **2020**, *15*, e0240855. [CrossRef]
43. Shafiei, J.; Heidari, F.; Khashen, C.; Ghandehari-Alavijeh, R.; Darmishonnejad, Z. Distinctive deregulation of miR-27a and miR-27b in relapsing remitting multiple sclerosis. *J. Bas. Res. Med. Sci.* **2020**, *7*, 1–6.
44. Ma, M.; Yin, Z.; Zhong, H.; Liang, T.; Guo, L. Analysis of the expression, function, and evolution of miR-27 isoforms and their responses in metabolic processes. *Genomics* **2019**, *111*, 1249–1257. [CrossRef] [PubMed]
45. Libby, P.; Ridker, P.M.; Hansson, G.K. Inflammation in Atherosclerosis. *J. Am. Coll. Cardiol.* **2009**, *54*, 2129–2138. [CrossRef]
46. Ross, R. Atherosclerosis—An Inflammatory Disease. *N. Engl. J. Med.* **1999**, *340*, 115–126. [CrossRef]
47. Kaur, A.; Mackin, S.T.; Schlosser, K.; Wong, F.L.; Elharram, M.; Delles, C.; Stewart, D.J.; Dayan, N.; Landry, T.; Pilote, L. Systematic review of microRNA biomarkers in acute coronary syndrome and stable coronary artery disease. *Cardiovasc. Res.* **2019**, *116*, 1113–1124. [CrossRef]
48. Cheng, H.S.; Sivachandran, N.; Lau, A.; Boudreau, E.; Zhao, J.L.; Baltimore, D.; Delgado-Olguin, P.; Cybulsky, M.I.; Fish, J.E. Micro RNA -146 represses endothelial activation by inhibiting pro-inflammatory pathways. *EMBO Mol. Med.* **2013**, *5*, 1017–1034. [CrossRef]
49. Wang, H.-J.; Huang-Joe, W.; Shih, Y.-Y.; Wu, H.-Y.; Peng, C.-T.; Lo, W.-Y. MicroRNA-146a Decreases High Glucose/Thrombin-Induced Endothelial Inflammation by Inhibiting NAPDH Oxidase 4 Expression. *Mediat. Inflamm.* **2014**, *2014*, 1–12. [CrossRef] [PubMed]
50. Lin, X.; Zhan, J.-K.; Wang, Y.-J.; Tan, P.; Chen, Y.-Y.; Deng, H.-Q.; Liu, Y.-S. Function, Role, and Clinical Application of MicroRNAs in Vascular Aging. *BioMed Res. Int.* **2016**, *2016*, 1–15. [CrossRef] [PubMed]

51. Li, J.; Zhao, L.; He, X.; Yang, T.; Yang, K. MiR-21 inhibits c-Ski signaling to promote the proliferation of rat vascular smooth muscle cells. *Cell. Signal.* **2014**, *26*, 724–729. [CrossRef]
52. Weber, M.; Baker, M.B.; Moore, J.P.; Searles, C.D. MiR-21 is induced in endothelial cells by shear stress and modulates apoptosis and eNOS activity. *Biochem. Biophys. Res. Commun.* **2010**, *393*, 643–648. [CrossRef]
53. Jin, C.; Zhao, Y.; Yu, L.; Xu, S.; Fu, G. MicroRNA-21 mediates the rapamycin-induced suppression of endothelial proliferation and migration. *FEBS Lett.* **2013**, *587*, 378–385. [CrossRef]
54. Zhou, J.; Wang, K.-C.; Wu, W.; Subramaniam, S.; Shyy, J.Y.-J.; Chiu, J.-J.; Li, J.Y.-S.; Chien, S. MicroRNA-21 targets peroxisome proliferators-activated receptor- in an autoregulatory loop to modulate flow-induced endothelial inflammation. *Proc. Natl. Acad. Sci. USA* **2011**, *108*, 10355–10360. [CrossRef]
55. Ulrich, V.; Rotllan, N.; Araldi, E.; Luciano, A.; Skroblin, P.; Abonnenc, M.; Perrotta, P.; Yin, X.; Bauer, A.; Leslie, K.L.; et al. Chronic miR-29 antagonism promotes favorable plaque remodeling in atherosclerotic mice. *EMBO Mol. Med.* **2016**, *8*, 643–653. [CrossRef]
56. Zhang, P.; Huang, A.; Ferruzzi, J.; Mecham, R.P.; Starcher, B.C.; Tellides, G.; Humphrey, J.D.; Giordano, F.J.; Niklason, L.E.; Sessa, W.C. Inhibition of MicroRNA-29 Enhances Elastin Levels in Cells Haploinsufficient for Elastin and in Bioengineered Vessels—Brief Report. *Arter. Thromb. Vasc. Biol.* **2012**, *32*, 756–759. [CrossRef] [PubMed]
57. Schober, A.; Nazari-Jahantigh, M.; Wei, Y.; Bidzhekov, K.; Gremse, F.; Grommes, J.; Megens, R.T.A.; Heyll, K.; Noels, H.; Hristov, M.; et al. MicroRNA-126-5p promotes endothelial proliferation and limits atherosclerosis by suppressing Dlk1. *Nat. Med.* **2014**, *20*, 368–376. [CrossRef]
58. Kumar, S.; Kim, C.W.; Simmons, R.D.; Jo, H. Role of Flow-Sensitive microRNAs in Endothelial Dysfunction and Atherosclerosis. *Arter. Thromb. Vasc. Biol.* **2014**, *34*, 2206–2216. [CrossRef] [PubMed]
59. Fernández-Hernando, C.; Suárez, Y. MicroRNAs in endothelial cell homeostasis and vascular disease. *Curr. Opin. Hematol.* **2018**, *25*, 227–236. [CrossRef]
60. Small, E.M.; Sutherland, L.B.; Rajagopalan, K.N.; Wang, S.; Olson, E.N. MicroRNA-218 Regulates Vascular Patterning by Modulation of Slit-Robo Signaling. *Circ. Res.* **2010**, *107*, 1336–1344. [CrossRef]
61. Huang, R.S.; Gamazon, E.R.; Ziliak, D.; Wen, Y.; Im, H.K.; Zhang, W.; Wing, C.; Duan, S.; Bleibel, W.K.; Cox, N.J.; et al. Population differences in microRNA expression and biological implications. *RNA Biol.* **2011**, *8*, 692–701. [CrossRef] [PubMed]
62. Rawlings-Goss, R.A.; Campbell, M.C.; Tishkoff, S.A. Global population-specific variation in miRNA associated with cancer risk and clinical biomarkers. *BMC Med. Genom.* **2014**, *7*, 53. [CrossRef]

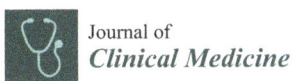

Article

# The Relationship between Cardiovascular Risk Scores and Several Markers of Subclinical Atherosclerosis in an Asymptomatic Population

Ovidiu Mitu [1,2,†], Adrian Crisan [2,\*], Simon Redwood [3], Ioan-Elian Cazacu-Davidescu [4], Ivona Mitu [5,\*], Irina-Iuliana Costache [1,2,†], Viviana Onofrei [1,2,†], Radu-Stefan Miftode [1,2], Alexandru-Dan Costache [1,6], Cristian Mihai Stefan Haba [1,2] and Florin Mitu [1,6]

1. 1st Medical Department, Faculty of Medicine, University of Medicine and Pharmacy "Grigore T. Popa", 700115 Iasi, Romania; mituovidiu@yahoo.co.uk (O.M.); ii.costache@yahoo.com (I.-I.C.); onofreiviana@gmail.com (V.O.); radu.miftode@yahoo.com (R.-S.M.); adcostache@yahoo.com (A.-D.C.); cristi.haba@gmail.com (C.M.S.H.); mitu.florin@yahoo.com (F.M.)
2. Department of Cardiology, Clinical Emergency Hospital "Sf. Spiridon", 700111 Iasi, Romania
3. Department of Cardiology, St. Thomas' Hospital, Westminster Bridge Road, London SE1 7EH, UK; simon.redwood@gstt.nhs.uk
4. Department of Cardiology, Clinical Emergency Hospital, 8 Calea Floreasca, 014475 Bucharest, Romania; elian.cazacu@gmail.com
5. Department of Morpho-Functional Sciences II, Faculty of Medicine, University of Medicine and Pharmacy "Grigore T. Popa", 700115 Iasi, Romania
6. Department of Cardiovascular Rehabilitation, Clinical Hospital of Rehabilitation, 700661 Iasi, Romania
\* Correspondence: crisanadrian93@yahoo.com (A.C.); ivonamitu@gmail.com (I.M.)
† Equal contribution.

**Abstract:** Background: The current cardiovascular disease (CVD) primary prevention guidelines prioritize risk stratification by using clinical risk scores. However, subclinical atherosclerosis may rest long term undetected. This study aimed to evaluate multiple subclinical atherosclerosis parameters in relation to several CV risk scores in asymptomatic individuals. Methods: A cross-sectional, single-center study included 120 asymptomatic CVD subjects. Four CVD risk scores were computed: SCORE, Framingham, QRISK, and PROCAM. Subclinical atherosclerosis has been determined by carotid intima-media thickness (cIMT), pulse wave velocity (PWV), aortic and brachial augmentation indexes (AIXAo, respectively AIXbr), aortic systolic blood pressure (SBPao), and ankle-brachial index (ABI). Results: The mean age was 52.01 ± 10.73 years. For cIMT—SCORE was more sensitive; for PWV—Framingham score was more sensitive; for AIXbr—QRISK and PROCAM were more sensitive while for AIXao—QRISK presented better results. As for SBPao—SCORE presented more sensitive results. However, ABI did not correlate with any CVD risk score. Conclusions: All four CV risk scores are associated with markers of subclinical atherosclerosis in asymptomatic population, except for ABI, with specific particularities for each CVD risk score. Moreover, we propose specific cut-off values of CV risk scores that may indicate the need for subclinical atherosclerosis assessment.

**Keywords:** subclinical atherosclerosis; SCORE; Framingham; QRISK; PROCAM; cardiovascular risk; pulse wave velocity; intima media thickness

## 1. Introduction

The current primary prevention guidelines for the management of cardiovascular diseases (CVD) prioritize risk identification, mostly through traditional CV risk factors and risk stratification by using clinical and risk scores [1–5]. Researchers have developed and validated multivariable risk prediction tools that synthesize CV risk-factor information to predict future CV events in different populations [5,6]. As CVD present a long asymptomatic phase, there has been support for the expansion of predictive studies of arterial disease from its clinical form to subclinical manifestation [7]. Several CVD predictive clinical tools have been developed, the most used being the SCORE risk for European countries [1], the Framingham risk score for USA [8], and the QRISK score for UK [9]. Nonetheless, the detection of subclinical atherosclerosis has been shown to be a useful method for predicting future CV events [10,11].

Atherosclerosis is widely recognized as a major cause of death and disability worldwide [12]. It manifests as a continuum from subclinical phase to patent clinical atherosclerotic CVD that starts early in life and remain clinically undetected until an acute CV event occurs [13,14]. Subclinical atherosclerosis is an early indicator of atherosclerotic burden and its timely recognition can slow or prevent the progression to overt CVD [15]. Thus, individuals with subclinical atherosclerosis require primary CVD prevention and, simultaneously, they represent a challenge in primary care setting. Further on, most people are at high risk for acute CV events but are not aware because their traditional risk-factor levels are not unusually high [16]. However, the current data is rather limited regarding the value of CV risk scores associated with the presence of subclinical atherosclerosis, especially in asymptomatic populations.

Thus, our study aimed to: (i) evaluate subclinical atherosclerosis in asymptomatic individuals using multiple risk prediction scores, (ii) establish cut-off values of the CVD risk scores in predicting the presence of subclinical atherosclerosis markers, and (iii) determine the variance and unit modifications of CVD risk scores in relationship to subclinical atherosclerosis parameters.

## 2. Materials and Methods

### 2.1. Study Design and Population

A cross-sectional, single-center, observational study was conducted over a two-year period and aimed to evaluate only asymptomatic CVD subjects. The "asymptomatic" status was defined as having no previous recordings of any acute or chronic diseases and not being under any chronic medical treatment. As inclusion criteria, only apparently healthy subjects, aged 35–75 years, were proposed for evaluation from the general practitioners' (GP) data lists. Moreover, pregnant or breastfeeding women were not eligible, as well as persons that refused or could not consent the study participation. Initially, 703 subjects were randomized from the GP data lists, resulting in 276 apparently healthy individuals that met the inclusion criteria. Further eligibility was ascertained by telephone interview, part of them refused or did not present to the study visit, resulting in 120 subjects that were finally evaluated.

The study protocol had been approved by the local Ethics Committee and all participants signed an informed written consent before enrolment. The protocol and the used methods adhered to the Helsinki Declaration.

At the study visit, a detailed medical interview was conducted in all participants. The traditional CV risk factors were analyzed along with a complete physical examination that assessed the anthropometric parameters as well. The office blood pressure was measured according to the ESC/ESH guidelines recommendations [17]. A fasting venous blood sample was collected for biochemical analysis that included lipid profile, plasma glucose, and renal and hepatic function.

### 2.2. CVD Risk Scores

Based on the CV risk factors obtained from the medical interview, physical examination and biochemical tests, four major CV risk scores were computed: HeartScore®, Framingham, QRISK®3, and PROCAM. HeartScore® was developed by applying the SCORE (Systematic Coronary Risk Evaluation Project) risk and derived from European population. We aimed to use different risk scores that were validated on different populations for a comprehensive overview. For a uniform analysis, all scores predict the 10-year CVD risk, but every score is based on different risk factors, the most facile being

HeartScore® while QRISK®3 presents the most exhaustive evaluation [1,8,9,18]. Table 1 summarizes the main characteristics of all four CV risk scores.

**Table 1.** Main characteristics of the cardiovascular disease (CVD) risk scores.

|  | HeartScore® | Framingham | QRISK®3 | PROCAM |
|---|---|---|---|---|
| Population assessed | European countries | USA | UK | Germany |
| Time prediction | 10 years | 10 years | 10 years | 10 years |
| Outcomes | Fatal CVD | Fatal and non-fatal CVD | Incident CVD | Fatal and non-fatal CVD |
| Number of risk factors | 5 | 8 | 20 (8—non CVD major risk factors) | 9 |
| Year of last developed model | 2003 | 2008 | 2017 | 2007 |

### 2.3. Subclinical Atherosclerosis Evaluation

The subclinical atherosclerosis was evaluated by several standardized methods: carotid ultrasound for carotid intima-media thickness (cIMT), arterial stiffness parameters, and ankle-brachial index (ABI).

cIMT and carotid plaques were assessed by using ultrasonography and performed by a physician blinded to all patient data and respecting the Mannheim criteria [19]. A cIMT value > 0.9 mm was considered abnormal.

Arterial stiffness was evaluated using an Arteriograph® system device which uses the oscillometric method for determination. Its results have been validated in previous studies [20,21]. Besides pulse wave velocity (PWV), the device also provided other arterial stiffness markers such as aortic and brachial augmentation indexes (AIXao, respectively AIXbr) or aortic systolic blood pressure (SBPao).

ABI was performed in a standardized method by a single trained operator. A ratio < 0.9 was considered pathological for defining peripheral artery disease. The lowest value from either leg was introduced into the final analysis.

### 2.4. Statistical Analysis

Statistical analysis was performed in IBM SPSS Statistics 22.0, US. The existence of a relationship between variables was evaluated by Pearson correlation coefficient and a linear regression equation was conducted to observe how two or more variables vary between them. To establish the most appropriate cut-off values of the CV risk scores in predicting the presence of subclinical atherosclerosis markers, ROC curves and the area under the curve (AUC) were used for the benefit of using the test(s) in question. Descriptive data is presented as mean ± standard deviation. A $p$-value < 0.05 was considered statistically significant.

## 3. Results

The clinical and biological characteristics of the study group are highlighted in Table 2. The mean age of patients was 52.01 ± 10.73 years, with one third being males and all of them had Caucasian ethnicity. Among traditional risk factors, more than 20% were smokers, 30% presented positive family history of CVD, mean body mass index (BMI) was 28 kg/m$^2$. Average blood pressure (BP) was in normal ranges, however, 28.3% of them had undiagnosed arterial hypertension. Mean lipid parameters were at the superior borderline limit while the plasma glucose level and renal function were mostly normal. Regarding subclinical atherosclerosis, about 40% of the subjects presented carotid ultrasound abnormalities, the majority had normal ABI, while 20% showed increased arterial stiffness parameters. Overall, average CV risk scores included population at intermediate risk.

Table 2. General characteristics of the study population.

| General Characteristics | Specific Characteristics | | All Subjects (n = 120) |
|---|---|---|---|
| Risk factors | Age, years | | 52.01 ± 10.73 |
| | Male, n (%) | | 40 (33.3) |
| | Smoking status | Current smoker, n (%) | 26 (21.6) |
| | | Former smoker, n (%) | 22 (18.3) |
| | | Never smoker, n (%) | 72 (60) |
| | Alcohol consumers, n (%) | | 15 (12.5) |
| | Family history of CVD *, n (%) | | 36 (30) |
| | Body mass index, kg/m$^2$ | | 28.50 ± 5.34 |
| | Waist circumference, male, cm | | 103.60 ± 10.29 |
| | Waist circumference, female, cm | | 97.2 ± 13.62 |
| | Systolic blood pressure, mmHg | | 127.30 ± 17.22 |
| | Diastolic blood pressure, mmHg | | 81.27 ± 13.07 |
| | Cholesterol total, mg/dL | | 209.77 ± 45.56 |
| | LDL cholesterol, mg/dL | | 129.96 ± 40.71 |
| | HDL cholesterol, mg/dL | | 52.49 ± 14.47 |
| | Non-HDL cholesterol, mg/dL | | 157.27 ± 44.89 |
| | Triglycerides, mg/dL | | 137.06 ± 81.42 |
| | Plasma glucose, mg/dL | | 97.21 ± 12.75 |
| | eGFR, ml/min/1.73 m$^2$ | | 89.35 ± 16.54 |
| Subclinical atherosclerosis | cIMT, mm | | 0.86 ± 0.13 |
| | cIMT > 0.9 mm, n (%) | | 44 (36.7) |
| | Carotid plaques, n (%) | | 48 (40) |
| | ABI | | 1.08 ± 0.13 |
| | PWV, m/s | | 8.28 ± 1.79 |
| | PWV > 10 m/s, n (%) | | 23 (20.9) |
| | Aortic systolic blood pressure, mmHg | | 128.14 ± 21.05 |
| | AIXbr, % | | −0.98 ± 31.03 |
| | AIXao, % | | 37.04 ± 15.60 |
| CVD risk charts | SCORE risk | | 2.95 ± 2.71 |
| | Framingham | | 10.29 ± 8.38 |
| | QRISK | | 7.23 ± 6.93 |
| | PROCAM | | 5.49 ± 7.83 |

ABI indicates ankle-brachial index; AIXao, aortic augmentation index; AIXbr, brachial augmentation index; cIMT, carotid intima-media thickness; CVD, cardiovascular diseases; eGFR, estimated glomerular filtration rate; HDL, high-density lipoprotein; LDL, low-density lipoproteins; PWV, pulse wave velocity; * acute atherosclerotic events for men <55 years of age and women <65 years of age in first degree relatives.

In univariate analysis, all four CV risk correlated significantly with cIMT, PWV, SBPao, AIXao, AIXbr ($p < 0.05$). As well, the presence of carotid plaques was associated with increased CV risk scores ($p < 0.001$). However, ABI alterations were not associated with increased CV risk scores.

Moreover, for each major determinant of subclinical atherosclerosis (cIMT, carotid plaques, PWV), the CV risk scores were introduced into the ROC curves (Figure 1), obtaining values with (AUC) more than 0.600 so we can consider our ROC curve significantly better than chance and relevant for a diagnostic. For cIMT, Framingham was the best score associated with increased values of this parameter, closely followed by SCORE and QRISK (Table 3). The same three scores presented rather similar values in predicting the presence of carotid plaques (Table 4). As for PWV, the AUC were a bit smaller, with QRISK and Framingham having the best performances (Table 5). Nonetheless, all CV risk scores significantly predicted the presence of subclinical atherosclerosis irrespective of the used method ($p < 0.05$).

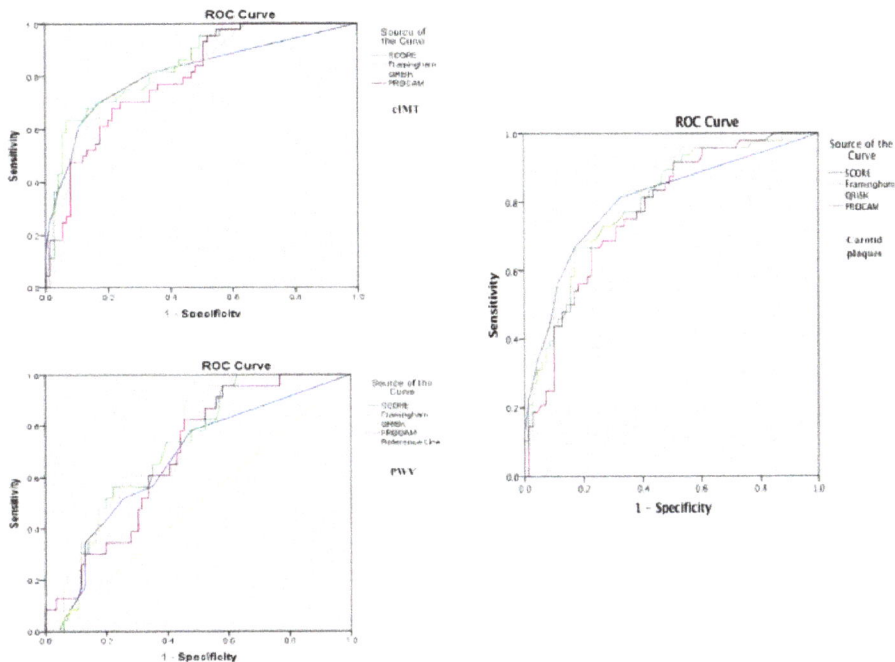

**Figure 1.** ROC curves of CV risk scores in association with subclinical atherosclerosis parameters (cIMT, carotid intima-media thickness; PWV, pulse wave velocity).

**Table 3.** Relationship between cIMT and CVD risk scores (by ROC analysis).

| Test Result Variable(s) | Area | Std. Error | Asymptotic Sig. | Asymptotic 95% Confidence Interval | |
|---|---|---|---|---|---|
| | | | | Lower Bound | Upper Bound |
| SCORE | 0.812 | 0.044 | 0.000 | 0.726 | 0.897 |
| Framingham | 0.845 | 0.036 | 0.000 | 0.774 | 0.916 |
| QRISK | 0.825 | 0.038 | 0.000 | 0.749 | 0.900 |
| PROCAM | 0.796 | 0.040 | 0.000 | 0.717 | 0.875 |

**Table 4.** Relationship between carotid plaques and CVD risk scores (by ROC analysis).

| Test Result Variable(s) | Area | Std. Error | Asymptotic Sig. | Asymptotic 95% Confidence Interval | |
|---|---|---|---|---|---|
| | | | | Lower Bound | Upper Bound |
| SCORE | 0.803 | 0.043 | 0.000 | 0.719 | 0.887 |
| Framingham | 0.799 | 0.041 | 0.000 | 0.720 | 0.879 |
| QRISK | 0.811 | 0.040 | 0.000 | 0.733 | 0.889 |
| PROCAM | 0.774 | 0.043 | 0.000 | 0.690 | 0.857 |

Table 5. Relationship between PWV and CVD risk scores (by ROC analysis).

| Test Result Variable(s) | Area | Std. Error | Asymptotic Sig. | Asymptotic 95% Confidence Interval | |
|---|---|---|---|---|---|
| | | | | Lower Bound | Upper Bound |
| SCORE | 0.666 | 0.062 | 0.015 | 0.545 | 0.787 |
| Framingham | 0.715 | 0.052 | 0.002 | 0.613 | 0.817 |
| QRISK | 0.733 | 0.050 | 0.001 | 0.635 | 0.832 |
| PROCAM | 0.688 | 0.054 | 0.006 | 0.582 | 0.794 |

Going into further analysis, we tried to obtain several cut-off points for CV risk scores that could predict the presence of subclinical atherosclerosis (Table 6). To investigate the cut-off points, we had to balance the importance of the false positive rate (FPR) in our analysis. Since we aimed the diagnosis for the presence of subclinical atherosclerosis, the repercussions for the FPR will only address the preventive concerns. That could only help the patient in order to prevent the development of subclinical atherosclerosis even though the patient is at low or intermediate CV risk. Thus, a higher FPR can be considered as necessary so that the result will not harm the patient under any circumstances. Assuming this hypothesis for identifying the most significant cut-off values that may suggest the screening for subclinical atherosclerosis, we considered that we could accept an increased value of FPR as long as the sensitivity is higher than 0.700, mostly 0.800, but with as lower specificity as possible. Nonetheless, for higher sensibility, we were willing to accept a moderate percentage of patients with FPR because the indicated tests are not invasive and widely available, and the subclinical atherosclerosis assessment could bring valuable information.

Table 6. Cut-off values of the CVD risk scores in predicting the presence of subclinical atherosclerosis markers.

| Risk Score | | cIMT | PWV | Carotid Plaques |
|---|---|---|---|---|
| SCORE | Cut-off value | 1.5 | 1.5 | 1.5 |
| | Sensitivity (%) | 81.8 | 78.3 | 81.3 |
| | Specificity (%) | 64.5 | 51.7 | 66.7 |
| | PPV (%) | 57.1 | 30 | 61.9 |
| | NPV (%) | 86 | 90 | 84.2 |
| Framingham | Cut-off value | 7.95 | 8.8 | 4.75 |
| | Sensitivity (%) | 81.8 | 73.9 | 89.6 |
| | Specificity (%) | 65.8 | 59.8 | 51.4 |
| | PPV (%) | 58.1 | 32.7 | 55.1 |
| | NPV (%) | 86.2 | 89.7 | 88.1 |
| QRISK | Cut-off value | 5.3 | 3.7 | 4.3 |
| | Sensitivity (%) | 81.8 | 95.7 | 83.3 |
| | Specificity (%) | 68.4 | 46 | 63.9 |
| | PPV (%) | 60 | 31.9 | 60.6 |
| | NPV (%) | 86.7 | 97.6 | 85.2 |
| PROCAM | Cut-off value | 2.11 | 2.05 | 1.62 |
| | Sensitivity (%) | 77.3 | 82.6 | 81.2 |
| | Specificity (%) | 63.2 | 54 | 58.3 |
| | PPV (%) | 54.8 | 32.2 | 56.5 |
| | NPV (%) | 82.8 | 92.2 | 82.4 |

cIMT indicates carotid intima-media thickness; NPV, negative predictive value; PPV, positive predictive value; PWV, pulse wave velocity.

Thus, a SCORE > 1.5 could indicate the presence of subclinical atherosclerosis regardless of the used method. Framingham values > 7.95 could indicate the presence of carotid modifications, while higher values are needed for an increase in PWV. For QRISK, the values are rather irregular, nonetheless values > 5.3 may represent a sign of subclinical atherosclerosis, while PROCAM values > 2.1 may trigger the attention towards subclinical changes.

By performing multivariate regression analysis for the relationship between different parameters of subclinical atherosclerosis and CV risks scores, a statistically significant correlation was obtained for all four CV risk scores. Thus, a regression equation was performed in order to predict the change in every risk score for detecting subclinical atherosclerosis parameters in the study group (Table 7). We interpret the results, from the point of view of sensitivity, as follows:

- For cIMT—SCORE is more sensitive (33% of the variance in cIMT was predictable from SCORE); each increase of SCORE with 1.16 signifies a further increase of cIMT with 0.1 mm. The prediction was closely followed by Framingham (29% variance) and QRISK (28% variance).
- For PWV—Framingham score is more sensitive (21% of the variance in PWV was predictable from Framingham score). This result can be translated that for each increase of Framingham value with 2.1, PWV increases as well with 1 m/s. The prediction was closely followed by QRISK (19% variance) and SCORE (17% variance).
- For AIXbr—QRISK and PROCAM are more sensitive, but all risk scores present a variance <10%.
- For AIXao—QRISK is more sensitive, but all risk scores present a variance <10%.
- For SBPao—SCORE is more sensitive (23% of the variance of SBPao was predictable from SCORE); each increase of SCORE with 0.6 signifies a further increase of SBPao with 10 mmHg. The prediction was closely followed by Framingham (21% variance) and QRISK (18% variance).
- For ABI—PROCAM score is more sensitive, but the overall prediction values are ≤0.1%.

Table 7. Variance and unit modifications of CVD risk scores in relationship to subclinical atherosclerosis parameters.

| | Linear Regression | PWV (Increase with One Unit) | cIMT Max (Increase with 0.1) | ABI (Increase with 0.1) | AIXbr (Increase with 1%) | AIXao (Increase with 1%) | SBPao (Increase with 1 mmHg) |
|---|---|---|---|---|---|---|---|
| SCORE | $r$ | 0.41 | 0.57 | −0.10 | 0.27 | 0.28 | 0.48 |
| | $p$ | <0.01 | <0.01 | <0.01 | 0.01 | <0.01 | <0.01 |
| | Increase/decrease | 0.6 | 1.16 | 0.2 | 0.025 | 0.05 | 0.06 |
| | $R^2$ | 0.17 | 0.33 | 0.01 | 0.07 | 0.07 | 0.23 |
| | Reg. ec. | $y = -2.27 + 0.65*x$ | $y = -6.96 + 11.46*x$ | $Y = 5.32 - 2.19*x$ | $Y = 3.11 + 0.02*x$ | $Y = 1.23 + 0.05*x$ | $Y = -5.06 + 0.06*x$ |
| Framingham | $r$ | 0.45 | 0.54 | −0.11 | 0.25 | 0.25 | 0.46 |
| | $p$ | <0.01 | <0.01 | <0.01 | <0.01 | <0.01 | <0.01 |
| | Increase/decrease | 2.1 | 3.3 | 0.6 | 0.069 | 0.14 | 0.18 |
| | $R^2$ | 0.21 | 0.29 | 0.01 | 0.06 | 0.06 | 0.21 |
| | Reg. ec. | $y = -7.49 + 2.19*x$ | $Y = -18.64 + 33.48*x$ | $Y = 17.71 - 6.86*x$ | $Y = 10.71 + 0.07*x$ | $Y = 5.46 + 0.14*x$ | $Y = -13.47 + 0.19*x$ |
| QRISK3 | $r$ | 0.44 | 0.53 | −0.07 | 0.27 | 0.28 | 0.42 |
| | $p$ | <0.01 | <0.01 | 0.04 | <0.01 | <0.01 | <0.01 |
| | Increase/decrease | 1.75 | 2.7 | 0.3 | 0.063 | 0.12 | 0.14 |
| | $R^2$ | 0.19 | 0.28 | 0.005 | 0.07 | 0.08 | 0.18 |
| | Reg. ec. | $y = -7.06 + 1.76*x$ | $Y = -16.11 + 27.01*x$ | $Y = 11.08 - 3.55*x$ | $Y = 2.75 + 0.13*x$ | $Y = 2.75 + 0.13*x$ | $Y = -10.84 + 0.14*x$ |
| PROCAM | $r$ | 0.37 | 0.42 | −0.15 | 0.27 | 0.28 | 0.29 |
| | $p$ | <0.01 | <0.01 | 0.04 | <0.01 | <0.01 | <0.01 |
| | Increase/decrease | 1.68 | 2.4 | 0.8 | 0.073 | 0.14 | 0.11 |
| | $R^2$ | 0.14 | 0.18 | 0.02 | 0.07 | 0.07 | 0.08 |
| | Reg. ec. | $y = -8.2 + 1.68*x$ | $Y = -15.56 + 24.32*x$ | $Y = 14.92 - 8.71*x$ | $Y = 0.22 + 0.15*x$ | $Y = 0.22 + 0.15*x$ | $Y = -8.6 + 0.11*x$ |

ABI indicates ankle-brachial index; AIXao, aortic augmentation index; AIXbr, brachial augmentation index; cIMT, carotid intima-media thickness; PWV, pulse wave velocity; SBPao, aortic systolic blood pressure; Reg. ec. = regression equation.

## 4. Discussion

The current guidelines for primary CVD prevention recommend initial assessment and risk stratification based on traditional risk factor scoring followed by therapeutic intervention when necessary [1,6,22–25]. However, risk scores have been developed to predict the risk of clinical evident CVD rather than subclinical changes. By comparing to other studies, our findings add novel data to the relationship between current CV risk evaluation based on risk scores and subclinical atherosclerotic evidence. It represents one of the fewest studies that correlated several risk scores with different markers of subclinical atherosclerosis, proposing specific cut-off values that would require a comprehensive CV evaluation in asymptomatic population.

Subclinical atherosclerosis parameters have proven their utility in clinical practice, both in primary and secondary CV prevention. In asymptomatic populations, increased values of coronary artery calcium score determined by computed tomography, several arterial stiffness markers, ABI or peripheral arterial modifications (carotid, aortic or iliofemoral) determined by ultrasound have been highly prevalent and detected as well in intermediate and low-risk subjects, not only in those with already high computed CV risk [26,27]. Moreover, increased subclinical atherosclerosis parameters have been correlated with CV risk events on long term.

According to current recommendations, the presence of carotid plaque is viewed as a high risk finding ($\geq$10% cardiovascular mortality risk at 10 years) [1]. In our study, all cardiovascular risk scores increased, in a directly proportional way, in patients with carotid plaques. Even if the sensibility was related to all four risk scores, the specificity was better for SCORE. These finding were similar with a study conducted by Romanens Michael et al., on 3.248 patients, aged 40–65, with no medication and no CV risk factors. The authors assessed the prevalence of "old" arteries (vascular age $\geq$70 years) using carotid plaque thickness. The results showed that most subjects with "old" arteries were classified as low risk according to PROCAM, while for SCORE only 20% of patients were in the low-risk group. Both scores correlated with carotid plaques, but the specificity and sensibility were better for SCORE [23]. Some studies assumed that the Framingham risk score underestimated subclinical atherosclerosis risk in asymptomatic individuals. In a carotid ultrasonography study, the echography assessment of subclinical CVD improved the reclassification of one-third of subjects with low or intermediate Framingham score into higher risk groups [24]. Rather similar, in a study on 662 patients without known CVD, 33.8% of patients who had been classified as low risk by the Framingham risk score presented subclinical coronary artery atherosclerosis detected by electron beam computed tomography. Despite this, they did not meet the criteria for pharmacologic therapy as defined by the score [25]. Another study aimed to investigate the features of subclinical carotid plaques in 166 asymptomatic patients with at least one CVD risk factor, by using multi-contrast weighted MRI and to correlate these findings with Framingham risk score. Sixty-six percent of the intraplaque hemorrhage occurred in low and intermediate-risk groups according to Framingham stratification. Therefore, Framingham risk score was not specific for carotid plaque because the stratification failed to identify more than half of individuals with complicated carotid plaque. Furthermore, nearly 1/3 of the individuals in the low-risk Framingham stratification had lipid rich necrotic core at the carotid assessment [6]. In our study all CV risk scores showed a directly proportional increase in patients with carotid plaques, but the specificity was superior for SCORE.

Carotid IMT is a strong predictor of CV events independent of conventional risk factors [28]. Juho RH Raiko et al. examined the carotid modifications in 2204 patients, aged 24–29 years, who were followed for 6 years. The authors used Framingham, SCORE, and PROCAM risk scores to predict subclinical atherosclerosis. All risk scores had equal performance in the prediction of 6-year increased cIMT and carotid plaques ($p < 0.05$) [29]. Another cohort study that followed 1348 subjects (18–99 years) over 12.7 years showed that 115 subjects developed nonfatal ischemic stroke, transient ischemic attack or vascular death. The inclusion of carotid findings (presence of cIMT > 1 mm or present plaque) resulted in a higher predictive power than Framingham risk score alone among those with a score > 20% [30,31]. In an observational, cross-sectional cohort study on 362 hypertensive subjects, cIMT correlated positively with the CV risk estimated by both SCORE ($r = 0.421$, $p < 0.01$) and Framingham ($r = 0.363$, $p < 0.01$) [32]. There was a significant positive correlation between cIMT and the Framingham risk score ($r$ for men = 0.571; $p < 0.001$; $r$ for women = 0.633; $p < 0.001$) and there was no significant gender difference between these two groups [33]. Furthermore, in a recent meta-analysis of 119 clinical trials involving 100.667 patients, the interventions reducing cIMT progression by 10, 20, 30, or 40 µm/year would yield CV relative risks of 0.84 (0.75–0.93), 0.76 (0.67–0.85), 0.69 (0.59–0.79), or 0.63 (0.52–0.74). In conclusion, the extent of interventions effects on cIMT progression predicted the degree of CV risk reduction [34]. We obtained similar results in our study, suggesting that the additional risk factors included in PROCAM (parental history of myocardial infarction and regional adjustment factor based on geographic prevalence) did not increase discrimination in our cohort. Moreover, although lacking HDL-cholesterol and diabetes status, SCORE showed an equal value in predicting high cIMT.

Regarding ABI evaluation, we did not find any associations with increased CV risk scores. A study conducted on 6091 patients aged ≥40 years, without any CVD, aimed to assess a link between subclinical atherosclerosis (determined by ABI) and different CV risk scores. Compared to individuals classified as low-risk by Framingham, individuals at intermediate-risk were not prone to have subclinical atherosclerosis, though individuals classified at high-risk had a two-fold increase of subclinical atherosclerosis (OR 2.31; 95%CI: 1.53–3.49). As for the sensitivity and specificity analysis, high-risk patients (vs. low-risk) had the lowest sensitivity (26.6%) and most specificity (87.4%) for identifying subclinical atherosclerosis. Intermediate-risk patients (vs. low-risk) had slightly better sensitivity (33.9%), but also lower specificity (64.9%) [5]. In a cross-sectional study on 6292 patients aged ≥40 years, without known CVD or diabetes, there was a close relation between abnormal ABI and Framingham risk score. 91.4% of patients were at < 20% Framingham risk score, and, out of these, only 2.7% (95%CI: 2.3–3.1%, $p < 0.0001$) had an abnormal ABI. The results showed that abnormal ABI is highly prevalent among individuals at low-intermediate Framingham risk score [35]. However, our results are divergent regarding the ABI screening possibly due to the sample size and the population characteristics.

As for PWV and CV risk scores, all four CV risk scores correlated significantly with PWV in our study. Similar results were obtained by L. Woźnicka-Leśkiewicz et al. where 200 patients were randomized into four different groups. In the group characterized by the lack of CV risk factors, PWV correlated significantly with the CV risk according to SCORE scale ($r = 0.45$, $p < 0.001$) and Framingham risk score ($r = 0.37$, $p < 0.001$) [36]. In a prospective study conducted on 177 subjects without evidence of significant CVD, the authors assessed the association between carotid augmentation index (CAI), carotid femoral PWV (cfPWV) and Framingham risk score. There was a significant association between cfPWV and Framingham score ($r = 0.417$, $p < 0.001$) and a weaker but also significant relation between CAI and Framingham score ($r = 0.267$, $p < 0.001$). cfPWV was significantly related to Framingham score in both men and women ($p < 0.001$ in both sexes), whereas the relation between CAI and Framingham score was significantly only in women ($p < 0.001$). The study suggested that cfPWV may be associated with CVD risk irrespective of sex, whereas CAI may be associated with CVD risk in women only [37]. Our study supports these results in terms of PWV (Framingham score was more sensitive) but not for AIX where QRISK and PROCAM were more sensitive, but all risk scores presented a variance <10%. Another study obtained slightly different results from our research, conducted with the aim to evaluate the association between SCORE risk and cfPWV, with a follow up of 4.9 years. A strong association between high CVD risk (SCORE ≥ 5%) and high PWV (OR 2.29; 95%CI 1.17–4.46) has been obtained [38].

Regarding AIXbr or AIXAo in our study, QRISK was the most sensitive. In another cross-sectional study on 81 young and middle-aged males (39.2 ± 6.3 years) without evidence of overt CVD or diabetes, the Framingham risk score was significantly correlated with AIXAo ($r = 0.266$, $p = 0.009$) [39]. Moreover, increased AIXAo was associated with a high Framingham risk score in patients that were referred to percutaneous coronary intervention (PCI) compared to non-PCI group (AIX was analyzed before coronary angiography) [40].

As CV risk scores are associated with subclinical atherosclerosis parameters, we defined specific cut-off values that may impose the screening for subclinical atherosclerosis. Thus, based on the results summarized in Table 6 and combined with the pre-defined risk categories for each CV score but taking into consideration the need for not abusing these methods, we suggest the screening of subclinical atherosclerosis in subjects with SCORE $\geq 3$, Framingham $\geq 10$, QRISK $\geq 10$ or PROCAM $\geq 5$, irrespective of used method.

Our study may present some limitations. Firstly, the moderate sample size population could represent a limiting factor for the divergent results obtained for ABI. As well, others novel markers of subclinical atherosclerosis could have been implemented as the coronary calcium score. However, we have used non-invasive methods that are easy for use in clinical practice and, added to the CV scores, could better refine the CV risk.

## 5. Conclusions

In the current study, all four CV risk scores were associated with markers of subclinical atherosclerosis in an asymptomatic population, except for ABI. The SCORE risk was better associated with carotid ultrasound abnormalities while Framingham and QRISK seemed more specific for increased arterial stiffness parameters. Moreover, we proposed specific cut-off values of CV risk scores that may indicate the need for subclinical atherosclerosis assessment. However, further research is needed for a tailored CV risk refinement based on risk scores and subclinical atherosclerosis markers.

**Author Contributions:** Conceptualization, O.M., A.C., I.-E.C.-D. and F.M.; methodology, O.M., A.C. and F.M.; software, A.C. and I.M.; investigation, I.M., R.-S.M., A.-D.C. and C.M.S.H.; resources, I.-I.C., V.O., and F.M.; data collection, O.M., A.C., I.-E.C.-D., I.M., R.-S.M., A.-D.C. and C.M.S.H.; writing—original draft preparation, O.M., A.C. and I.M.; writing—review and editing, I.-I.C., V.O. and F.M.; visualization, S.R., I.-I.C. and V.O.; supervision, F.M. and S.R. All authors have read and agreed to the published version of the manuscript.

**Funding:** This research received no external funding.

**Institutional Review Board Statement:** The study was conducted according to the guidelines of the Declaration of Helsinki, and approved by the Ethics Committee of the University of Medicine and Pharmacy "Grigore T. Popa" Iasi, Romania.

**Informed Consent Statement:** Informed consent was obtained from all subjects involved in the study.

**Data Availability Statement:** The data presented in this study are available on request from the corresponding author.

**Conflicts of Interest:** The authors declare no conflict of interest.

## References

1. Piepoli, M.F.; Hoes, A.W.; Agewall, S.; Albus, C.; Brotons, C.; Catapano, A.L.; Cooney, M.T.; Corrà, U.; Cosyns, B.; Deaton, C.; et al. Guidelines: Editor's choice: 2016 European Guidelines on cardiovascular disease prevention in clinical practice: The Sixth Joint Task Force of the European Society of Cardiology and Other Societies on Cardiovascular Disease Prevention in Clinical Practice (constituted by representatives of 10 societies and by invited experts) Developed with the special contribution of the European Association for Cardiovascular Prevention & Rehabilitation (EACPR). *Eur. Heart J.* **2016**, *37*, 2315. [PubMed]
2. Stone, N.J.; Robinson, J.G.; Lichtenstein, A.H. 2013 ACC/AHA guideline on the treatment of blood cholesterol to reduce atherosclerotic cardiovascular risk in adults: A report of the American College of Cardiology/American Heart Association Task Force on Practice Guidelines. *Circulation* **2014**, *129* (Suppl. 2), S1–S45. [CrossRef] [PubMed]
3. Goff, D.C., Jr.; Lloyd-Jones, D.M.; Bennett, G. 2013 ACC/AHA guideline on the assessment of cardiovascular risk: A report of the American College of Cardiology/American Heart Association Task Force on Practice Guidelines. *Circulation* **2014**, *129* (Suppl. 2), S49–S73. [CrossRef] [PubMed]
4. Bibbins-Domingo, K.; Grossman, D.C.; Curry, S.J.; Davidson, K.W.; Epling, J.W.; García, F.A.; Gillman, M.W.; Kemper, A.R.; Krist, A.H.; Kurth, A.E.; et al. Statin Use for the Primary Prevention of Cardiovascular Disease in Adults: US Preventive Services Task Force Recommendation Statement. *JAMA* **2016**, *316*, 1997–2007. [PubMed]
5. Singh, S.S.; Pilkerton, C.S.; Shrader, C.D.; Frisbee, S.J. Subclinical atherosclerosis, cardiovascular health, and disease risk: Is there a case for the Cardiovascular Health Index in the primary prevention population? *BMC Public Health* **2018**, *18*, 429. [CrossRef] [PubMed]

29. RH Raiko, J.; Magnussen, C.G.; Kivimäki, M.; Taittonen, L.; Laitinen, T.; Kähönen, M.; Hutri-Kähönen, N.; Jula, A.; Loo, B.M.; Thomson, R.J.; et al. Cardiovascular risk scores in the prediction of subclinical atherosclerosis in young adults: Evidence from the cardiovascular risk in a young Finns study. *Eur. J. Cardiovasc. Prev. Rehabil.* **2010**, *17*, 549–555. [CrossRef]
30. Prati, P.; Tosetto, A.; Vanuzzo, D.; Bader, G.; Casaroli, M.; Canciani, L.; Castellani, S.; Touboul, P.J. Carotid intima media thickness and plaques can predict the occurrence of ischemic cerebrovascular events. *Stroke* **2008**, *39*, 2470–2476. [CrossRef]
31. Mookadam, F.; Tanasunont, W.; Jalal, U.; Mookadam, M.; Wilansky, S. Carotid intima-media thickness and cardiovascular risk. *Future Cardiol.* **2011**, *7*, 173–182. [CrossRef] [PubMed]
32. Hermida, A.; Novo, J.; Marcos Ortega, J.E. Distribution of carotid intima-media thickness based on cardiovascular risk stratification according to the Framingham-REGICOR and SCORE functions. *Hypertens. Vasc. Risk* **2016**, *33*, 51–57.
33. Yao, F.; Liu, Y.; Liu, D.; Wu, S.; Lin, H.; Fan, R.; Li, C. Sex differences between vascular endothelial function and carotid intima-media thickness by Framingham Risk Score. *J. Ultrasound Med.* **2014**, *33*, 281–286. [CrossRef]
34. Willeit, P.; Tschiderer, L.; Allara, E.; Reuber, K.; Seekircher, L.; Gao, L.; Liao, X.; Lonn, E.; Gerstein, H.C.; Yusuf, S.; et al. Carotid Intima-Media Thickness Progression as Surrogate Marker for Cardiovascular Risk: Meta-Analysis of 119 Clinical Trials Involving 100,667 Patients. *Circulation* **2020**, *142*, 621–642. [CrossRef] [PubMed]
35. Dhangana, R.; Murphy, T.P.; Pencina, M.J.; Zafar, A.M. Prevalence of low ankle-brachial index, elevated plasma fibrinogen and CRP across Framingham risk categories: Data from the National Health and Nutrition Examination Survey (NHANES) 1999–2004. *Atherosclerosis* **2011**, *216*, 174–179. [CrossRef] [PubMed]
36. Woznicka-Leskiewicz, L.; Posadzy-Małaczyńska, A.; Juszkat, R. The impact of ankle brachial index and pulse wave velocity on cardiovascular risk according to SCORE and Framingham scales and sex differences. *J. Hum. Hypertens.* **2015**, *29*, 502–510. [CrossRef]
37. Song, B.G.; Park, J.B.; Cho, S.J.; Lee, S.Y.; Kim, J.H.; Choi, S.M.; Park, J.H.; Park, Y.H.; Choi, J.-O.; Lee, S.-C.; et al. Pulse wave velocity is more closely associated with cardiovascular risk than augmentation index in the relatively low-risk population. *Heart Vessels* **2009**, *24*, 413. [CrossRef]
38. Podolec, M.; Siniarski, A.; Pająk, A.; Rostoff, P.; Gajos, G.; Nessler, J.; Olszowska, M.; Nowakowski, M.; Szafraniec, K.; Kopeć, G. Association between carotid-femoral pulse wave velocity and overall cardiovascular risk score assessed by the SCORE system in urban Polish population. *Kardiol. Pol.* **2019**, *77*, 363–370. [CrossRef] [PubMed]
39. Stamatelopoulos, K.S.; Kalpakos, D.; Protogerou, A.D.; Papamichael, C.M.; Ikonomidis, I.; Tsitsirikos, M.; Revela, I.; Papaioannou, T.G.; Lekakis, J.P. The combined effect of augmentation index and carotid intima-media thickness on cardiovascular risk in young and middle-aged men without cardiovascular disease. *J. Hum. Hypertens.* **2006**, *20*, 273–279. [CrossRef] [PubMed]
40. Choi, J.; Kim, S.Y.; Joo, S.J.; Kim, K.S. Augmentation index is associated with coronary revascularization in patients with high Framingham risk scores: A hospital-based observational study. *BMC Cardiovasc. Disord.* **2015**, *15*, 131. [CrossRef]

6. Li, F.; Wang, X. Relationship between Framingham risk score and subclinical atherosclerosis in carotid plaques: An in vivo study using multi-contrast MRI. *Sci. China Life Sci.* **2017**, *60*, 23–27. [CrossRef] [PubMed]
7. Simon, A.; Levenson, J. May subclinical arterial disease help to better detect and treat high-risk asymptomatic individuals? *J. Hypertens.* **2005**, *23*, 1939–1945. [CrossRef]
8. D'Agostino, R.B.; Vasan, R.S.; Pencina, M.J.; Wolf, P.A.; Cobain, M.; Massaro, J.M.; Kannel, W.B. General cardiovascular risk profile for use in primary care: The framingham heart study. *Circulation* **2008**, *117*, 743–753. [CrossRef]
9. Hippisley-Cox, J.; Coupland, C.; Brindle, P. Development and validation of QRISK3 risk prediction algorithms to estimate future risk of cardiovascular disease: Prospective cohort study. *BMJ* **2017**, *357*, j2099. [CrossRef]
10. Simon, A.; Chironi, G.; Levenson, J. Performance of subclinical arterial disease detection as a screening test for coronary heart disease. *Hypertension* **2006**, *48*, 392–396. [CrossRef]
11. Plantinga, Y.; Dogan, S.; Grobbee, D.E.; Bots, M.L. Carotid intima-media thickness measurement in cardiovascular screening programmes. *Eur. J. Cardiovasc. Prev. Rehabil.* **2009**, *16*, 639–644. [CrossRef]
12. Roger, V.L.; Go, A.S.; Lloyd-Jones, D.M.; Benjamin, E.J.; Berry, J.D.; Borden, W.B.; Bravata, D.M.; Dai, S.; Ford, E.S.; Fox, C.S.; et al. Executive summary: Heart disease and stroke statistics—2012 update: A report from the American Heart Association. *Circulation* **2012**, *125*, 188–197. [PubMed]
13. Herrington, W.; Lacey, B.; Sherliker, P.; Armitage, J.; Lewington, S. Epidemiology of Atherosclerosis and the Potential to Reduce the Global Burden of Atherothrombotic Disease. *Circ. Res.* **2016**, *118*, 535–546. [CrossRef] [PubMed]
14. Frostegard, J. Immunity, atherosclerosis and cardiovascular disease. *BMC Med.* **2013**, *11*, 117. [CrossRef] [PubMed]
15. Resnick, H.E.; Lindsay, R.S.; McDermott, M.M.; Devereux, R.B.; Jones, K.L.; Fabsitz, R.R.; Howard, B.V. Relationship of high and low ankle brachial index to all-cause and cardiovascular disease mortality: The Strong Heart Study. *Circulation* **2004**, *109*, 733–739. [CrossRef]
16. Muntendam, P.; McCall, C.; Sanz, J.; Falk, E.; Fuster, V.; Fuster, V. The BioImage Study: Novel approaches to risk assessment in the primary prevention of atherosclerotic cardiovascular disease—Study design and objectives. *Am. Heart J.* **2010**, *160*, 49–57.e1. [CrossRef]
17. Williams, B.; Mancia, G.; Spiering, W.; Rosei, E.A.; Azizi, M.; Burnier, M.; Clement, D.L.; Coca, A.; De Simone, G.; Dominiczak, A.; et al. 2018 ESC/ESH Guidelines for the management of arterial hypertension: The Task Force for the management of arterial hypertension of the European Society of Cardiology (ESC) and the European Society of Hypertension (ESH). *Eur. Heart J.* **2018**, *39*, 3021–3104. [CrossRef] [PubMed]
18. Assmann, G.; Cullen, P.; Schulte, H. Simple scoring scheme for calculating the risk of acute coronary events based on the 10-year follow-up of the prospective cardiovascular Munster (PROCAM) study. *Circulation* **2002**, *105*, 310–315. [CrossRef]
19. Touboul, P.J.; Hennerici, M.G.; Meairs, S.; Adams, H.; Amarenco, P.; Bornstein, N.; Csiba, L.; Desvarieux, M.; Ebrahim, S.; Hernandez, R.; et al. Mannheim carotid intima-media thickness and plaque consensus (2004–2006–2011). *Cerebrovasc. Dis.* **2012**, *34*, 290–296. [CrossRef]
20. Horvath, I.G.; Nemeth, A.; Lenkey, Z.; Alessandri, N.; Tufano, F.; Kis, P.; Balázs, G.; Attila, C. Invasive validation of a new oscillometric device (Arteriograph) for measuring augmentation index, central blood pressure and aortic pulse wave velocity. *J. Hypertens.* **2010**, *28*, 2068–2075. [CrossRef]
21. Rajzer, M.W.; Wojciechowska, W.; Klocek, M.; Palka, I.; Brzozowska-Kiszka, M.; Kawecka-Jaszcz, K. Comparison of aortic pulse wave velocity measured by three techniques: Complior, SphygmoCor and Arteriograph. *J. Hypertens.* **2008**, *26*, 2001–2007. [CrossRef] [PubMed]
22. Naghavi, M.; Falk, E.; Hecht, H.S.; Jamieson, M.J.; Kaul, S.; Berman, D.; Fayad, Z.; Budoff, M.J.; Rumberger, J.; Naqvi, T.Z.; et al. From vulnerable plaque to vulnerable patient–Part III: Executive summary of the Screening for Heart Attack Prevention and Education (SHAPE) Task Force report. *Am. J. Cardiol.* **2006**, *98*, 2H–15H. [CrossRef] [PubMed]
23. Romanens, M.; Sudano, I.; Adams, A.; Warmuth, W. Advanced carotid atherosclerosis in middle-aged subjects: Comparison with PROCAM and SCORE risk categories, the potential for reclassification and cost-efficiency of carotid ultrasound in the setting of primary care. *SWISS Med. Wkly.* **2019**, *149*, w20006. [CrossRef] [PubMed]
24. Abe, Y.; Rundek, T.; Sciacca, R.R.; Jin, Z.; Sacco, R.L.; Homma, S.; Di Tullio, M.R. Ultrasound assessment of subclinical cardiovascular disease in a community-based multiethnic population and comparison to the framingham score. *Am. J. Cardiol.* **2006**, *98*, 1374–1378. [CrossRef] [PubMed]
25. Canpolat, U.; Yorgun, H.; Aytemir, K.; Hazrolan, T.; Kaya, E.B.; Ateş, A.H.; Dural, M.; Gürses, K.M.; Sunman, H.; Tokgözoğlu, L.; et al. Cardiovascular risk and coronary atherosclerotic plaques detected by multidetector computed tomography. *Coron. Artery Dis.* **2012**, *23*, 195–200. [CrossRef] [PubMed]
26. Fernández-Friera, L.; Peñalvo, J.L.; Fernández-Ortiz, A.; Ibañez, B.; López-Melgar, B.; Laclaustra, M.; Olive, B.; Mocoroa, A.; Mendiguren, J.; de Vega Martínez, V.; et al. Prevalence, Vascular Distribution, and Multiterritorial Extent of Subclinical Atherosclerosis in a Middle-Aged Cohort: The PESA (Progression of Early Subclinical Atherosclerosis) Study. *Circulation* **2015**, *131*, 2104–2113. [CrossRef]
27. Bonarjee, V.V.S. Arterial Stiffness: A Prognostic Marker in Coronary Heart Disease. Available Methods and Clinical Application. *Front. Cardiovasc. Med.* **2018**, *5*, 64. [CrossRef]
28. Lorenz, M.W.; Markus, H.S.; Bots, M.L.; Rosvall, M.; Sitzer, M. Prediction of clinical cardiovascular events with carotid intima-media thickness: A systematic review and meta-analysis. *Circulation* **2007**, *115*, 459–467. [CrossRef]

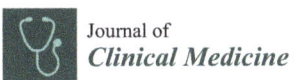 

Article

# Increased Circulating Malondialdehyde-Modified Low-Density Lipoprotein Level Is Associated with High-Risk Plaque in Coronary Computed Tomography Angiography in Patients Receiving Statin Therapy

Keishi Ichikawa [1], Toru Miyoshi [1,*], Kazuhiro Osawa [2], Takashi Miki [1] and Hiroshi Ito [1]

[1] Department of Cardiovascular Medicine, Okayama University Graduate School of Medicine, Dentistry and Pharmaceutical Sciences, Okayama 700-8558, Japan; ichikawa1987@gmail.com (K.I.); tm.f20c.2000@gmail.com (T.M.); itomd@md.okayama-u.ac.jp (H.I.)
[2] Department of Cardiovascular Medicine, Japanese Red Cross Okayama Hospital, Okayama 700-8607, Japan; rohiwasa@yahoo.co.jp
* Correspondence: miyoshit@cc.okayama-u.ac.jp

**Abstract:** Objective: To evaluate the association of serum malondialdehyde low-density lipoprotein (MDA-LDL), an oxidatively modified LDL, with the prevalence of high-risk plaques (HRP) determined with coronary computed tomography angiography (CTA) in statin-treated patients. Methods: This study was a single-center retrospective cohort comprising 268 patients (mean age 67 years, 58% men) with statin therapy and who underwent coronary CTA for suspected stable coronary artery disease. Patients were classified into two groups according to median MDA-LDL level or median LDL-C level. Coronary CTA-verified HRP was defined when two or more characteristics, including positive remodeling, low-density plaques, and spotty calcification, were present. Results: Patients with HRP had higher MDA-LDL ($p = 0.011$), but not LDL-C ($p = 0.867$) than those without HRP. High MDA-LDL was independently associated with HRP (odds ratio 1.883, 95% confidential interval 1.082–3.279) after adjustment for traditional risk factors. Regarding incremental value of MDA-LDL for predicting CTA-verified HRP, addition of serum MDA-LDL levels to the baseline model significantly increased global chi-square score from 26.1 to 32.8 ($p = 0.010$). Conclusions: A high serum MDA-LDL level is an independent predictor of CTA-verified HRP, which can lead to cardiovascular events in statin-treated patients.

**Keywords:** malondialdehyde low-density lipoprotein; high-risk plaque; coronary computed tomography angiography; statin

**Citation:** Ichikawa, K.; Miyoshi, T.; Osawa, K.; Miki, T.; Ito, H. Increased Circulating Malondialdehyde-Modified Low-Density Lipoprotein Level Is Associated with High-Risk Plaque in Coronary Computed Tomography Angiography in Patients Receiving Statin Therapy. *J. Clin. Med.* **2021**, *10*, 1480. https://doi.org/10.3390/jcm10071480

Academic Editor: Anna Kabłak-Ziembicka

Received: 17 March 2021
Accepted: 30 March 2021
Published: 2 April 2021

**Publisher's Note:** MDPI stays neutral with regard to jurisdictional claims in published maps and institutional affiliations.

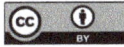

**Copyright:** © 2021 by the authors. Licensee MDPI, Basel, Switzerland. This article is an open access article distributed under the terms and conditions of the Creative Commons Attribution (CC BY) license (https://creativecommons.org/licenses/by/4.0/).

## 1. Introduction

Cardiovascular disease is the leading global cause of adult mortality and morbidity [1]. Many studies have demonstrated a beneficial effect of low-density lipoprotein (LDL)-lowering therapies by statins on cardiovascular outcomes [2,3]. Lowering low-density lipoprotein cholesterol (LDL-C) is the primary target in cardiovascular disease prevention; however, despite effective LDL-lowering treatment, substantial patients remain at cardiovascular risk [4]. Among several lipid markers, serum malondialdehyde low-density lipoprotein (MDA-LDL), which is an oxidatively modified LDL, has been reported to be associated with coronary plaque vulnerability [5], adverse clinical outcomes after percutaneous coronary intervention [6], and the incidence of acute coronary syndrome [7]. However, the clinical relevance of serum MDA-LDL levels in patients receiving statin therapy for cardiovascular events has not been fully elucidated.

Coronary computed tomography angiography (CTA) is used to noninvasively evaluate coronary artery disease [8]. In addition to the evaluation of stenosis, coronary CTA identifies characteristics of plaque composition. Many observational follow-up studies have demonstrated the association between high-risk plaques (HRP) by coronary CTA and cardiovascular events [9,10]. Although statins contribute to the stabilization of plaques [11], HRP is often detected by coronary CTA even in patients receiving statin therapy.

Therefore, we hypothesized that serum MDA-LDL levels in patients with statin therapy is involved in the prevalence of HRP by coronary CTA. The aim of this study was to clarify the association between serum MDA-LDL levels and the prevalence of HRP, which increases the likelihood of acute coronary events in patients with suspected stable coronary artery disease receiving statin therapy.

## 2. Materials and Methods

### 2.1. Study Population and Risk Assessment

This single-center retrospective study included 268 outpatients who underwent coronary CTA from August 2011 to December 2018 at Okayama University Hospital. A flow diagram of this study is shown in Figure 1. Participants had no history of coronary artery disease but had been taking statins.

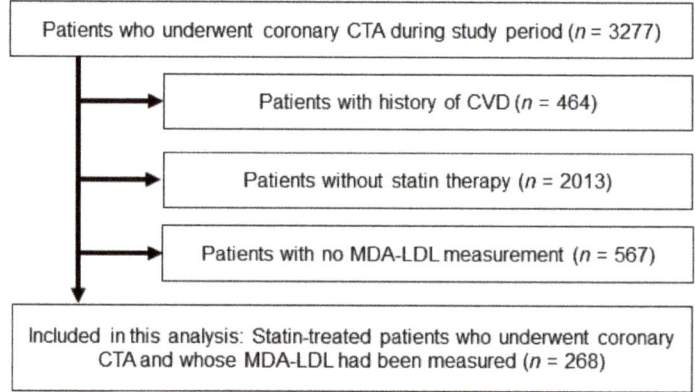

**Figure 1.** Study flowchart. CTA, computed tomography angiography; CVD, cardiovascular disease; MDA-LDL, malondialdehyde-modified low-density lipoprotein.

Hypertension was defined as systolic blood pressure (BP) $\geq$140 mmHg or diastolic BP $\geq$90 mmHg, and/or the use of antihypertensive medication. Diabetes mellitus was defined as a fasting blood glucose concentration of $\geq$126 mg/dL or postprandial blood glucose concentration of $\geq$200 mg/dL, and/or the use of insulin or oral hypoglycemic medication. medication. Smoking was defined as a self-reported history of current smoking. This study was conducted according to the principles of the Declaration of Helsinki and approved by the ethics committees of Okayama University Graduate School of Medicine, Dentistry and Pharmaceutical Sciences. All patients enrolled in the study provided written informed consent.

### 2.2. Blood Sampling and the Measurement of MDA-LDL

Blood samples were collected from the antecubital vein after fasting overnight on the day of coronary CTA. MDA-LDL levels were measured using an enzyme-linked immunosorbent assay kit (Sekisui Medical Co., Tokyo, Japan), as described previously [12].

### 2.3. Acquisition and Analyses of Coronary CTA Image

CT images were acquired using a Somatom Definition Flash scanner (Siemens Medical Solutions, Munich, Germany) as described previously [13]. Coronary artery plaques were evaluated on axial and curved multiplanar reformatted images using commercially available cardiac reconstruction software (Virtual Place, Raijin; AZE Inc., Tokyo, Japan).

Interpretation of coronary CTA was evaluated by two experienced cardiologists. Significant coronary artery stenosis was defined as a luminal narrowing of >50%. Coronary plaque was defined as a structure >1 mm$^2$ located within the vessel wall, and plaque density was calculated for all lesions [14]. Plaques with a CT attenuation number <50 Hounsfield units were defined as low-density plaques. Positive remodeling, which indicates an enlarged vessel to compensate for atherosclerotic change, was assessed visually on multiplanar reformatted images that were reconstructed in long-axis and short-axis views of the vessel. Positive remodeling was defined as a threshold of 1.1 for the maximal diameter of the vessel. Spotty calcification was defined as a calcium burden length <1.5 times the vessel diameter and a width of less than two-thirds of the vessel diameter. CT-verified high-risk plaques were defined when two or more plaque characteristics, including positive remodeling, low-density plaques, and spotty calcification, were present [14].

### 2.4. Outcome Data

Follow-up clinical information was obtained from a review of the medical records or telephone interviews by attending physicians. Cardiovascular events were defined as a composite of cardiac death and acute coronary syndrome. Cardiac death was defined as death from myocardial infarction, cardiogenic shock, cardiac failure, or ventricular arrhythmias. Acute coronary syndrome included myocardial infarction and unstable angina. Non-fatal myocardial infarction was defined using the criteria of typical acute chest pain and persistent ST-segment elevation or positive cardiac enzymes. Unstable angina pectoris was defined as typical acute chest pain with negative cardiac enzymes if coronary artery disease could not be excluded as the cause of symptoms in accordance with current guidelines [15].

### 2.5. Statistical Analysis

Continuous variables were expressed as mean ± standard deviation or median with interquartile range. Dichotomous variables were expressed as numbers and percentages. Differences in continuous variables between the two groups were analyzed using Student's $t$-test and the Mann–Whitney U-test, as appropriate. Categorical data were compared by $\chi^2$ analysis and Fisher's test, as appropriate. Patients were classified into two groups based on the median serum MDA-LDL level (93 U/L): high MDA-LDL group ($\geq$93 U/L, $n$ = 139) and low MDA-LDL group (<93 U/L, $n$ = 129), or LDL-C level (104 mg/dL): high LDL-C group ($\geq$104 mg/dL, $n$ = 136) and low MDA-LDL group (<104 mg/dL, $n$ = 132). Associations between serum MDA-LDL and each variable were assessed using Pearson's correlation coefficient. Univariate and multivariate logistic regression analyses were performed to evaluate the association between serum MDA-LDL levels and CTA-verified HRP. A receiver operating characteristic (ROC) curve was generated to evaluated diagnostic value to predict the presence of HRP. The increased discriminative value after the addition of serum MDA-LDL levels to the baseline model in predicting the presence of HRP was assessed by the global chi-square test and ROC curve analysis. ROC curves were built based on a logistic regression model, and the Delong test was used to compare the C-statistics. The net reclassification improvement and integrated discrimination improvement were also calculated. The baseline model consisted of established clinical risk factors with $p < 0.05$ by univariate logistic regression analysis. Cumulative survival estimates were calculated using the Kaplan–Meier method and compared with the log-rank test. A Cox proportional hazard model was used to identify whether serum MDA-LDL was associated with cardiovascular events. All reported $p$-values were two-sided, and $p < 0.05$ was considered statistically significant. Statistical analyses were performed using SPSS statistical software (Version 24; IBM Corp., Armonk, NY, USA).

## 3. Results

### 3.1. Patient Characteristics

The baseline characteristics of the patients are summarized in Table 1. The mean age was 67 years, and 58% of the patients were men. A share of 76% of patients had hypertension and 46% had diabetes mellitus. Age, sex, prevalence of hypertension, diabetes mellitus, current smoking status, medications, renal function, hemoglobin A1c, and high-sensitivity CRP did not differ between the high and low MDA-LDL groups. Patients with high MDA-LDL had greater body mass index ($p = 0.016$), and higher levels of LDL-C ($p < 0.001$) and triglyceride ($p < 0.001$), than those with low MDA-LDL. Patients with high MDA-LDL had greater body mass index ($p = 0.016$), and higher levels of LDL-C ($p < 0.001$) and triglyceride ($p < 0.001$), and a lower proportion of patients achieved LDL-C <70 mg/dL, than those with low MDA-LDL.

**Table 1.** Baseline patient demographic and clinical characteristics according to high or low levels of MDA-LDL.

|  | All Patients | High MDA-LDL (≥93 U/L) | Low MDA-LDL (<93 U/L) | *p*-Value |
|---|---|---|---|---|
| n | 268 | 139 | 129 |  |
| Age, year | 67 ± 11 | 67 ± 11 | 68 ± 11 | 0.521 |
| Male sex | 154 (58) | 76 (55) | 78 (61) | 0.338 |
| Body mass index, kg/m$^2$ | 24.6 ± 4.1 | 25.2 ± 3.9 | 24.0 ± 4.2 | 0.016 |
| Hypertension | 203 (76) | 109 (78) | 94 (73) | 0.290 |
| Diabetes mellitus | 122 (46) | 59 (42) | 63 (49) | 0.294 |
| Current Smoker | 70 (26) | 36 (26) | 34 (26) | 0.932 |
| Medications |  |  |  |  |
| Beta blockers | 71 (27) | 37 (27) | 34 (26) | 0.933 |
| CCBs | 122 (46) | 70 (50) | 52 (40) | 0.099 |
| ACE-Is or ARBs | 135 (50) | 73 (53) | 62 (48) | 0.466 |
| Oral antihyperglycemic drugs | 86 (32) | 45 (32) | 41 (32) | 0.918 |
| Ezetimibe | 15 (6) | 10 (7) | 5 (4) | 0.293 |
| Statin intensity, low/moderate * | 160 (60)/108 (40) | 76 (55)/63 (45) | 84 (65)/45 (35) | 0.082 |
| Statin type, dosage |  |  |  |  |
| Atorvastatin, 5 mg/10 mg | 18/49 | 5/26 | 13/23 |  |
| Fluvastatin, 20 mg/40 mg | 4/1 | 3/1 | 1/0 |  |
| Pitavastatin, 1 mg/2 mg/4 mg | 14/28/4 | 6/13/3 | 8/15/1 |  |
| Pravastatin, 5 mg/10 mg | 9/36 | 5/21 | 4/15 |  |
| Rosuvastatin, 2.5 mg/5 mg/10 mg | 68/24/2 | 30/19/2 | 38/5/0 |  |
| Simvastatin, 5 mg/10 mg | 8/3 | 4/1 | 4/2 |  |
| Laboratory findings |  |  |  |  |
| Creatinine, mg/dL | 0.89 ± 0.78 | 0.85 ± 0.64 | 0.93 ± 0.92 | 0.397 |
| eGFR, mL/min/1.73 m$^2$ | 68 ± 18 | 68 ± 17 | 69 ± 19 | 0.665 |
| Total cholesterol, mg/dL | 186 ± 40 | 203 ± 40 | 168 ± 31 | <0.001 |
| LDL cholesterol, mg/dL | 107 ± 32 | 122 ± 33 | 90 ± 22 | <0.001 |
| HDL cholesterol, mg/dL | 58 ± 17 | 57 ± 17 | 60 ± 17 | 0.080 |
| Triglyceride, mg/dL | 121 (88, 171) | 150 (104, 198) | 101 (76, 130) | <0.001 |
| MDA-LDL, U/L | 96 ± 35 | 122 ± 28 | 69 ± 15 | <0.001 |
| HbA1c, % | 6.6 ± 1.3 | 6.6 ± 1.4 | 6.6 ± 1.3 | 0.968 |
| hsCRP, mg/dL | 0.08 (0.05, 0.18) | 0.08 (0.04, 0.16) | 0.08 (0.05, 0.20) | 0.608 |
| Patients achieving LDLcholesterol <70 mg/dL | 24 (9) | 1 (1) | 23 (18) | <0.001 |

Data are presented as mean ± standard deviation, number (%), or median (25th, 75th percentile). MDA-LDL, malondialdehyde low-density lipoprotein cholesterol; CCBs, calcium channel blockers; ACE-Is, angiotensin-converting enzyme inhibitors; ARBs, angiotensin receptor blockers; eGFR, estimated glomerular filtration rate; LDL, low-density lipoprotein; HDL, high-density lipoprotein; HbA1c, glycated hemoglobin A1c; hsCRP, high-sensitivity C-reactive protein. * No patients received high-intensity statins.

In addition, simple correlation coefficients for the association between serum MDA-LDL and other lipid variables were analyzed. Serum MDA-LDL levels were significantly positively associated with total cholesterol ($r = 0.52$, $p < 0.001$), LDL-C ($r = 0.60$, $p < 0.001$), and log-transformed triglyceride ($r = 0.34$, $p < 0.001$), and were significantly inversely associated with high-density lipoprotein cholesterol (HDL) ($r = -0.14$, $p = 0.025$).

*3.2. MDA-LDL and Coronary CTA Findings*

Among all patients, the prevalence of HRP and significant stenosis presented in 87 patients (32%) and 120 patients (45%), respectively. As shown in Figure 2A, the prevalence of HRP in the high MDA-LDL group was significantly greater than that in the low MDA-LDL group ($p = 0.040$). However, no differences in the prevalence of calcified plaques ($p = 0.904$), non-calcified plaques ($p = 0.267$), low-density plaque ($p = 0.344$), positive remodeling ($p = 0.057$), spotty calcification ($p = 0.883$), and significant stenosis ($p = 0.355$) were found between the high and low MDA-LDL groups. Figure 2B shows no differences in the prevalence of HRP ($p = 0.4111$) and significant stenosis ($p = 0.229$), or other plaque features, between the high and low LDL-C groups.

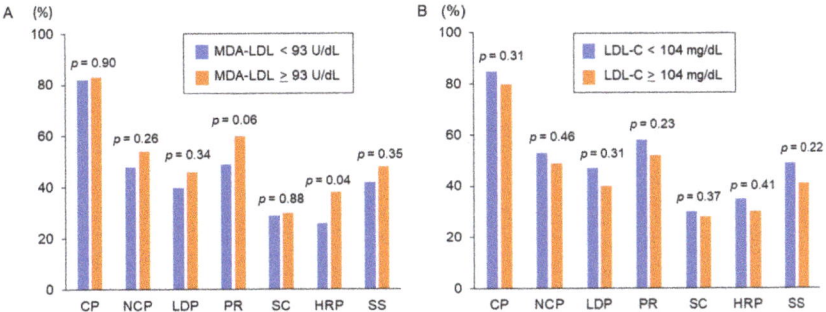

**Figure 2.** The prevalence of coronary plaque characteristics according to MDA-LDL and LDL-C. (**A**) Patients were divided into two groups based on the median value of MDA-LDL. (**B**) Patients were divided into two groups based on the median value of LDL-C. MDA-LDL, malondialdehyde-modified low-density lipoprotein; LDL-C, low-density lipoprotein cholesterol; CP, calcified plaque; NCP, non-calcified plaque; LDP, low density plaque; PR, positive remodeling; SC, spotty calcification; HRP, high-risk plaque: SS, significant stenosis.

As shown in Table 2, patients with HRP had a higher prevalence of male gender ($p < 0.001$), hypertension ($p = 0.031$), and diabetes mellitus ($p = 0.028$) compared with patients without HRP. Patients with HRP had lower HDL-C levels ($p = 0.014$) and serum MDA-LDL levels ($p = 0.011$), whereas LDL-C levels did not differ between patients with and without HRP. Although patients with significant stenosis had higher prevalence of male gender ($p < 0.001$) and diabetes mellitus ($p = 0.039$) compared with patients without significant stenosis, serum levels of LDL-C and MDA-LDL did not differ between patients with and without significant stenosis.

As shown in Table 3, in univariate logistic regression analysis, male sex, hypertension, diabetes mellitus, HDL, and MDA-LDL, but not LDL-C, were significantly associated with the presence of HRP. In multivariate logistic regression analysis, MDA-LDL was independently associated with the presence of HRP with an odds ratio of 1.883 (95% confidence interval 1.082–3.279, $p = 0.025$). When serum MDA-LDL levels were added to the baseline model, global chi-square scores significantly increased from 24.0 to 31.6 ($p = 0.006$). The net reclassification improvement and integrated discrimination improvement were significantly improved by 0.282 ($p = 0.029$) and 0.030 ($p = 0.008$), respectively. However, the increase in the C-statistic was not significant (0.68 to 0.70, $p = 0.352$).

Table 2. Comparison of patient characteristics according to coronary CTA findings.

| Variables | High-Risk Plaque | | | Significant Stenosis | | |
|---|---|---|---|---|---|---|
| | Present | Absent | p Value | Present | Absent | p Value |
| n | 87 | 181 | | 119 | 148 | |
| Age, year | 68 ± 10 | 67 ± 12 | 0.747 | 68 ± 11 | 67 ± 12 | 0.489 |
| Male sex | 64 (74) | 90 (50) | <0.001 | 84 (70) | 70 (47) | <0.001 |
| Body mass index, kg/m$^2$ | 24.7 ± 3.4 | 24.5 ± 4.4 | 0.718 | 24.4 ± 4.1 | 24.7 ± 4.1 | 0.450 |
| Hypertension | 73 (84) | 130 (76) | 0.031 | 93 (78) | 110 (74) | 0.546 |
| Diabetes mellitus | 48 (55) | 74 (41) | 0.028 | 63 (53) | 59 (40) | 0.039 |
| Current smoker | 29 (33) | 41 (23) | 0.062 | 32 (27) | 38 (25) | 0.854 |
| Oral antihyperglycemic drugs | 32 (37) | 54 (30) | 0.254 | 42 (35) | 44 (30) | 0.333 |
| Creatinine, mg/dL | 1.00 ± 0.99 | 0.83 ± 0.65 | 0.087 | 0.91 ± 0.71 | 0.88 ± 0.83 | 0.066 |
| Total cholesterol, mg/dL | 186 ± 45 | 187 ± 38 | 0.834 | 183 ± 41 | 188 ± 38 | 0.300 |
| LDL cholesterol, mg/dL | 107 ± 37 | 107 ± 30 | 0.867 | 106 ± 34 | 107 ± 31 | 0.728 |
| HDL cholesterol, mg/dL | 55 ± 16 | 60 ± 17 | 0.014 | 58 ± 18 | 58 ± 16 | 0.905 |
| Triglyceride, mg/dL | 130 (90, 182) | 117 (85, 170) | 0.206 | 118 (86, 158) | 122 (89, 183) | 0.155 |
| MDA-LDL, U/L | 105 ± 40 | 92 ± 32 | 0.011 | 96 ± 33 | 96 ± 36 | 0.979 |
| HbA1c, % | 6.7 ± 1.3 | 6.5 ± 1.4 | 0.347 | 6.6 ± 1.3 | 6.5 ± 1.4 | 0.122 |
| hsCRP, mg/dL | 0.08 (0.05, 0.16) | 0.08 (0.04, 0.19) | 0.907 | 0.09 (0.05, 0.200) | 0.07 (0.040, 0.160) | 0.132 |

Table 3. Univariate and multivariate predictors of the presence of HRP.

| | Univariate | | Multivariate | |
|---|---|---|---|---|
| | Odds Ratio (95%CI) | p Value | Odds Ratio (95%CI) | p Value |
| Age, per 1 year | 1.004 (0.981–1.028) | 0.746 | | |
| Male | 2.814 (1.609–4.918) | <0.001 | 2.749 (1.502–1.502) | 0.001 |
| Hypertension | 2.046 (1.060–3.947) | 0.033 | 2.027 (1.022–4.019) | 0.049 |
| Diabetes Mellitus | 1.780 (1.062–2.982) | 0.029 | 1.630 (0.941–2.824) | 0.081 |
| Current smoker | 1.707 (0.970–3.006) | 0.064 | | |
| HDL cholesterol, per 1 mg/dL | 0.980 (0.964–0.996) | 0.015 | 0.994 (0.977–1.012) | 0.531 |
| LDL cholesterol, >104 mg/dL | 0.807 (0.483–1.347) | 0.412 | | |
| Triglyceride *, per 1 index | 1.454 (0.854–2.475) | 0.168 | | |
| MDA-LDL, >93 U/L | 1.722 (1.024–2.897) | 0.041 | 1.883 (1.082–3.279) | 0.025 |
| hsCRP *, per 1 index | 0.983 (0.793–1.219) | 0.878 | | |

HRP, high-risk plaques; LDL, low-density lipoprotein; HDL-C, high-density lipoprotein; MDA-LDL, malondialdehyde low-density lipoprotein cholesterol; hsCRP, high sensitivity C-reactive protein. * Triglyceride and hsCRP were logarithm-transformed.

### 3.3. Prognostic Impact of HRP and MDA-LDL for Cardiovascular Events

During a median follow-up period of 2.5 years, 11 cardiovascular events (two cardiac deaths, nine acute coronary syndrome) occurred. Kaplan–Meier curves showed that the high MDA-LDL group had more cardiovascular events than the low MDA-LDL group ($p = 0.012$, log-rank test) (Figure 3A), whereas no significant difference in the incidence of cardiovascular events was observed between patients with the high and low LDL-C groups (Figure 3B). Cox univariate regression analysis showed that high MDA-LDL (HR 5.717, 95%CI 1.225–26.670, $p = 0.027$), but not high LDL-C (hazard ratio 2.697, 95% confidence interval 0.715–10.183, $p = 0.143$), was significantly associated with cardiovascular events. In age and sex adjusted Cox multivariate regression analysis, high MDA-LDL was independently associated with cardiovascular events (hazard ratio 5.865, 95% confidence interval 1.250–27.512, $p = 0.025$).

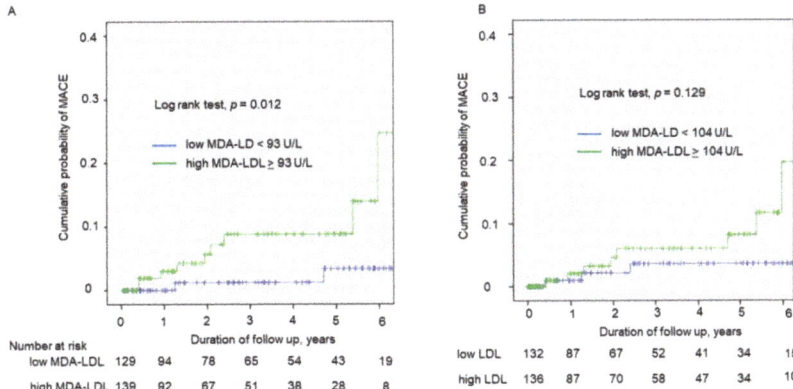

**Figure 3.** Kaplan–Meier curves of cumulative incidence of cardiovascular events. Kaplan–Meier curves (**A**) according to low or high MDA-LDL, and (**B**) according to low or high LDL-C. MDA-LDL, malondialdehyde-modified low-density lipoprotein; LDL-C, low-density lipoprotein cholesterol.

## 4. Discussion

This study demonstrated that serum MDA-LDL, but not LDL-C, was significantly associated with the presence of HRP and had a moderate incremental value to predict HRP over traditional risk factors in statin-treated patients with suspected coronary artery disease. In addition, high MDA-LDL was shown to be a possible predictor for cardiovascular events defined as a composite of cardiac death and ACS in statin-treated patients.

Although increased oxidized LDL, including serum MDA-LDL, is known to be a predictor for atherosclerotic cardiovascular diseases [16], the clinical impact of serum MDA-LDL in patients receiving statin therapy has not been clarified. High triglyceride levels and low HDL levels have been known as risk markers in patients treated with lipid-lowering therapy [17]. These lipid abnormalities are associated with an increase in small dense LDL [18], which are more susceptible to oxidative modification compared with LDL. Even after considering triglyceride and HDL-C, this study clearly demonstrated that serum MDA-LDL is a relevant biomarker for the presence of HRP in statin-treated patients.

Oxidized LDL plays a critical role in plaque vulnerability. Oxidized LDL through lectin-like oxidized LDL receptor-1, which is the major receptor for oxidized LDL in endothelial cells, contributes to increased matrix metalloproteinase activity [19]. In addition, elevated concentrations of oxidized LDL induce apoptosis in vascular smooth muscle cells [20]. Enhanced matrix metalloproteinase production and apoptosis of vascular smooth muscle cells contribute to plaque instability [21]. Several previous clinical studies reported that serum MDA-LDL levels have been associated with thin-cap fibroatheroma identified by frequency-domain optical coherence tomography or with tissue characteristics evaluated by integrated backscatter intravascular ultrasound, both of which are considered to be indicators of plaque vulnerability [5,22]. However, these studies only included patients with obstructive coronary artery disease. In addition, previous studies have reported an association between serum MDA-LDL and plaque vulnerability in lesions targeted for revascularization.

Our findings suggest that serum MDA-LDL is an independent factor for cardiovascular events such as cardiac death and acute coronary syndrome. Similar to our results, a recent clinical study demonstrated that small dense LDL, which is easily oxidized to MDA-LDL, was strongly associated with myocardial infarction [23]. In fact, oxidized LDL is also reported to be involved in platelet activation [24]. The significant association between MDA-LDL and HRP shown in this study may partly explain the role of MDA-LDL as a predictor of cardiovascular events; nevertheless, further studies are required to clarify whether there is a causal relationship.

Statin therapies have been shown to decrease not only LDL but also serum MDA-LDL [25]. In fact, the current study demonstrated that LDL-C had a significant correlation with serum MDA-LDL, and the proportion of patients achieving LDL-C < 70 mg/dL in the low MDA-LDL group was significantly greater than that in the high MDA-LDL group. In addition, inflammation has been considered as a residual risk in statin-treated patients, and a previous study reported that oxidized LDL-induced interleukins (IL)-1β secretion promotes foam cell formation [26]. Recently, a clinical trial showed that antibody therapy against IL-1β significantly reduced cardiovascular events without lowering lipid or blood pressure [27]. Further studies are needed to investigate whether additional anti-inflammatory treatment in patients with high MDA-LDL will reduce cardiovascular events.

Our study has some limitations that need to be addressed. First, this was a single-center study and the number of patients was relatively small. Patient selection may have been biased and a prospective study would be preferable. Second, we included only Japanese patients with suspected stable coronary artery diseasse; the results cannot be applied to other ethnic groups and the general population. Third, the follow-up study was relatively short and a small number of cardiovascular events were documented. To determine the impact of MDA-LDL on cardiovascular death and acute coronary syndrome in statin-treated patients, a large long-term study is warranted.

## 5. Conclusions

Our study demonstrated that serum MDA-LDL was significantly associated with HRP and had an incremental value to predict HRP over traditional risk factors in statin-treated patients with suspected stable coronary artery disease. Our results suggest the measurement of serum MDA-LDL is useful in identifying patients likely to have HRP who are at high risk. Further studies with larger sample size are needed to prove the association between serum MDA-LDL and cardiovascular events in statin-treated patients.

**Author Contributions:** Conceptualization, K.I., T.M. (Toru Miyoshi) and H.I.; methodology, K.I. and T.M. (Takashi Miki); formal analysis, K.I., T.M. (Toru Miyoshi) and K.O.; investigation, K.I., K.O. and T.M. (Takashi Miki); writing—original draft preparation, K.I., T.M. (Toru Miyoshi) and T.M. (Takashi Miki).; writing—review and editing, H.I. All authors have read and agreed to the published version of the manuscript.

**Funding:** This research received no external funding.

**Institutional Review Board Statement:** This study was conducted according to the principles of the Declaration of Helsinki and approved by the ethics committees of Okayama University Graduate School of Medicine, Dentistry and Pharmaceutical Sciences.

**Informed Consent Statement:** Patient consent was waived due to the low-risk nature of the study and the inability to obtain consent directly from all the study subjects.

**Data Availability Statement:** The data presented in this study are available on request from the corresponding author. The data are not publicly available due to privacy.

**Conflicts of Interest:** The authors declare no conflict of interest.

## References

1. Timmis, A.; Townsend, N.; Gale, C.; Grobbee, R.; Maniadakis, N.; Flather, M.; Wilkins, E.; Wright, L.; Vos, R.; Bax, J.; et al. European Society of Cardiology: Cardiovascular Disease Statistics 2017. *Eur. Heart J.* **2018**, *39*, 508–579. [CrossRef]
2. Ridker, P.M.; Pradhan, A.; MacFadyen, J.G.; Libby, P.; Glynn, R.J. Cardiovascular benefits and diabetes risks of statin therapy in primary prevention: An analysis from the JUPITER trial. *Lancet* **2012**, *380*, 565–571. [CrossRef]
3. Mills, E.J.; Rachlis, B.; Wu, P.; Devereaux, P.J.; Arora, P.; Perri, D. Primary prevention of cardiovascular mortality and events with statin treatments: A network meta-analysis involving more than 65,000 patients. *J. Am. Coll. Cardiol.* **2008**, *52*, 1769–1781. [CrossRef]
4. Reith, C.; Armitage, J. Management of residual risk after statin therapy. *Atherosclerosis* **2016**, *245*, 161–170. [CrossRef] [PubMed]

5. Matsuo, Y.; Kubo, T.; Okumoto, Y.; Ishibashi, K.; Komukai, K.; Tanimoto, T.; Ino, Y.; Kitabata, H.; Hirata, K.; Imanishi, T.; et al. Circulating malondialdehyde-modified low-density lipoprotein levels are associated with the presence of thin-cap fibroatheromas determined by optical coherence tomography in coronary artery disease. *Eur. Heart J. Cardiovasc. Imaging* **2013**, *14*, 43–50. [CrossRef] [PubMed]
6. Ito, T.; Fujita, H.; Tani, T.; Ohte, N. Malondialdehyde-modified low-density lipoprotein is a predictor of cardiac events in patients with stable angina on lipid-lowering therapy after percutaneous coronary intervention using drug-eluting stent. *Atherosclerosis* **2015**, *239*, 311–317. [CrossRef] [PubMed]
7. Holvoet, P.; Collen, D.; Van de Werf, F. Malondialdehyde-modified LDL as a marker of acute coronary syndromes. *JAMA* **1999**, *281*, 1718–1721. [CrossRef] [PubMed]
8. Xie, J.X.; Cury, R.C.; Leipsic, J.; Crim, M.T.; Berman, D.S.; Gransar, H.; Budoff, M.J.; Achenbach, S.; Hartaigh, B.O.; Callister, T.Q.; et al. The Coronary Artery Disease-Reporting and Data System (CAD-RADS): Prognostic and Clinical Implications Associated With Standardized Coronary Computed Tomography Angiography Reporting. *JACC Cardiovasc. Imaging* **2018**, *11*, 78–89. [CrossRef] [PubMed]
9. Bamberg, F.; Sommer, W.H.; Hoffmann, V.; Achenbach, S.; Nikolaou, K.; Conen, D.; Reiser, M.F.; Hoffmann, U.; Becker, C.R. Meta-analysis and systematic review of the long-term predictive value of assessment of coronary atherosclerosis by contrast-enhanced coronary computed tomography angiography. *J. Am. Coll. Cardiol.* **2011**, *57*, 2426–2436. [CrossRef]
10. Versteylen, M.O.; Kietselaer, B.L.; Dagnelie, P.C.; Joosen, I.A.; Dedic, A.; Raaijmakers, R.H.; Wildberger, J.E.; Nieman, K.; Crijns, H.J.; Niessen, W.J.; et al. Additive value of semiautomated quantification of coronary artery disease using cardiac computed tomographic angiography to predict future acute coronary syndrome. *J. Am. Coll. Cardiol.* **2013**, *61*, 2296–2305. [CrossRef]
11. Puri, R.; Nicholls, S.J.; Shao, M.; Kataoka, Y.; Uno, K.; Kapadia, S.R.; Tuzcu, E.M.; Nissen, S.E. Impact of statins on serial coronary calcification during atheroma progression and regression. *J. Am. Coll. Cardiol.* **2015**, *65*, 1273–1282. [CrossRef] [PubMed]
12. Amioka, N.; Miyoshi, T.; Otsuka, H.; Yamada, D.; Takaishi, A.; Ueeda, M.; Hirohata, S.; Ito, H. Serum malondialdehyde-modified low-density lipoprotein levels on admission predict prognosis in patients with acute coronary syndrome undergoing percutaneous coronary intervention. *J. Cardiol.* **2019**, *74*, 258–266. [CrossRef] [PubMed]
13. Osawa, K.; Miyoshi, T.; Yamauchi, K.; Koyama, Y.; Nakamura, K.; Sato, S.; Kanazawa, S.; Ito, H. Nonalcoholic Hepatic Steatosis Is a Strong Predictor of High-Risk Coronary-Artery Plaques as Determined by Multidetector CT. *PLoS ONE* **2015**, *10*, e0131138. [CrossRef] [PubMed]
14. Ichikawa, K.; Miyoshi, T.; Osawa, K.; Miki, T.; Nakamura, K.; Ito, H. Prognostic Value of Coronary Computed Tomographic Angiography in Patients With Nonalcoholic Fatty Liver Disease. *JACC Cardiovasc. Imaging* **2020**, *13*, 1628–1630. [CrossRef]
15. Anderson, J.L.; Adams, C.D.; Antman, E.M.; Bridges, C.R.; Califf, R.M.; Casey, D.E., Jr.; Chavey, W.E., 2nd; Fesmire, F.M.; Hochman, J.S.; Levin, T.N.; et al. 2011 ACCF/AHA Focused Update Incorporated Into the ACC/AHA 2007 Guidelines for the Management of Patients With Unstable Angina/Non-ST-Elevation Myocardial Infarction: A report of the American College of Cardiology Foundation/American Heart Association Task Force on Practice Guidelines. *Circulation* **2011**, *123*, e426–e579. [CrossRef]
16. Gao, S.; Zhao, D.; Wang, M.; Zhao, F.; Han, X.; Qi, Y.; Liu, J. Association Between Circulating Oxidized LDL and Atherosclerotic Cardiovascular Disease: A Meta-analysis of Observational Studies. *Can. J. Cardiol.* **2017**, *33*, 1624–1632. [CrossRef] [PubMed]
17. Matsuura, Y.; Kanter, J.E.; Bornfeldt, K.E. Highlighting Residual Atherosclerotic Cardiovascular Disease Risk. *Arterioscler. Thromb. Vasc. Biol.* **2019**, *39*, e1–e9. [CrossRef]
18. Fan, J.; Liu, Y.; Yin, S.; Chen, N.; Bai, X.; Ke, Q.; Shen, J.; Xia, M. Small dense LDL cholesterol is associated with metabolic syndrome traits independently of obesity and inflammation. *Nutr. Metab.* **2019**, *16*, 7. [CrossRef]
19. Hu, C.; Dandapat, A.; Sun, L.; Chen, J.; Marwali, M.R.; Romeo, F.; Sawamura, T.; Mehta, J.L. LOX-1 deletion decreases collagen accumulation in atherosclerotic plaque in low-density lipoprotein receptor knockout mice fed a high-cholesterol diet. *Cardiovasc. Res.* **2008**, *79*, 287–293. [CrossRef]
20. Kume, N.; Kita, T. Apoptosis of vascular cells by oxidized LDL: Involvement of caspases and LOX-1 and its implication in atherosclerotic plaque rupture. *Circ. Res.* **2004**, *94*, 269–270. [CrossRef]
21. Kattoor, A.J.; Pothineni, N.V.K.; Palagiri, D.; Mehta, J.L. Oxidative Stress in Atherosclerosis. *Curr. Atheroscler. Rep.* **2017**, *19*, 42. [CrossRef]
22. Ikenaga, H.; Kurisu, S.; Kono, S.; Sumimoto, Y.; Watanabe, N.; Shimonaga, T.; Higaki, T.; Iwasaki, T.; Mitsuba, N.; Ishibashi, K.; et al. Impact of Malondialdehyde-Modified Low-Density Lipoprotein on Tissue Characteristics in Patients With Stable Coronary Artery Disease- Integrated Backscatter-Intravascular Ultrasound Study. *Circ. J.* **2016**, *80*, 2173–2182. [CrossRef] [PubMed]
23. Duran, E.K.; Aday, A.W.; Cook, N.R.; Buring, J.E.; Ridker, P.M.; Pradhan, A.D. Triglyceride-Rich Lipoprotein Cholesterol, Small Dense LDL Cholesterol, and Incident Cardiovascular Disease. *J. Am. Coll. Cardiol.* **2020**, *75*, 2122–2135. [CrossRef] [PubMed]
24. Marwali, M.R.; Hu, C.P.; Mohandas, B.; Dandapat, A.; Deonikar, P.; Chen, J.; Cawich, I.; Sawamura, T.; Kavdia, M.; Mehta, J.L. Modulation of ADP-induced platelet activation by aspirin and pravastatin: Role of lectin-like oxidized low-density lipoprotein receptor-1, nitric oxide, oxidative stress, and inside-out integrin signaling. *J. Pharmacol. Exp. Ther.* **2007**, *322*, 1324–1332. [CrossRef] [PubMed]
25. Nishikido, T.; Oyama, J.; Keida, T.; Ohira, H.; Node, K. High-dose statin therapy with rosuvastatin reduces small dense LDL and MDA-LDL: The Standard versus high-dose therApy with Rosuvastatin for lipiD lowering (SARD) trial. *J. Cardiol.* **2016**, *67*, 340–346. [CrossRef] [PubMed]

26. Liu, W.; Yin, Y.; Zhou, Z.; He, M.; Dai, Y. OxLDL-induced IL-1 beta secretion promoting foam cells formation was mainly via CD36 mediated ROS production leading to NLRP3 inflammasome activation. *Inflamm. Res.* **2014**, *63*, 33–43. [CrossRef]
27. Ridker, P.M.; Everett, B.M.; Thuren, T.; MacFadyen, J.G.; Chang, W.H.; Ballantyne, C.; Fonseca, F.; Nicolau, J.; Koenig, W.; Anker, S.D.; et al. Antiinflammatory Therapy with Canakinumab for Atherosclerotic Disease. *N. Engl. J. Med.* **2017**, *377*, 1119–1131. [CrossRef]

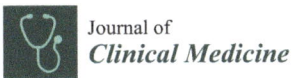 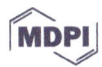

Article

# Importance of Increased Arterial Resistance in Risk Prediction in Patients with Cardiovascular Risk Factors and Degenerative Aortic Stenosis

Jakub Baran [1], Paweł Kleczyński [1], Łukasz Niewiara [1,2], Jakub Podolec [1], Rafał Badacz [1], Andrzej Gackowski [3,4], Piotr Pieniążek [1,5], Jacek Legutko [1], Krzysztof Żmudka [1], Tadeusz Przewłocki [1,5] and Anna Kabłak-Ziembicka [1,4,*]

[1] Department of Interventional Cardiology, Institute of Cardiology, Jagiellonian University Medical College, John Paul II Hospital, 31-202 Krakow, Poland; jakub_baran@yahoo.pl (J.B.); kleczu@interia.pl (P.K.); lniewiara@gmail.com (Ł.N.); jjpodolec@gmail.com (J.P.); rbadacz@gmail.com (R.B.); kardio@kki.krakow.pl (P.P.); jacek.legutko@uj.edu.pl (J.L.); zmudka@icloud.com (K.Ż.); tadeuszprzewlocki@op.pl (T.P.)
[2] Department of Emergency Medicine, Faculty of Health Sciences, Jagiellonian University Medical College, 31-126 Krakow, Poland
[3] Department of Coronary Disease and Heart Failure, Institute of Cardiology, Jagiellonian University Medical College, John Paul II Hospital, 31-202 Krakow, Poland; agackowski@gmail.com
[4] Noninvasive Cardiovascular Laboratory, John Paul II Hospital, 31-202 Krakow, Poland
[5] Department of Cardiac and Vascular Diseases, Institute of Cardiology, Jagiellonian University Medical College, John Paul II Hospital, 31-202 Krakow, Poland
* Correspondence: kablakziembicka@op.pl

**Citation:** Baran, J.; Kleczyński, P.; Niewiara, Ł.; Podolec, J.; Badacz, R.; Gackowski, A.; Pieniążek, P.; Legutko, J.; Żmudka, K.; Przewłocki, T.; et al. Importance of Increased Arterial Resistance in Risk Prediction in Patients with Cardiovascular Risk Factors and Degenerative Aortic Stenosis. *J. Clin. Med.* **2021**, *10*, 2109. https://doi.org/10.3390/jcm10102109

Academic Editor: Vanessa Bianconi

Received: 20 April 2021
Accepted: 11 May 2021
Published: 13 May 2021

**Publisher's Note:** MDPI stays neutral with regard to jurisdictional claims in published maps and institutional affiliations.

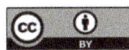

**Copyright:** © 2021 by the authors. Licensee MDPI, Basel, Switzerland. This article is an open access article distributed under the terms and conditions of the Creative Commons Attribution (CC BY) license (https://creativecommons.org/licenses/by/4.0/).

**Abstract:** Background: Cardiovascular disease is a leading cause of heart failure (HF) and major adverse cardiac and cerebral events (MACCE). Objective: To evaluate impact of vascular resistance on HF and MACCE incidence in subjects with cardiovascular risk factors (CRF) and degenerative aortic valve stenosis (DAS). Methods: From January 2016 to December 2018, in 404 patients with cardiovascular disease, including 267 patients with moderate-to-severe DAS and 137 patients with CRF, mean values of resistive index (RI) and pulsatile index (PI) were obtained from carotid and vertebral arteries. Patients were followed-up for 2.5 years, for primary outcome of HF and MACCE episodes. Results: RI and PI values in patients with DAS compared to CRF were significantly higher, with optimal cut-offs discriminating arterial resistance of $\geq 0.7$ for RI (sensitivity: 80.5%, specificity: 78.8%) and $\geq 1.3$ for PI (sensitivity: 81.3%, specificity: 79.6%). Age, female gender, diabetes, and DAS were all independently associated with increased resistance. During the follow-up period, 68 (16.8%) episodes of HF-MACCE occurred. High RI (odds ratio 1.25, 95% CI 1.13–1.37) and PI (odds ratio 1.21, 95% CI 1.10–1.34) were associated with risk of HF-MACCE. Conclusions: An accurate assessment of vascular resistance may be used for HF-MACCE risk stratification in patients with DAS.

**Keywords:** cardiovascular risk factors; heart failure; major cardiac and cerebral ischemic events; degenerative aortic stenosis; risk stratification; vascular resistance

## 1. Introduction

With ageing, a reduction in the elastin content and an increase in the collagen content lead to increased arterial stiffness and elevated central as well as peripheral arterial blood pressure [1]. Similarly, chronic low-grade inflammation or metabolic disorders, e.g., glycation of vessel wall proteins, contribute to the stiffening process of large arteries [2–4]. Arterial stiffness is a well-known predictor of all-cause mortality, including cardiovascular mortality [5].

Degenerative aortic valve stenosis (DAS) is another condition in which prevalence increases with age [6]. DAS progression, similar to arterial stiffening, is accelerated by common cardiovascular risk factors (CRF) and ageing [6–8].

Ultrasonography can easily and non-invasively provide information on vascular resistance indices (resistive index; RI and pulsatile index; PI), that are surrogate markers of arterial stiffness. Peripheral flow parameters can be particularly important in patients with DAS, in whom severely reduced left-ventricle outflow has an impact on the altered vascular system flow pattern [9].

Although both chronological and vascular ageing processes progress in time, they are often not parallel [10]. In patients with CRF, cardiac, and/or arterial disease, vascular ageing outruns the normal ageing process [1,10].

Patients with increased arterial stiffness tend to develop cardiovascular events at a younger age and with a higher mortality rate [1]. However, there are scarce data available as to whether DAS relates to vascular resistance at a higher extent as compared to the ageing process and CRF, and more importantly, whether vascular resistance can contribute to heart failure (HF) episodes and major adverse cardiac and cerebral events (MACCE) in patients with DAS.

We aimed to evaluate impact of vascular resistance on HF and MACCE events in subjects with cardiovascular risk factors and degenerative aortic valve stenosis.

## 2. Materials and Methods

### 2.1. Study Population and Cardiovascular Risk Factors

In this single-center prospective study, from January 2016 to December 2018, 517 consecutive patients with either CRF or DAS were assessed. A flowchart of this study is presented in Figure 1.

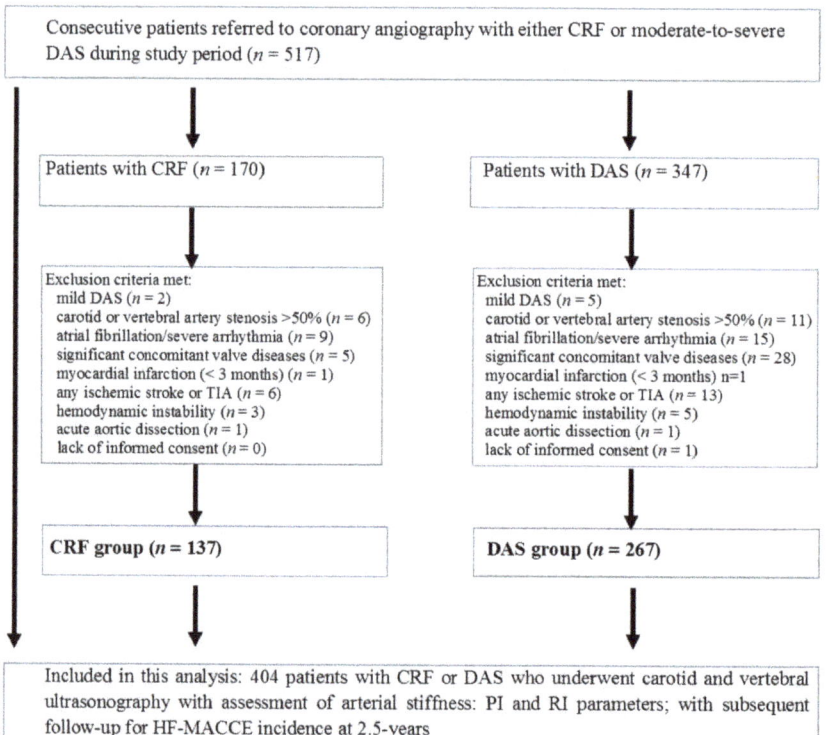

**Figure 1.** Study flowchart. CRF, cardiovascular risk factors; DAS, degenerative aortic valve stenosis; HF, heart failure; MACCE, major adverse cardiac and cerebral events; PI, pulsatile index; RI, resistive index.

CRF group was enrolled from patients with suspected or known stable coronary artery disease, with preserved LVEF ≥ 50% admitted to our department for coronary angiography.

Subjects with DAS were eligible if (1) aortic valve area was less than 1.5 cm$^2$; they (2) had left ventricular ejection fraction (LVEF) ≥ 50%; and (3) underwent coronary angiography.

The exclusion criteria for both study and control groups included: significant stenosis of any carotid or vertebral artery (exceeding 50% lumen reduction), persistent atrial fibrillation or other severe arrhythmia, significant concomitant valve diseases, ongoing or recent myocardial infarction (<3 months), ischemic stroke or TIA, hemodynamic instability: NYHA class IV or acute heart failure, LVEF < 50%, aortic dissection, and lack of informed consent.

Finally, in 404 study patients, including 267 patients with moderate-to-severe DAS and 137 patients with CRF, distribution of RI and PI registered at carotid and vertebral arteries was evaluated. Patients were followed-up for mean 2.5 years, with primary outcome of HF and MACCE episodes.

The prevalence of CRF, including age, gender, hypertension, diabetes and dyslipidemia, and coronary artery disease was evaluated in both groups. Cardiovascular risk factors were defined as: hypertension (treated, or newly recognized, based on average on three measurements; SBP ≥ 140 mm Hg and/or DBP ≥ 90 mm Hg), diabetes mellitus (treated or newly recognized > 11 mmol/l (200 mg/d) in oral glucose tolerance test, hyperlipidemia (treated or newly recognized—total cholesterol > 4.9 mmol/L (190 mg/dL) and/or LDL > 3.0 mmol/L (115 mg/dL) and/or HDL men < 1.0 mmol/L (40 mg/dL), HDL women < 1.2 mmol/L (46 mg/dL) and/or triglycerides > 1.7 mmol/L (150 mg/dL) [11]. Coronary artery disease was defined as presence on coronary angiography of at least one main coronary artery lumen reduction exceeding 50%.

The study protocol was consistent with the requirements of the Helsinki Declaration, and approved by the local Institutional Ethics Committee. All subjects gave informed consent for participation in the study.

### 2.2. Echocardiography, Carotid and Vertebral Artery Ultrasonography

All patients underwent a complete echocardiographic study in compliance with the guidelines of the European Association of Cardiovascular Imaging [12]. Peak and the mean gradient across aortic valve, aortic valve area (AVA), LVEF were assessed in all subjects.

High-resolution B-Mode, color Doppler, and pulse Doppler ultrasonography of both carotid and vertebral arteries were performed with an ultrasound machine (TOSHIBA APLIO 450) equipped with a linear-array 5–10 MHz transducer in a patient lying in supine position with head tilted slightly backward. Exam was performed by two experienced sonographers who were blinded to subjects' clinical, echocardiographic, and angiographic characteristics.

Vascular resistance parameters were expressed as averaged RI and PI values calculated bilaterally from internal carotid and vertebral arteries. For this purpose, the peak-systolic (PSV) and the end-diastolic velocities (EDV), as well as vessel diameters were measured within 1.0 to 1.5 cm proximal segment of the internal carotid artery (ICA), and proximal V2 segment of vertebral artery, with a calculation of the pulsatile (PI) and resistive (RI) indexes in each evaluated segment, according to the following equations:

Resistive Index (RI) = PSV − EDV/PSV

Pulsatile Index (PI) = PSV − EDV/[(PSV + 2 × EDV)/3]

The averaged value of RI and PI from four arterial segments was taken into further statistical analysis.

### 2.3. Outcome Data, Follow-Up, and Adverse Cardiovascular Events

During mean observation period of 2.5 years, the incidences of HF episodes and MACCE were recorded.

MACCE was defined as fatal or non-fatal ischemic stroke, myocardial infarction, acute heart failure episode, or cardiovascular death (i.e., any sudden or unexpected death unless proven as non-cardiovascular on autopsy). HF episode was defined as new-onset acute HF incidence or any exacerbation of chronic heart failure requiring in-hospital stay and administration of intravenous medications such as diuretics, dopamine, adrenaline, or dobutamine.

Final visit was conducted through the telephone contact with a patient or pointed family member. For patients lost to follow-up ($n = 4$), the data on patient vital status were obtained from the national health registry.

### 2.4. Statistical Analysis

Data are presented as mean ± standard deviation for continuous variables and as proportions for categorical variables. Differences between mean values were verified using the T-Student, analysis of variance (ANOVA) test, and frequencies were compared by the chi-2 test for independence, as appropriate. The normal distribution of studied variables was determined by the Shapiro–Wilk test. The Spearman's rank-order correlation was performed for correlation between RI and PI. A receiver-operating characteristic (ROC) analysis was performed to determine the optimal cut-off values (common point of the most distant $y = x$ line with ROC curve) for vascular resistance as potentially associated with DAS. The area under the curve (AUC), cut-offs sensitivity and specificity were calculated. The C statistic with comparison of AUCs was performed for evaluation of models with and without DAS to assess the probability of obtaining arterial stiffness parameters above thresholds. The analysis of risk factors associated with increased PI and RI values was performed with univariate regression analysis. We included age, gender, diabetes mellitus, hypertension, hyperlipidemia, coronary artery disease, LVEF, and DAS as factors potentially associated with vascular resistance. After identification of parameters potentially associated with increased vascular resistance, the multivariable logistic backward regression analysis was used to calculate odds ratio (OR) and 95% confidence interval (95% CI). We used Z-scores to standardize the raw values of age to a normal distribution. We also assessed incidence of HF-MACCE events in groups classified by high versus low PI and RI using univariate logistic regression analysis, followed by the multivariable regression models, with the PI $\geq$ 1.3 and the RI $\geq$ 0.7 as referent in all study participants. A 2-sided value of $p < 0.05$ was considered statistically significant. Statistical analyses were performed with Statistica version 13.3 software (TIBCO Software, Palo Alto, CA, USA) and with R Studio 3.6.3 [13].

## 3. Results

### 3.1. Patient Characteristics

The baseline characteristics of the patients are summarized in Table 1. Patients with DAS in comparison to patients with CRFs were significantly older (74.5 vs. 70.0 years, $p = 0.001$) and more often had hyperlipidemia (95.9 vs. 79.6%, $p < 0.001$), while history of myocardial infarction was more frequent in CRF group (31.4 vs. 20.2%, $p = 0.002$). Gender distribution, prevalence of hypertension, diabetes mellitus, and significant coronary artery disease did not differ between the CRF and DAS groups. On echocardiography, baseline LVEF was similar in both study groups, while peak and systolic aortic gradients were significantly higher in DAS vs. CRF groups.

Table 1. Baseline groups characteristics.

| | DAS Group N = 267 | CRF Group N = 137 | p-Value |
|---|---|---|---|
| **Demographic data** | | | |
| Age (years) ± SD | 74.5 (8.8) | 70.0 (11) | 0.001 |
| Female, n (%) | 172 (64.4) | 87 (63.5) | 0.305 |
| Hypertension, n (%) | 239 (89.5) | 114 (83.2) | 0.157 |
| Diabetes, n (%) | 86 (32.7) | 41 (29.9) | 0.556 |
| Hyperlipidemia (%) | 256 (95.9) | 109 (79.6) | <0.001 |
| Coronary artery disease (%) | 111 (41.6) | 54 (39.4) | 0.054 |
| Previous myocardial infarction, n (%) | 54 (20.2) | 43 (31.4) | 0.002 |
| **Selected echocardiographic data** | | | |
| Aortic valve area (cm2) ± SD | 0.82 ± 0.28 | 2.5 ± 0.24 | <0.001 |
| Peak aortic gradient (mmHg) ± SD | 87.8 ± 29 | 9.6 ± 4.5 | <0.001 |
| Mean aortic gradient (mmHg) ± SD | 50.5 ± 18.7 | 4.3 ± 4.2 | <0.001 |
| Left ventricular ejection fraction (%) ± SD | 60.1 ± 6.6 | 60 ± 10 | 0.263 |
| **Carotid and vertebral ultrasonography** | | | |
| Mean Resistive Index ± SD | 0.73 ± 0.06 | 0.64 ± 0.05 | <0.001 |
| Mean Pulsatile Index ± SD | 1.45 ± 0.23 | 1.14 ± 0.16 | <0.001 |
| **Left internal carotid artery** | | | |
| Resistive Index ± SD | 0.75 ± 0.07 | 0.64 ± 0.06 | < 0.001 |
| Pulsatile Index ± SD | 1.52 ± 0.28 | 1.12 ± 0.17 | < 0.001 |
| **Right internal carotid artery** | | | |
| Resistive Index ± SD | 0.75 ± 0.07 | 0.64 ± 0.06 | < 0.001 |
| Pulsatile Index ± SD | 1.52 ± 0.28 | 1.14 ± 0.17 | < 0.001 |
| **Left Vertebral artery** | | | |
| Resistive Index ± SD | 0.72 ± 0.07 | 0.65 ± 0.07 | <0.001 |
| Pulsatile Index ± SD | 1.40 ± 0.25 | 1.16 ± 0.21 | <0.001 |
| **Right vertebral artery** | | | |
| Resistive Index ± SD | 0.72 ± 0.06 | 0.64 ± 0.08 | <0.001 |
| Pulsatile Index ± SD | 1.38 ± 0.23 | 1.12 ± 0.23 | <0.001 |

CRF, cardiovascular risk factors; DAS, degenerative aortic stenosis.

*3.2. Study Groups and Arterial Stiffness Findings*

The RI values were significantly positively correlated with the PI values (r = 0.99, $p < 0.001$).

The RI and PI values in both carotid and vertebral arteries differed significantly between patients with DAS vs. CRF (Table 1). Moreover, mean values of the RI (0.73 ± 0.06 vs. 0.64 ± 0.05, $p < 0.001$) and the PI (1.45 ± 0.23 vs. 1.14 ± 0.16, $p < 0.001$) were significantly higher in patients with DAS, compared to CRF (Table 1).

In line, in patients with moderate (n = 32) vs. severe (n = 235) DAS, mean values of RI (0.70 ± 0.06 vs. 0.74 ± 0.06; $p = 0.001$) and PI (1.34 ± 0.21 vs. 1.47 ± 0.23; $p = 0.002$) differed significantly.

The optimal cut-off values obtained from ROC analysis best discriminating vascular resistance in CRF vs. DAS patients were RI of 0.7 or higher (sensitivity of 80.5%, specificity of 78.8%) and PI value of 1.3 or higher (sensitivity of 81.3%, specificity of 79.6%).

Univariate regression backward analysis, followed by the multivariate regression analysis, showed associations with the RI ≥ 0.7 and the PI ≥ 1.3 for age, female gender, diabetes, and DAS (Table 2). There was also association between increased arterial stiffness and hyperlipidemia and hypertension in univariate analysis (Table 2).

In multivariable logistic regression backward analysis, DAS confirmed its independent association with high RI and high PI in the multivariate analysis, both in unadjusted and Z-score age-adjusted analysis (Table 2).

**Table 2.** Factors associated with increased arterial resistance.

|  | Univariate OR (95% CI), *p*-Value | Multivariate OR (95% CI), *p*-Value | Multivariate Age-Adjusted OR (95% CI), *p*-Value |
| --- | --- | --- | --- |
| **Predictors of RI ≥ 0.7** |  |  |  |
| Age | 1.22 (1.12–1.33), <0.001 | 1.29 (1.20–1.40), <0.001 | 1.29 (1.20–1.40), <0.001 |
| Female gender | 1.10 (1.01–1.19), 0.025 | 1.07 (0.99–1.16), 0.070 | 1.07 (0.99–1.16), 0.071 |
| Diabetes | 1.15 (1.04–1.27), 0.004 | 1.10 (1.02–1.18), 0.018 | 1.10 (1.02–1.19), 0.018 |
| Hypertension | 1.17 (1.06–1.29), 0.002 | 1.07 (0.99–1.16), 0.076 | 1.07 (0.99–1.16), 0.076 |
| Hyperlipidemia | 1.27 (1.15–1.39), <0.001 | 1.06 (0.98–1.55), 0.155 | 1.06 (0.98–1.15), 0.155 |
| Coronary artery disease | 1.07 (0.97–1.18), 0.173 | - | - |
| Previous myocardial infarction | 1.00 (0.91–1.10), 0.944 | - | - |
| Left ventricular ejection fraction | 1.05 (0.95–1.16), 0.319 | - | - |
| Aortic valve stenosis | 2.49 (1.64–3.78), <0.001 | 1.65 (1.53–1.79), <0.001 | 1.66 (1.53–1.79), <0.001 |
| **Predictors of PI ≥ 1.3** |  |  |  |
| Age | 1.44 (1.32–1.58), <0.001 | 1.25 (1.16–1.35), <0.001 | 1.25 (1.16–1.35), <0.001 |
| Female gender | 1.16 (1.05–1.28), 0.002 | 1.12 (1.04–1.20), 0.004 | 1.12 (1.04–1.21), 0.004 |
| Diabetes | 1.17 (1.06–1.29), 0.001 | 1.11 (1.03–1.19), 0.009 | 1.11 (1.03–1.19), 0.009 |
| Hypertension | 1.18 (1.07–1.29), 0.001 | 1.06 (0.98–1.15), 0.117 | 1.06 (0.98–1.15), 0.118 |
| Hyperlipidemia | 1.29 (1.18–1.42), <0.001 | 1.09 (1.01–1.18), 0.027 | 1.09 (1.01–1.18), 0.027 |
| Coronary artery disease | 1.10 (1.00–1.21), 0.059 | - | - |
| Previous myocardial infarction | 1.01 (0.92–1.11), 0.934 | - | - |
| Left ventricular ejection fraction | 1.04 (0.95–1.15), 0.388 | - | - |
| Aortic valve stenosis | 1.79 (1.65–1.94), <0.001 | 1.67 (1.54–1.80), <0.001 | 1.67 (1.54–1.80), <0.001 |

Adding DAS to the model with CRF resulted in a higher predicted probability of the RI ≥ 0.7 (AUC: 0.843 vs. 0.754, $p$ = 0.014) and the PI ≥ 1.3 (AUC: 0.891 vs. 0.789; $p$ = 0.002) (Figure 2A,B).

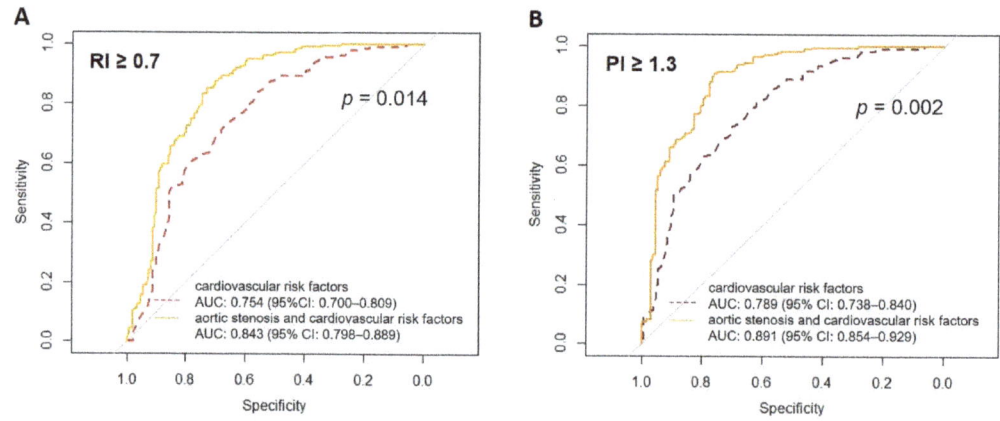

**Figure 2.** Comparison of area under the curve (AUC) for multivariate models to detect increased Resistive Index (panel (**A**)) and Pulsatile Index (panel (**B**)). Baseline models AUCs for CRF are presented as dashed lines, AUCs for degenerative aortic stenosis are presented as solid lines. Abbreviations: AUC—area under the curve; PI—Pulsatile Index; RI—Resistive Index.

### 3.3. Vascular Resistance Properties and the Outcomes

During follow-up period, 68 (16.8%) episodes of HF-MACCE occurred, including 16 (11.7%) in CRF group and 52 (19.5%) in DAS group, $p$ = 0.047.

HF-MACCEs were observed in 9 out of 172 patients with RI values below 0.7, as compared to 59 of 232 with RI ≥ 0.7 (5.2% vs. 25.4%, $p$ < 0.001), whereas in 9 of 161 patients with PI < 1.3 vs. 59 of 245 patients with PI ≥ 1.3 (5.6% vs. 24.1%, $p$ < 0.001).

In both study groups, patients who had HF-MACCE were older, and had higher prevalence of high RI and PI values.

Age, female gender, diabetes, hypertension, DAS, RI ≥ 0.7, and PI ≥ 1.3 showed association with HF-MACCE in univariable analysis (Table 3). In multivariable analysis, high RI (OR, 1.25; 95% CI 1.13–1.37) and PI (OR, 1.21; 95% CI 1.10–1.34), similar to age were independently associated with the risk of HF-MACCE.

Table 3. Univariate and multivariate logistic regression analysis of factors associated with heart failure episodes (HF) and major adverse cardiac and cerebral events (MACCE).

| Parameter | Univariate Analysis OR (95% CI), p-Value | Multivariate Analysis with RI OR (95% CI), p-Value | Multivariate Analysis with PI OR (95% CI), p-Value |
|---|---|---|---|
| Age | 1.23 (1.12–1.35), 0.001 | 1.13 (1.03–1.25), 0.014 | 1.16 (1.04–1.26), 0.008 |
| Female gender | 1.12 (1.02–1.23), 0.019 | 1.07 (0.98–1.18), 0.133 | 1.07 (0.97–1.18), 0.163 |
| Diabetes | 1.11 (1.01–1.23), 0.029 | 1.05 (0.96–1.16), 0.293 | 1.06 (0.96–1.16), 0.269 |
| Hypertension | 1.12 (1.02–1.23), 0.025 | 1.07 (0.97–1.17), 0.169 | 1.07 (0.97–1.18) 0.162 |
| Hyperlipidemia | 1.01 (0.92–1.12), 0.783 | - | - |
| Coronary artery disease | 1.07 (0.97–1.18), 0.172 | - | - |
| Previous myocardial infarction | 1.01 (0.91–1.11), 0.919 | - | - |
| Left ventricle ejection fraction | 1.04 (0.95–1.15), 0.384 | - | - |
| Aortic valve stenosis | 1.10 (1.00–1.21), 0.047 | 1.07 (0.95–1.19), 0.253 | 1.05 (0.94–1.18), 0.407 |
| Peak aortic gradient | 1.10 (0.98–1.24), 0.106 | - | - |
| RI ≥ 0.7 | 1.30 (1.19–1.43), 0.001 | 1.25 (1.13–1.37), <0.001 | - |
| PI ≥ 1.3 | 1.28 (1.16–1.40), <0.001 | - | 1.21 (1.10–1.34), <0.001 |

## 4. Discussion

In the present study, in a subset of patients with moderate-to-severe DAS, similar to patients with CRF, we showed associations between increased carotid arterial resistance, defined as the PI ≥ 1.3 and the RI ≥ 0.7 with heart failure exacerbation episodes and adverse cardiovascular events in mid-term observational period. Therefore, high carotid PI and RI values could be used as surrogate markers of poor cardiovascular prognosis in patients with advanced DAS. The advantage of our concept is that carotid stiffness parameters are easily obtainable non-invasively and are reproducible [14].

Furthermore, ultrasonographic assessment of vascular resistance was also used in former studies, in the setting of large arteries disease or renovascular disease, as the prognostic marker of the outcome [15,16]. Lately, arterial stiffness was also used for risk assessment in patients with COVID infection [17].

Our study demonstrated that about three quarters of patients with DAS and cardiovascular risk factors had high RI and PI values, compared to ~ 20% of patients with CRF only. This high distribution of increased arterial stiffness parameters in DAS, as compared to CRF patients, corresponds to ~21–25% relative risk increase of HF-MACCE in mean 2.5-years follow-up period, compared to patients with lower PI and RI values.

We found that moderate-to-severe DAS independently relates to higher vascular resistance, likewise age, female gender, and diabetes. In a study by Yan et al., hypertension (HR 1.71; 95% CI: 1.66–1.76), diabetes (HR: 1.49; 95% CI: 1.44–1.54), and dyslipidemia (HR: 1.17; 95% CI: 1.14–1.21) were all significantly associated with increased risk of developing severe DAS [6]. There was a positive relationship between the severity, number and duration of cardiac risk factors, and risk of DAS [6]. Moreover, gender plays an important role in DAS pathogenesis, development and progression of valvular calcification processes, fibrosis, and hemodynamic severity, left ventricle hypertrophy, and cardiovascular outcomes in men and women [18,19]. Patients with DAS are often older and have more cardiovascular risk factors, systemic hypertension and atherosclerosis, which all show association with increased aortic stiffness and cognitive decline [20–23].

In contrast to overwhelming studies in favor of an independent role for arterial stiffness in predicting cardiovascular events in healthy elderly and diseased hypertensive, diabetic, or end stage renal disease subjects [24,25], studies concerning potential application of vascular resistance parameters in patients with advanced DAS are innumerous [26,27].

In one research study enrolling 103 asymptomatic patients with moderate-to-severe DAS, arterial stiffness assessed with femoral-carotid pulse wave velocity (PWV) method, showed significantly lower event-free survival in patients with PWV $\geq$ 10 m/s compared to those with lower PWV [26]. In line, the Simvastatin and Ezetimibe in Aortic Stenosis study during median 4.3 years observation period demonstrated a higher cardiovascular morbidity rate (hazard ratio 2.13; 95% CI 1.34–3.40) in patients with initially mild-to-moderate DAS and echocardiographically established low systemic arterial compliance [27].

There is some uncertainty about sequence of developing aortic valve calcifications, exposure to atherosclerosis risk factors, and arterial stiffening [1,28]. More recent data demonstrated that increasing arterial stiffness initiates systemic hypertension; thus, it is a cause, not an effect. However, once induced, hypertension leads to further arterial stiffening [28]. In addition, arterial stiffening reflects the vascular ageing process, and the latter one is at least as important as chronological age in cardiovascular events and mortality prediction [29,30].

In fact, the results of our study demonstrate that both chronological and vascular age were the only independent risk predictors of HF-MACCE in multivariate analysis.

It is important to realize that DAS is not only a disease of the valve (or heart), but this is a disease of the whole vascular system, and the latter contributes to adverse events. A decrease in elasticity is associated with a multitude of complications, including increased stress on the left ventricle, a gradual increase in blood pressure and, eventually, even end-organ damage through the transmission of harmful pulsation into the microcirculation. Thus, the increase in pulsatility associated with loss of elastic recoil in large blood vessels has detrimental effects on global cardiovascular health [9].

Biological vascular age should be used to select individuals for early prevention of cardiovascular complications with intensification of pharmacotherapy and earlier intervention on the valve [30–32].

Hypothetically, the risk prediction models may help clinicians develop personalized treatments, i.e., in patients with PI $\geq$ 1.3 or RI $\geq$ 0.7, early intervention on DAS could be considered. The treatment of choice could perhaps be transcatheter aortic valve implantation in such a subset of patients, as surgical aortic valve replacement may lead to further significant increase in PWV [31,32].

## 5. Conclusions

Patients with DAS have greater vascular resistance compared to controls with cardiovascular risk factors. Moreover, RI $\geq$ 0.7 and PI $\geq$ 1.3 may be used for cardiovascular risk stratification.

## 6. Study Limitations

Our study has obvious limitations, as it consisted of a single-center observational design. Secondly, in general, DAS patients are elderly, which caused difficulties when matching with a control group. For this reason, age-adjustment in multivariate analyses was performed.

**Author Contributions:** Conceptualization, J.B., A.G., T.P. and A.K.-Z.; data curation, Ł.N., R.B., A.G., P.P., J.L., K.Ż. and A.K.-Z.; formal analysis, J.P., A.G. and P.P.; funding acquisition, J.P. and A.K.-Z.; investigation, P.K., Ł.N., R.B., P.P. and A.K.-Z.; methodology, J.B., Ł.N., R.B., T.P. and A.K.-Z.; project administration, K.Ż.; resources, J.B. and T.P.; software, J.B. and Ł.N.; supervision, A.K.-Z.; validation, A.G., J.L. and K.Ż.; visualization, J.B., Ł.N. and R.B.; writing—original draft, J.B., P.K. and J.P.; writing—review and editing, J.L., K.Ż., T.P. and A.K.-Z. All authors have read and agreed to the published version of the manuscript.

**Funding:** This research was funded by grants from the Jagiellonian University (grant numbers: N41/DBS/000038 and N41/DBS/000437).

**Institutional Review Board Statement:** The study was conducted according to the guidelines of the Declaration of Helsinki, and approved by the Institutional Ethics Committee of the Jagiellonian University (KBET/118/B/2014 and KBET/1072.6120.148.2018).

**Informed Consent Statement:** Informed consent was obtained from all subjects involved in the study.

**Data Availability Statement:** The data presented in this study are available on request from the corresponding author. The data are not publicly available due to privacy.

**Conflicts of Interest:** The authors declare no conflict of interest.

# References

1. Nilsson, P.M.; Boutouyrie, P.; Cunha, P.; Kotsis, V.; Narkiewicz, K.; Parati, G.; Rietzschel, E.; Scuteri, A.; Laurent, S. Early vascular ageing in translation: From laboratory investigations to clinical applications in cardiovascular prevention. *J. Hypertens.* **2013**, *31*, 1517–1526. [CrossRef]
2. Stehouwer, C.D.; Henry, R.M.; Ferreira, I. Arterial stiffness in diabetes and the metabolic syndrome: A pathway to cardiovascular disease. *Diabetologia* **2008**, *51*, 527–539. [CrossRef]
3. Alonso-Fernández, P.; De la Fuente, M. Role of the immune system in aging and longevity. *Curr. Aging Sci.* **2011**, *4*, 78–100. [CrossRef] [PubMed]
4. Scuteri, A.; Orru, M.; Morrell, C.; Taub, D.; Schlessinger, D.; Uda, M.; Lakatta, E.G. Independent and additive effects of cytokine patterns and the metabolic syndrome on arterial aging in the SardiNIA Study. *Atherosclerosis* **2011**, *215*, 459–464. [CrossRef]
5. Sutton-Tyrrell, K.; Najjar, S.S.; Boudreau, R.M.; Venkitachalam, L.; Kupelian, V.; Simonsick, E.M.; Havlik, R.; Lakatta, E.G.; Spurgeon, H.; Kritchevsky, S.; et al. Elevated Aortic Pulse Wave Velocity, a Marker of Arterial Stiffness, Predicts Cardiovascular Events in Well-Functioning Older Adults. *Circulation* **2005**, *111*, 3384–3390. [CrossRef] [PubMed]
6. Yan, A.T.; Koh, M.; Chan, K.K.; Guo, H.; Alter, D.A.; Austin, P.C.; Tu, J.V.; Wijeysundera, H.C.; Ko, D.T. Association between Cardiovascular Risk Factors and Aortic Stenosis: The CANHEART Aortic Stenosis Study. *J. Am. Coll. Cardiol.* **2017**, *69*, 1523–1532. [CrossRef] [PubMed]
7. Podolec, J.; Baran, J.; Siedlinski, M.; Urbanczyk, M.; Krupinski, M.; Bartus, K.; Niewiara, L.; Podolec, M.; Guzik, T.; Tomkiewicz-Pajak, L.; et al. Serum rantes, transforming growth factor-β1 and interleukin-6 levels correlate with cardiac muscle fibrosis in patients with aortic valve stenosis. *J. Physiol. Pharmacol.* **2018**, *69*, 615–623.
8. Baran, J.; Podolec, J.; Tomala, M.T.; Nawrotek, B.; Niewiara, Ł.; Gackowski, A.; Przewłocki, T.; Żmudka, K.; Kabłak-Ziembicka, A. Increased risk profile in the treatment of patients with symptomatic degenerative aortic valve stenosis over the last 10 years. *Adv. Interv. Cardiol.* **2018**, *14*, 276–284. [CrossRef]
9. Bardelli, M.; Cavressi, M.; Furlanis, G.; Pinamonti, B.; Leone, M.; Albani, S.; Korcova, R.; Fabris, B.; Sinagra, G. Relationship between aortic valve stenosis and the hemodynamic pattern in the renal circulation, and restoration of the flow wave profile after correction of the valvular defect. *J. Int. Med. Res.* **2020**, *48*, 1–14. [CrossRef]
10. Hamczyk, M.R.; Nevado, R.M.; Barettino, A.; Fuster, V.; Andrés, V. Biological Versus Chronological Aging. *J. Am. Coll. Cardiol.* **2020**, *75*, 919–930. [CrossRef]
11. Mach, F.; Baigent, C.; Catapano, A.L.; Koskinas, K.C.; Casula, M.; Badimon, L.; Chapman, M.J.; De Backer, G.G.; Delgado, V.; Ference, B.A.; et al. 2019 ESC/EAS Guidelines for the management of dyslipidaemias: Lipid modification to reduce cardiovascular risk. *Eur. Heart J.* **2020**, *41*, 111–188. [CrossRef] [PubMed]
12. Baumgartner, H.; Hung, J.; Bermejo, J.; Chambers, J.B.; Edvardsen, T.; Goldstein, S.; Lancellotti, P.; LeFevre, M.; Miller, F., Jr.; Otto, C.M. Recommendations on the echocardiographic assessment of aortic valve stenosis: A focused update from the European Association of Cardiovascular Imaging and the American Society of Echocardiography. *J. Am. Soc. Echocardiogr.* **2017**, *30*, 372–392. [CrossRef] [PubMed]
13. Robin, X.A.; Turck, N.; Hainard, A.; Tiberti, N.; Lisacek, F.; Sanchez, J.-C.; Muller, M.J. pROC: An open-source package for R and S+ to analyze and compare ROC curves. *BMC Bioinform.* **2011**, *12*, 77. [CrossRef] [PubMed]
14. Frauchiger, B.; Schmid, H.P.; Roedel, C.; Moosmann, P.; Staub, D. Comparison of carotid arterial resistive indices with intima-media thickness as sonographic markers Atherosclerosis. *Stroke* **2001**, *32*, 836–841. [CrossRef] [PubMed]
15. Kabłak-Ziembicka, A.; Rosławiecka, A.; Badacz, R.; Sokołowski, A.; Rzeźnik, D.; Trystuła, M.; Musiałek, P.; Przewłocki, T. Simple clinical scores to predict blood pressure and renal function response to renal artery stenting for atherosclerotic renal artery stenosis. *Pol. Arch. Intern. Med.* **2020**, *130*, 953–959. [CrossRef] [PubMed]
16. Wielicka, M.; Neubauer-Geryk, J.; Kozera, G.; Bieniaszewski, L. Clinical application of pulsatility index. *Med. Res. J.* **2020**, *5*, 201–210. [CrossRef]
17. Nakano, H.; Shiina, K.; Tomiyama, H. Cardiovascular Outcomes in the Acute Phase of COVID-19. *Int. J. Mol. Sci.* **2021**, *22*, 4071. [CrossRef]
18. Summerhill, V.; Moschetta, D.; Orekhov, A.; Poggio, P.; Myasoedova, V. Sex-Specific Features of Calcific Aortic Valve Disease. *Int. J. Mol. Sci.* **2020**, *21*, 5620. [CrossRef]
19. Thomassen, H.K.; Cioffi, G.; Gerdts, E.; Einarsen, E.; Midtbø, H.B.; Mancusi, C.; Cramariuc, D. Echocardiographic aortic valve calcification and outcomes in women and men with aortic stenosis. *Heart* **2017**, *103*, 1619–1624. [CrossRef]

20. Weisz, S.H.; Magne, J.; Dulgheru, R.; Caso, P.; Piérard, L.A.; Lancellotti, P. Carotid Artery and Aortic Stiffness Evaluation in Aortic Stenosis. *J. Am. Soc. Echocardiogr.* **2014**, *27*, 385–392. [CrossRef]
21. Kablak-Ziembicka, A.; Przewlocki, T.; Tracz, W.; Podolec, P.; Stopa, I.; Kostkiewicz, M.; Sadowski, J.; Mura, A.; Kopeć, G. Prognostic Value of Carotid Intima-Media Thickness in Detection of Coronary Atherosclerosis in Patients with Calcified Aortic Valve Stenosis. *J. Ultrasound Med.* **2005**, *24*, 461–467. [CrossRef] [PubMed]
22. Safar, M.E.; Nilsson, P.M.; Blacher, J.; Mimran, A. Pulse Pressure, Arterial Stiffness, and End-Organ Damage. *Curr. Hypertens. Rep.* **2012**, *14*, 339–344. [CrossRef] [PubMed]
23. Baran, J.; Przewłocki, T.; Podolec, J.; Gryglicka, K.; Badacz, R.; Gackowski, A.; Pieniążek, P.; Legutko, J.; Żmudka, K.; Kabłak-Ziembicka, A. Assessment of the Willis circle flow changes with the severity of degenerative aortic stenosis and cognitive impairment. *Kardiol. Pol.* **2021**, *79*, 46–52. [PubMed]
24. Sequí-Domínguez, I.; Cavero-Redondo, I.; Álvarez-Bueno, C.; Pozuelo-Carrascosa, D.P.; De Arenas-Arroyo, S.N.; Martínez-Vizcaíno, V. Accuracy of Pulse Wave Velocity Predicting Cardiovascular and All-Cause Mortality. A Systematic Review and Meta-Analysis. *J. Clin. Med.* **2020**, *9*, 2080. [CrossRef]
25. Zoungas, S.; Asmar, R.P. Arterial stiffness and cardiovascular outcome. *Clin. Exp. Pharmacol. Physiol.* **2007**, *34*, 647–651. [CrossRef] [PubMed]
26. Saeed, S.; Saeed, N.; Grigoryan, K.; Chowienczyk, P.; Chambers, J.B.; Rajani, R. Determinants and clinical significance of aortic stiffness in patients with moderate or severe aortic stenosis. *Int. J. Cardiol.* **2020**, *315*, 99–104. [CrossRef]
27. Bahlmann, E.; Cramariuc, D.; Saeed, S.; Chambers, J.B.; A Nienaber, C.; Kuck, K.-H.; Lønnebakken, M.T.; Gerdts, E. Low systemic arterial compliance is associated with increased cardiovascular morbidity and mortality in aortic valve stenosis. *Heart* **2019**, *105*, 1507–1514. [CrossRef]
28. Ungvari, Z.; Tarantini, S.; Donato, A.J.; Galvan, V.; Csiszar, A. Mechanisms of Vascular Aging. *Circ. Res.* **2018**, *123*, 849–867. [CrossRef]
29. Humphrey, J.D.; Harrison, D.G.; Figueroa, C.A.; Lacolley, P.; Laurent, S. Central Artery Stiffness in Hypertension and Aging: A Problem with Cause and Consequence. *Circ. Res.* **2016**, *118*, 379–381. [CrossRef]
30. Janić, M.; Lunder, M.; Šabovič, M. Arterial Stiffness and Cardiovascular Therapy. *BioMed Res. Int.* **2014**, *2014*, 621437. [CrossRef]
31. Musa, T.A.; Uddin, A.; Fairbairn, T.A.; Dobson, L.E.; Sourbron, S.P.; Steadman, C.D.; Motwani, M.; Kidambi, A.; Ripley, D.P.; Swoboda, P.P.; et al. Assessment of aortic stiffness by cardiovascular magnetic resonance following the treatment of severe aortic stenosis by TAVI and surgical AVR. *J. Cardiovasc. Magn. Reson.* **2016**, *18*, 37. [CrossRef] [PubMed]
32. Bruschi, G.; Maloberti, A.; Sormani, P.; Colombo, G.; Nava, S.; Vallerio, P.; Casadei, F.; Bruno, J.; Moreo, A.; Merlanti, B. Arterial Stiffness in Aortic Stenosis: Relationship with Severity and Echocardiographic Procedures Response. *High Blood Press. Cardiovasc. Prev.* **2017**, *24*, 19–27. [CrossRef] [PubMed]

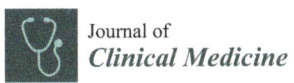

*Review*

# OCT Findings in MINOCA

Krzysztof Bryniarski [1], Pawel Gasior [2], Jacek Legutko [1], Dawid Makowicz [3], Anna Kedziora [4], Piotr Szolc [1], Leszek Bryniarski [5], Pawel Kleczynski [1] and Ik-Kyung Jang [6,7,*]

1. Jagiellonian University Medical College, Institute of Cardiology, Department of Interventional Cardiology, John Paul II Hospital, 31-202 Krakow, Poland; kbrynia@gmail.com (K.B.); jacek.legutko@uj.edu.pl (J.L.); piotr.szolc4@gmail.com (P.S.); kleczu@interia.pl (P.K.)
2. Division of Cardiology and Structural Heart Diseases, Medical University of Silesia, 40-635 Katowice, Poland; p.m.gasior@gmail.com
3. Interventional Cardiology, Electrotherapy and Angiology Department, John Paul II Hospital, 38-400 Krosno, Poland; david1990@onet.pl
4. Department of Cardiovascular Surgery and Transplantation, John Paul II Hospital, 31-202 Krakow, Poland; kdzra.a@gmail.com
5. 2nd Department of Cardiology and Cardiovascular Interventions, University Hospital, Institute of Cardiology, Jagiellonian University Medical College, 31-501 Krakow, Poland; l_bryniarski@poczta.fm
6. Cardiology Division, Massachusetts General Hospital, Harvard Medical School, 55 Fruit Street l GRB 800, Boston, MA 02114, USA
7. Department of Cardiology, School of Medicine, Kyung Hee University, Dongdaemoon-gu, Seoul 130-701, Korea
* Correspondence: ijang@mgh.harvard.edu; Tel.: +1-617-726-9226; Fax: +1-617-726-7419

**Abstract:** Myocardial infarction with non-obstructive coronary artery disease (MINOCA) is a working diagnosis for patients presenting with acute myocardial infarction without obstructive coronary artery disease on coronary angiography. It is a heterogenous entity with a number of possible etiologies that can be determined through the use of appropriate diagnostic algorithms. Common causes of a MINOCA may include plaque disruption, spontaneous coronary artery dissection, coronary artery spasm, and coronary thromboembolism. Optical coherence tomography (OCT) is an intravascular imaging modality which allows the differentiation of coronary tissue morphological characteristics including the identification of thin cap fibroatheroma and the differentiation between plaque rupture or erosion, due to its high resolution. In this narrative review we will discuss the role of OCT in patients presenting with MINOCA. In this group of patients OCT has been shown to reveal abnormal findings in almost half of the cases. Moreover, combining OCT with cardiac magnetic resonance (CMR) was shown to allow the identification of most of the underlying mechanisms of MINOCA. Hence, it is recommended that both OCT and CMR can be used in patients with a working diagnosis of MINOCA. Well-designed prospective studies are needed in order to gain a better understanding of this condition and to provide optimal management while reducing morbidity and mortality in that subset patients.

**Keywords:** cardiovascular disease; acute myocardial infarction; intravascular imaging

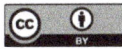

## 1. Introduction

Atherosclerotic cardiovascular disease is one of the leading causes of death around the world [1,2]. Advances in the understanding of the underlying pathobiology, diagnosis, and treatment of atherosclerosis have been made during the past century. This progress has significantly lowered the mortality rate in patients presenting with acute myocardial infarction (AMI) with obstructive coronary artery disease (CAD). However, in recent years challenges in the diagnosis and treatment of patients who presented with symptoms of AMI but did not have obstructive CAD have been recognized.

First reports of AMI without obstructive CAD go back 80 years [3,4]. This phenomenon was observed in the late 1970s by one of the pioneers in the field of interventional cardiology—DeWood. In his studies, he performed coronary angiography in patients presenting with ST elevation myocardial infarction (STEMI) and non-ST elevation myocardial infarction (NSTEMI) [5,6]. Surprisingly, about 10% of patients presenting with AMI had no significant CAD on coronary angiography. His initial observations were later confirmed in several large AMI registries in which 13% of patients presenting with AMI did not have obstructive CAD [7,8].

Important questions were raised regarding the underlying pathophysiological mechanism and treatment of this presentation. This led to the creation of new terminology for this phenomenon, myocardial infarction with non-obstructive coronary artery disease (MINOCA). The first position papers regarding MINOCA were published by the European Society of Cardiology (ESC) in 2018, followed by the American Heart Association in 2019 [9,10]. According to both position papers, the diagnosis of MINOCA should be made immediately upon coronary angiography in a patient presenting with features consistent with AMI [11]. Although chest pain and elevated troponin levels are not specific for AMI, MINOCA is an umbrella term for several different conditions, thus should only be a working diagnosis requiring further evaluation. MINOCA can be confirmed only after the investigation of other underlying causes of elevated troponin levels. Ascertaining the pathophysiological mechanism and prognostic markers in order to provide proper management strategies is vital in patients with a diagnosis of MINOCA. In this narrative review we will discuss the role of optical coherence tomography (OCT) in patients presenting with MINOCA.

## 2. Discussion

### 2.1. MINOCA: Is It a Serious Condition?

Significantly, patients presenting with MINOCA have comparable, or only a slightly lower, incidence of major adverse cardiac events (MACE) during follow-up as compared to those presenting with AMI, despite their younger age and less comorbidities [12,13].

Kang et al. showed that the 12-month MACE rate in patients with MINOCA was comparable to patients with AMI with single or double vessel CAD (7.8% vs. 12.2%; $p = 0.359$) (Table 1) [14]. Ishi et al. observed that MINOCA was associated with a high risk of in-hospital mortality compared with MI with obstructive CAD [15]. In a study which included 4793 consecutive patients presenting with STEMI, patients without obstructive CAD had a long-term risk of death similar to, or higher than, patients with obstructive CAD, although their causes of death were less often cardiovascular [16]. Lindahl et al., in a retrospective study involving almost 10,000 patients, observed a 13% mortality rate for MINOCA patients during four-year follow-up [17]. Gasior et al., in a retrospective study of over 6000 patients, demonstrated higher mortality at 12-month follow-up in the MINOCA group when compared to the MI-CAD group (10.94% vs. 9.54%, $p < 0.001$), with no statistical difference in mortality at three-year follow up [18].

Contrary to those findings, Pasupathy et al. in a metaanalysis including 28 publications, demonstrated that patients with MINOCA had lower one-year all-cause mortality [12]. However, it should be emphasized that even though patients with AMI had a higher one-year mortality rate at 6.7%, the mortality of patients with MINOCA was still high (4.7%). Considering that patients with stable chest pain (without previous AMI) and non-obstructed coronary arteries had 0.2% one-year mortality, the mortality in MINOCA patients was markedly elevated [22].

It is of the utmost importance to optimize the management of patients with MINOCA based on the underlying mechanism. Montone et al. observed that patients with vasospastic angina who had a reduction in their dosing of calcium channel blockers (CCB) had increased mortality during follow-up compared to those who continued to take high doses of CCB [23,24]. Of note, more than one third of patients with MINOCA did not receive an optimal cardioprotective pharmacotherapy [25,26].

Table 1. Selected studies with outcomes of patients with myocardial infarction with non-obstructive coronary artery disease.

| Study | No. of Patients with Non-Significant CAD, n | No. of Patients with Significant CAD, n | Follow-Up Length | Mortality | MACE | Other | STEMI at Admission | Notes |
|---|---|---|---|---|---|---|---|---|
| Safdar et al. [19] | <50% CAS-299 | ≥50% CAS-2374 | 12 months | 1 month: 1.1% vs. 1.7% ($p$ = 0.43) 12 months: 0.6% vs. 2.3% ($p$ = 0.68) | NA | SAQ: 76.5 vs. 73.5 ($p$ = 0.06) | 21.4% vs. 52.1% $p$ = 0.001 | NA |
| Kang et al. [14] | <50% CAS-372 ([A]) | >50% CAS (one or two-vessel disease)-6136 ([B]) >50% CAS (three-vessel disease or LM disease)-2002 ([C]) | 12 months | In hospital: 2.2% ([A]) vs. 2.6% ([B]) vs. 6.9% ([C]); $p$ = 0.952 ([A] vs. [B]). | 12 months 7.8% ([A]) vs. 12.2% ([B]) vs. 23.3% ([C]); $p$ = 0.359 ([A] vs. [B]). | Repeat PCI at 12 months: 2.4% ([A]) vs. 2.4% ([B]) vs. 14.0% ([C]); $p$ = 0.180 ([A] vs. [B]). | 36.3% ([A]) vs. 63.8% ([B]) vs. 52.0% ([C]); $p$ < 0.001 ([A] vs. [B]). | NA |
| Ishii et al. [15] | <50% CAS-14,045 | ≥50% CAS-123,633 | 30 days | In hospital: 6.4% vs. 6.2% | NA | NA | NA | NA |
| Andersson et al. [16] | Normal CA-256 ([A]) Non-obstructive CAS-298 ([B]) | ≥50% CAS-4239 ([C]) | 2.2 years | CVD 3.5% ([A]) vs. 5.0% ([B]) vs. 9.8% ([C]) Non-CVD 7.4% ([A]) vs. 8.4% ([B]) vs. 4.2% | NA | NA | NA | NA |
| Lindahl et al. [17] | 9466 (9136 after one month) | | 4.1 years | 13.4% | 23.9% | NA | 17.1% | NA |
| Larsen et al. [20] | <30% CAS-127 | ≥30% CAS-3475 | 3 years | CVD 0.8% vs. 4.0% ($p$ = 0.12) | 7.7% vs. 22.2% ($p$ = 0.002) | Re-infarction: 0% vs. 1.9% ($p$ = 0.12) | 100% | Study included only patients with STEMI |
| Gasior et al. [18] | <50% CAS-6063 | >50% CAS-160886 | 36 months | 16.8% vs. 14.93% ($p$ = 0.081) | NA | PCI at 36 months: 5.82% vs. 23.9% ($p$ < 0.01) | NA | NA |
| Grodzinsky et al. [21] | ≤70% CAS-381 | >70% or >50% in LM CAS-4941 | 12 months | 3.9% vs. 3.1% ($p$ = 0.08) | NA | Angina prevalence at 12 months: 24.6% vs. 21.4% ($p$ = 0.199) SAQ QOL 60.5 vs. 63.8 ($p$ = 0.006) | 13.4% vs. 49.0% ($p$ < 0.001) | NA |

CA indicates coronary artery; CAS, coronary artery stenosis; CVD, cardiovascular disease; LM, left main; MACE, major adverse cardiovascular events; NA, not available; PCI, percutaneous coronary intervention; SAQ, Seattle Angina Questionnaire; STEMI, ST-elevation myocardial infarction; and QOL, quality of life. [A], [B] and [C] stand for different groups. When not indicated, results of patients with myocardial infarction with non-obstructive coronary artery disease are given first.

## 2.2. Etiology of MINOCA

Myocardial infarction with non-obstructive coronary artery disease is a heterogenous entity with many possible etiologies that need to be clarified by proper diagnostics algorithm. Over the past several years, a few algorithms were developed in order to optimize the care of MINOCA patients [9,11,27]. Rigorous algorithms are crucial for effective treatment for certain conditions (for example, vasospasm) but may not be effective for another group of patients with MINOCA caused by a different mechanism (for example, plaque rupture) [11]. Common causes of a MINOCA working diagnosis may include plaque disruption, spontaneous coronary artery dissection (SCAD), coronary artery spasm, coronary thromboembolism, Takotsubo cardiomyopathy, and myocarditis. Importantly, due to the low resolution of coronary angiography, plaque disruption may occur in areas of coronary arteries which appear normal on the angiogram [28]. A large thrombus may result in severe narrowing or occlusion of the artery visible on angiogram, whereas smaller thrombi may either result in insignificant stenosis not visible on the angiogram or embolization to distal segments. Information regarding the exact pathogenic mechanism responsible for MINOCA, plaque vulnerability, or plaque burden cannot be obtained from angiography alone [29,30]. Spontaneous coronary artery dissection is another diagnosis which cannot be completely ruled out with angiography alone [31]. Two intravascular imaging modalities have been proposed to surpass the limitations of angiography: intravascular ultrasound (IVUS) and optical coherence tomography (OCT). IVUS studies showed that plaque rupture or ulceration may be identified in about 40% patients presenting with MINOCA [32,33]. Optical coherence tomography with a resolution of 10–20µm allows the visualization of intraluminal and superficial coronary artery structures in detail [34]. It has the ability to differentiate tissue morphological characteristics including the detection of lipid-rich, calcified, and fibrous plaques, thin cap fibroatheroma, and the differentiation between plaque rupture and erosion, red and white thrombi, as well as the identification of even small spontaneous dissections (Figure 1) [35,36]. It can function as a type of optical biopsy and is a powerful imaging technology for medical diagnostics. Unlike conventional histopathology, which requires removal of a tissue specimen and processing for microscopic examination,

OCT can provide images of the vascular wall in situ and in real time. Its higher resolution undoubtedly can confirm findings such as plaque erosion or calcified nodule which may cause AMI and usually are not visible on both conventional angiography and IVUS.

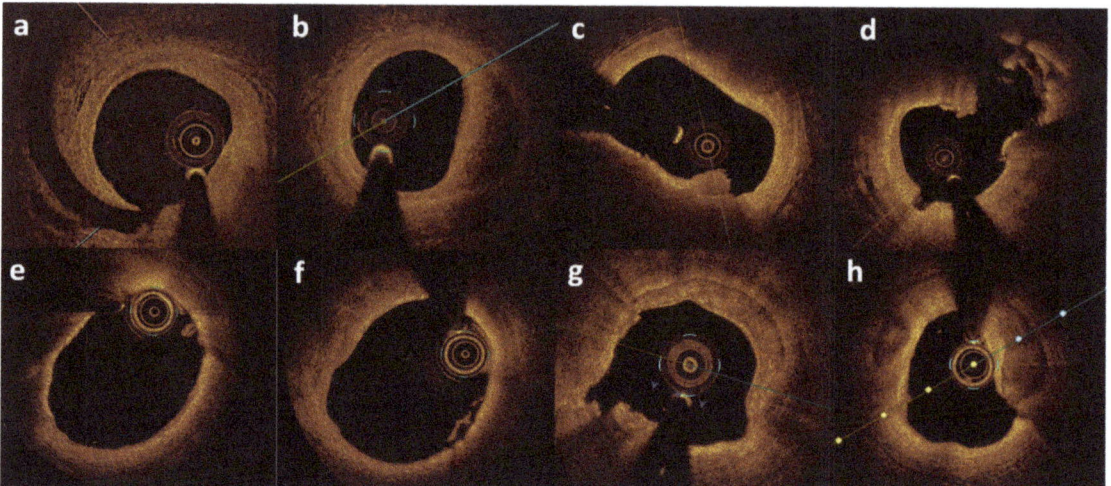

**Figure 1.** Optical coherence tomography images from patients with MINOCA. Spontaneous dissection (**a,b**), plaque erosion (**c**), plaque rupture (**d**), thin-cap fibroatheroma (**e**), small white thrombi (**f**), and calcified nodule erosion (**g,h**). Figures from authors' library.

Howbeit, it should be emphasized that OCT also has several drawbacks [37]. First, its greater resolution as compared to IVUS comes with a lower penetration depth. In the case of large arteries such as the left main, visualization of the whole coronary artery may not be possible. Moreover, when performing pullback in ostial lesions incomplete blood clearance may lead to suboptimal image quality. Second, the need for contrast agents to clear blood may increase risk of contrast-induced nephropathy. Third, OCT images cannot penetrate lipid plaque and red thrombi.

According to a recent metaanalysis, up to 33% of patients with the diagnosis of MINOCA may have myocarditis [38]. In a recent prospective study, cardiac magnetic resonance (CMR) showed evidence of myocarditis in 25% of patients presenting with MINOCA, an MI in 25%, and cardiomyopathy in 25% [39]. Recent studies demonstrated the value of combined CMR and OCT imaging in MINOCA patients. Moreover, it should be stressed that finding one cause of MINOCA does not necessarily mean that others have been excluded. Several studies have emphasized the importance of coronary artery vasospasm in Takotsubo cardiomyopathy and myocarditis [40,41]. An OCT study including 23 patients found that those with Takotsubo cardiomyopathy have high plaque vulnerability [42].

### 2.3. OCT in MINOCA

Coronary thrombosis is the most frequent final event leading to an acute coronary syndrome in patients with AMI with obstructive coronary disease. Plaque rupture, plaque erosion, and calcified plaque are believed to be the most common underlying mechanisms contributing to AMI with the former being the most frequent in both autopsy and in vivo studies [43,44].

While angiographic images of haziness or minor filling may suggest plaque disruption, it can be definitively diagnosed using intracoronary imaging, with OCT being the preferable modality due to its higher resolution. However, IVUS may be considered as an alternative to OCT to a lesser extent [45]. One of the first OCT studies in MINOCA patients showed that plaque disruption or thrombi were visible in 39% of 38 patients included in the study [46] (Table 2). Notably, during hospitalization 82% patients underwent CMR. In a detailed assessment of infarct-related arteries (i.e., those where infarct-related artery was identified on the basis of the association between coronary artery distribution and myocardial segments with late gadolinium-enhancement of ischemic origin), the authors found that 40% had plaque rupture and 30% had plaque erosion. Importantly, 30% of lesions had plaque disruption without thrombus. The latter might have resulted, as stated by the authors, either by resolution of thrombi from the initial antithrombotic therapy or by distal embolization during advancement of the OCT catheter. It could have also been an incidental finding after silent plaque rupture which occurred in the near past [47]. Findings by Opolski et al. led to the modification of the initial treatment in six patients. One of the main limitations of this study was the relatively small number of patients recruited which could present bias. Moreover, only 21% of the patients had three-vessel OCT.

**Table 2.** Myocardial infarction with non-obstructive coronary artery disease selected studies with use of optical coherence tomography.

| Study | No. of Patients | Modalities Used, n | Three-Vessel OCT, n | Two-Vessel OCT, n | Abnormal Image in OCT, n | Plaque Rupture, n | Plaque Erosion, n | Calcified Nodule, n | Lone Thrombus, n | SCAD, n | Other, n | Abnormal Image in CMR, n | Abnormal Image OCT or CMR, n |
|---|---|---|---|---|---|---|---|---|---|---|---|---|---|
| Opolski et al. [46] | 38 | OCT-38 (100%) CMR-31 (82%) | 8 (21%) | 26 (68%) | 15 (39%) | 8 (21%) | 4 (11%) | 2 (11%) | 2 (5%) | NA | Takotsubo-5 (13%) Myocarditis-3 (8%) | 16 (52%) * | NA |
| Mas-Lladó et al. [48] | 27 | OCT-27 (100%) | 0 | 1 (4%) | 21 (78%) | 8 (30%) | 11 (41%) | 2 (7%) | NA | NA | NA | NA | NA |
| Gerbaud et al. [38] | 40 | OCT-40 (100%) CMR-40 (100%) | 5 (13%) | 11 (28%) | 32 (80%) | 14 (35%) | 12 (30%) | 1 (3%) | 3 (8%) | 2 (5%) | NA | 31 (78%) | 40 (100%) |
| Reynolds et al. [49] | 145 | OCT-145 (100%) CMR-116 (80%) | 86 (59%) | 47 (32%) | 67 (46%) | 8 (6%) | NA | 0 (0%) | Thrombus without plaque rupture-5 (4%) | 1 (1%) | Intra plaque cavity-31 (21%) Layered plaque-19 (13%) Intimal bump-3 (2%) | 86 (74%) | 98 (85%) |

CMR indicates cardiac magnetic resonance; OCT, optical coherence tomography; SCAD, spontaneous coronary artery dissection; and TCFA, thin cap fibroatheroma. * T1-weighted imaging.

In a small study by Mas-Lladó et al. involving 27 patients with MINOCA who had mostly one-vessel OCT, an abnormal image was found in 78% of patients [48]. Patients predominantly had either plaque erosion (41%) or plaque rupture (30%).

In a more recent study presented by Gerabaud et al. 40 patients with MINOCA underwent both OCT and CMR [50]. Optical coherence tomography provided a diagnosis of AMI in 80% of patients including 35% with plaque rupture, 30% with plaque erosion, 7.5% with lone thrombus, 5% with SCAD, and 2.5% with calcified nodule. Acute myocardial infarction was evident in CMR in 77.5% of patients. Over half the patients (57.5%) had a substrate and/or diagnosis supported by both modalities, 22.5% of patients had a mechanism specified only by OCT, and 20% of patients had a clear diagnosis only by CMR. One of the major findings of this study was that combination of both CMR and OCT provided a much higher yield in diagnosing MINOCA as compared to using only one of the mentioned modalities. The limitations of this study were similar to the study of Opolski et al.—the small number of patients and the low number of patients with three-vessel OCT (12.5%). Moreover, OCT was not always done at the index procedure, and an older CMR imaging protocol was used.

Reynolds et al. presented the biggest study to date, involving 145 women with a diagnosis of MINOCA [49]. In this study CMR was interpretable in 116 patients. Over half of the patients had three-vessel OCT (59.3%) and a possible culprit lesion was identified in 46.2% of patients. Plaque rupture, intra-plaque cavity, or a layered plaque phenotype were evident in 39% of patients, whereas thrombus without plaque rupture was found in 3.5% of patients and one patient had SCAD. Moreover, 2.1% of patients had intimal bumping suggestive of coronary artery spasm. Combining both OCT and CMR allowed the identification of the cause of MINOCA in 84.5% of patients. A lesion visible on OCT could be identified in 42% of patients with CMR-detected infarction and in 79% of patients with CMR-detected regional injury. Hypothetically, patients who had CMR evidence of infarction or regional injury without abnormalities identified by OCT could suffer from coronary spasm or thromboembolism as the mechanism of MI. Importantly, 40% of patients without abnormal CMR had an OCT identified culprit lesion—this finding underlines the importance of OCT in the diagnosis of MINOCA and strengthens the guidelines which suggest multimodality imaging in patients with MINOCA. Reynolds et al. confirmed previous findings that multi imaging modalities, including both OCT and CMR, should be used in patients with MINOCA—the identification of the etiology of MINOCA may have potential to guide optimal medical therapy; however, new studies are warranted. Limitations of this study were the lack of three-vessel OCT in all patients and the inclusion of layered plaque phenotype and intra-plaque cavity as causes of MINOCA. Layered plaque phenotype is a consequence and not an etiology of plaque destabilization. The process of lesion progression to a layered plaque phenotype may take from weeks to months. Moreover, a recent OCT study reported that a layered plaque phenotype may be found in more than 50% of patients with stable angina [51]. To our knowledge, there was only one case report for the OCT finding of intraplaque hemorrhage. It should be emphasized that there is a difference in methodology used for OCT interpretation between the presented studies. Some studies include lone thrombus which in these authors' opinion may not always be easy to distinguish from plaque erosion. Also, other definitions were introduced, such as layered plaque phenotype. This may cause differences in incidence of OCT findings between different studies.

Although pathogenesis of SCAD remains unclear there is some evidence that it is related to connective/collagen tissue alterations. In-hospital mortality of patients with SCAD is similar to those with obstructive CAD. On angiogram, SCAD may be missed or misdiagnosed as vasospasm due to low resolution of the image, even though there may be a life-threatening condition [52]. In the recent OCT and CMR study, the incidence of SCAD was up to 5%. It is therefore crucial to perform both OCT and CMR in patients with a working diagnosis of MINOCA [53].

Coronary artery spasm reflects a vascular smooth muscle hyper-reactivity to endogenous vasospastic substance, but may also occur in the context of exogenous vasospastic agents [11,54]. Prevalence of coronary artery spasm in patients with MINOCA may vary between 3% and 95% [55]. Moreover, previous studies have shown that about one quarter of the patients with MINOCA have evidence of microvascular spasm [56]. In a recent study, Montone et al. showed that out of 80 enrolled patients presenting with MINOCA, a provocative test was positive in almost half of the patients [23]. Furthermore, a thrombus was found by OCT in 28.8% of patients presenting with vasospastic angina [57]. In patients presenting with vasospasm-induced AMI intimal tear, intra luminal thrombi and plaque erosion were significantly more frequent compared to patients with chronic stable vasospastic angina [58]. Thus, OCT may be a useful modality when assessing MINOCA patients suspected for coronary artery spasm. Coronary artery spasm on OCT is characterized by intimal bumping with a larger medial area and medial thickness [59].

Most of the current studies support the necessity of OCT in the diagnosis of patients presenting with MINOCA. Proper management of every patient with suspected myocardial infarction should include several different imaging modalities. A proposed approach to the proper diagnosis of patients with MINOCA is presented in Figure 2. In the authors' opinion, the first step starts with proper analysis of trans thoracic echocardiography (TTE) performed before angiography. Next, during coronary angiography when MINOCA is identified, angiography of the left ventricle (LV) could be of help for assessment of regional wall abnormalities. A combination of both TTE and LV angiography could be used to identify Takotsubo cardiomyopathy or myocarditis. OCT can be used to evaluate coronary arteries based on findings in the electrocardiogram, TTE, or LV angiography. If no abnormalities, such as plaque disruption or SCAD, are found on OCT, CMR should be performed [60]. Finally, other tests such as the intracoronary acetylcholine provocation test could be considered for further evaluation of MINOCA patients in order to identify abnormalities, such as coronary artery spasm or microvascular dysfunction.

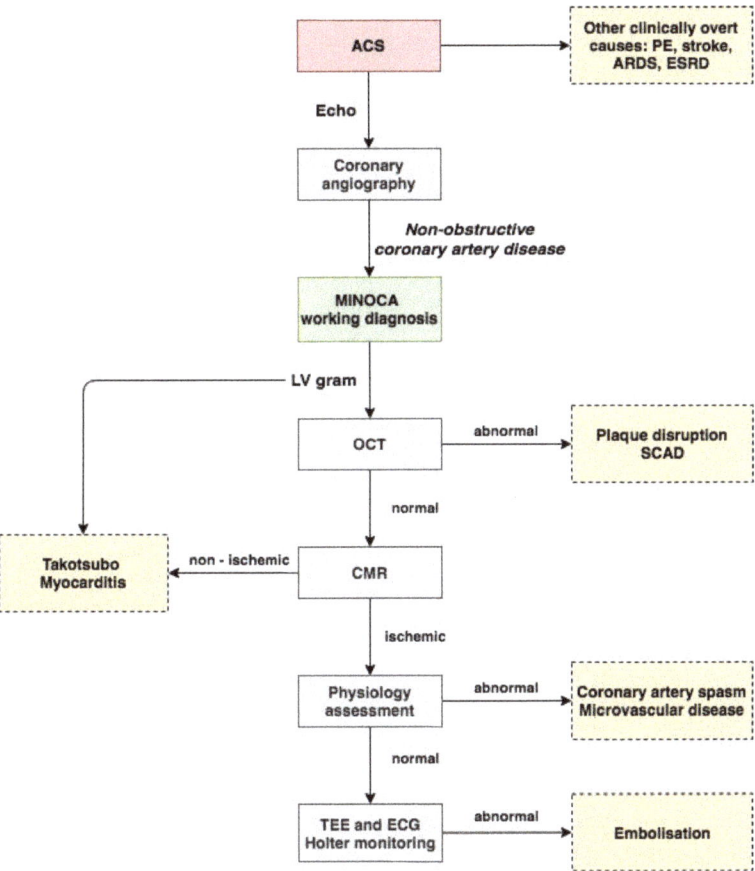

**Figure 2.** Proposed approach to myocardial infarction with non-obstructive coronary artery disease diagnosis. Flowchart is explained in the text. ACS indicates acute coronary syndrome; ARDS, acute respiratory distress syndrome; CMR, cardiac magnetic resonance; ESRD, end stage renal disease; MINOCA, myocardial infarction with non-obstructive coronary artery disease; OCT, optical coherence tomography; SCAD, spontaneous coronary artery dissection; and TEE, trans esophageal echocardiography.

## 3. Conclusions

Although AMI and non-obstructive coronary artery disease have been known for more than five decades, our knowledge is limited and many challenges still remain. Current studies show the importance of using OCT and CMR in patients with a working diagnosis of MINOCA. Moreover, when no abnormal findings are present on OCT, other tests should be performed in order to assess the coronary flow reserve (CFR) and microcirculatory resistance (iMR). Although recent studies shed light on the pathogenesis of MINOCA, well-designed prospective studies are needed in order to gain a better understanding of this condition and to provide optimal management while reducing morbidity and mortality in patients with MINOCA.

**Author Contributions:** Conceptualization, I.-K.J. and K.B.; methodology, I.-K.J., K.B., J.L., L.B., A.K., D.M., P.S., P.G. and P.K.; resources, K.B., P.S., D.M., A.K. and P.G.; data curation, K.B., P.G., P.S. and P.K.; writing—original draft preparation, K.B.; writing—review and editing, K.B., I.-K.J., D.M., P.G., P.S., J.L. and P.K.; visualization, K.B. and I.-K.J.; supervision, P.K., J.L. and I.-K.J.; project administration, K.B. and I.-K.J.; All authors have read and agreed to the published version of the manuscript.

**Funding:** This research received no external funding.

**Institutional Review Board Statement:** Not applicable.

**Informed Consent Statement:** Not applicable.

**Conflicts of Interest:** Jang's research was supported by the Allan Gray Fellowship Fund and by Michael and Kathryn Park. Jang has received educational grants from Abbott Vascular and a consulting fee from Svelte Medical Systems Inc. (NJ, USA) and Mitobridge Inc. (MA, USA).

## References

1. Murray, C.J.; Lopez, A.D. Global mortality, disability, and the contribution of risk factors: Global Burden of Disease Study. *Lancet* **1997**, *349*, 1436–1442. [CrossRef]
2. Barton, M.; Grüntzig, J.; Husmann, M.; Rösch, J. Balloon Angioplasty—The Legacy of Andreas Grüntzig, M.D. (1939–1985). *Front. Cardiovasc. Med.* **2014**, *1*, 15. [CrossRef]
3. Miller, R.D.; Burchell, H.B.; Edwards, J.E. Myocardial Infarction with and without Acute Coronary Occlusion: A Pathologic Study. *AMA Arch. Intern. Med.* **1951**, *88*, 597–604. [CrossRef]
4. Bean, W.B. Infarction of the heart. III. clinical course and morphological findings. *Ann. Intern. Med.* **1938**, *12*, 71–94.
5. DeWood, M.A.; Spores, J.; Notske, R.; Mouser, L.T.; Burroughs, R.; Golden, M.S.; Lang, H.T. Prevalence of total coronary occlusion during the early hours of transmural myocardial infarction. *N. Engl. J. Med.* **1980**, *303*, 897–902. [CrossRef]
6. DeWood, M.A.; Stifter, W.F.; Simpson, C.S.; Spores, J.; Eugster, G.S.; Judge, T.P.; Hinnen, M.L. Coronary arteriographic findings soon after non-Q-wave myocardial infarction. *N. Engl. J. Med.* **1986**, *315*, 417–423. [CrossRef] [PubMed]
7. Gehrie, E.R.; Reynolds, H.R.; Chen, A.Y.; Neelon, B.H.; Roe, M.T.; Gibler, W.B.; Ohman, E.M.; Newby, L.K.; Peterson, E.D.; Hochman, J.S. Characterization and outcomes of women and men with non-ST-segment elevation myocardial infarction and nonobstructive coronary artery disease: Results from the Can Rapid Risk Stratification of Unstable Angina Patients Suppress Adverse Outcomes with Early Implementation of the ACC/AHA Guidelines (CRUSADE) quality improvement initiative. *Am. Heart J.* **2009**, *158*, 688–694.
8. Larsen, A.I.; Galbraith, P.D.; Ghali, W.A.; Norris, C.M.; Graham, M.M.; Knudtson, M.L.; APPROACH Investigators. Characteristics and outcomes of patients with acute myocardial infarction and angiographically normal coronary arteries. *Am. J. Cardiol.* **2005**, *95*, 261–263. [CrossRef] [PubMed]
9. Tamis-Holland, J.E.; Jneid, H.; Reynolds, H.R.; Agewall, S.; Brilakis, E.S.; Brown, T.M.; Lerman, A.; Cushman, M.; Kumbhani, D.J.; Arslanian-Engoren, C.; et al. Contemporary Diagnosis and Management of Patients With Myocardial Infarction in the Absence of Obstructive Coronary Artery Disease: A Scientific Statement From the American Heart Association. *Circulation* **2019**, *139*, e891–e908. [CrossRef] [PubMed]
10. Scalone, G.; Niccoli, G.; Crea, F. Pathophysiology, diagnosis and management of MINOCA: An update. *Eur. Heart J. Acute Cardiovasc. Care* **2018**, *8*, 54–62. [CrossRef] [PubMed]
11. Agewall, S.; Beltrame, J.F.; Reynolds, H.R.; Niessner, A.; Rosano, G.; Caforio, A.L.P.; De Caterina, R.; Zimarino, M.; Roffi, M.; Kjeldsen, K.; et al. WG on Cardiovascular Pharmacotherapy. ESC working group position paper on myocardial infarction with non-obstructive coronary arteries. *Eur. Heart J.* **2017**, *38*, 143–153.
12. Pasupathy, S.; Air, T.; Dreyer, R.P.; Tavella, R.; Beltrame, J.F. Systematic review of patients presenting with suspected myocardial infarction and nonobstructive coronary arteries. *Circulation* **2015**, *131*, 861–870. [CrossRef]
13. Von Korn, H.; Graefe, V.; Ohlow, M.-A.; Yu, J.; Huegl, B.; Wagner, A.; Gruene, S.; Lauer, B. Acute coronary syndrome without significant stenosis on angiography: Characteristics and prognosis. *Tex. Heart Inst. J.* **2008**, *35*, 406–412.
14. Kang, W.Y.; Jeong, M.H.; Ahn, Y.K.; Kim, J.H.; Chae, S.C.; Kim, Y.J.; Hur, S.H.; Seong, I.W.; Hong, T.J.; Choi, D.H.; et al. Korea Acute Myocardial Infarction Registry Investigators. Are patients with angiographically near-normal coronary arteries who present as acute myocardial infarction actually safe? *Int. J. Cardiol.* **2011**, *146*, 207–212. [CrossRef] [PubMed]
15. Ishii, M.; Kaikita, K.; Sakamoto, K.; Seki, T.; Kawakami, K.; Nakai, M.; Sumita, Y.; Nishimura, K.; Miyamoto, Y.; Noguchi, T.; et al. Characteristics and in-hospital mortality of patients with myocardial infarction in the absence of obstructive coronary artery disease in super-aging society. *Int. J. Cardiol.* **2020**, *301*, 108–113. [CrossRef]
16. Andersson, H.B.; Pedersen, F.; Engstrøm, T.; Helqvist, S.; Jensen, M.K.; Jørgensen, E.; Kelbæk, H.; Räder, S.B.E.W.; Saunamäki, K.; Bates, E.; et al. Long-term survival and causes of death in patients with ST-elevation acute coronary syndrome without obstructive coronary artery disease. *Eur. Heart J.* **2018**, *39*, 102–110. [CrossRef] [PubMed]
17. Lindahl, B.; Baron, T.; Erlinge, D.; Hadziosmanovic, N.; Nordenskjöld, A.; Gard, A.; Jernberg, T. Medical Therapy for Secondary Prevention and Long-Term Outcome in Patients with Myocardial Infarction with Nonobstructive Coronary Artery Disease. *Circulation* **2017**, *135*, 1481–1489. [CrossRef] [PubMed]

18. Gasior, P.; Desperak, A.; Gierlotka, M.; Milewski, K.; Wita, K.; Kalarus, Z.; Fluder, J.; Kazmierski, M.; Buszman, P.E.; Gasior, M.; et al. Clinical Characteristics, Treatments, and Outcomes of Patients with Myocardial Infarction with Non-Obstructive Coronary Arteries (MINOCA): Results from a Multicenter National Registry. *J. Clin. Med.* **2020**, *9*, 2779. [CrossRef] [PubMed]
19. Safdar, B.; Spatz, E.S.; Dreyer, R.P.; Beltrame, J.F.; Lichtman, J.H.; Spertus, J.A.; Reynolds, H.R.; Geda, M.; Bueno, H.; Dziura, J.D.; et al. Presentation, Clinical Profile, and Prognosis of Young Patients with Myocardial Infarction With Nonobstructive Coronary Arteries (MINOCA): Results From the VIRGO Study. *J. Am. Heart Assoc.* **2018**, *7*, e009174. [CrossRef]
20. Larsen, A.I.; Nilsen, D.W.T.; Yu, J.; Mehran, R.; Nikolsky, E.; Lansky, A.J.; Caixeta, A.; Parise, H.; Fahy, M.; Cristea, E.; et al. Long-term prognosis of patients presenting with ST-segment elevation myocardial infarction with no significant coronary artery disease (from the HORIZONS-AMI trial). *Am. J. Cardiol.* **2013**, *111*, 643–648. [CrossRef]
21. Grodzinsky, A.; Arnold, S.V.; Gosch, K.; Spertus, J.A.; Foody, J.M.; Beltrame, J.; Maddox, T.M.; Parashar, S.; Kosiborod, M. Angina Frequency After Acute Myocardial Infarction In Patients Without Obstructive Coronary Artery Disease. *Eur. Heart J. Qual. Care Clin. Outcomes* **2015**, *1*, 92–99. [CrossRef]
22. Di Fiore, D.P.; Beltrame, J.F. Chest pain in patients with "normal angiography": Could it be cardiac? *Int. J. Evid. Based Healthc.* **2013**, *11*, 56–68. [CrossRef]
23. Montone, R.A.; Niccoli, G.; Fracassi, F.; Russo, M.; Gurgoglione, F.; Cammà, G.; Lanza, G.A.; Crea, F. Patients with acute myocardial infarction and non-obstructive coronary arteries: Safety and prognostic relevance of invasive coronary provocative tests. *Eur. Heart J.* **2018**, *39*, 91–98. [CrossRef] [PubMed]
24. Kaski, J.C. Provocative tests for coronary artery spasm in MINOCA: Necessary and safe? *Eur. Heart J.* **2018**, *39*, 99–101. [CrossRef]
25. Hjort, M.; Lindahl, B.; Baron, T.; Jernberg, T.; Tornvall, P.; Eggers, K.M. Prognosis in relation to high-sensitivity cardiac troponin T levels in patients with myocardial infarction and non-obstructive coronary arteries. *Am. Heart J.* **2018**, *200*, 60–66. [CrossRef] [PubMed]
26. Pitts, R.; Daugherty, S.L.; Tang, F.; Jones, P.; Ho, P.M.; Tsai, T.T.; Spertus, J.; Maddox, T.M. Optimal Secondary Prevention Medication Use in Acute Myocardial Infarction Patients with Non-Obstructive Coronary Artery Disease is Modified by Management Strategy: Insights from the TRIUMPH Registry. *Clin. Cardiol.* **2017**, *40*, 347–355. [CrossRef] [PubMed]
27. Poku, N.; Noble, S. Myocardial infarction with non obstructive coronary arteries (MINOCA): A whole new ball game. *Expert Rev. Cardiovasc. Ther.* **2017**, *15*, 7–14. [CrossRef]
28. Iqbal, S.N.; Feit, F.; Mancini, G.B.J.; Wood, D.; Patel, R.; Pena-Sing, I.; Attubato, M.; Yatskar, L.; Slater, J.N.; Hochman, J.S.; et al. Characteristics of plaque disruption by intravascular ultrasound in women presenting with myocardial infarction without obstructive coronary artery disease. *Am. Heart J.* **2014**, *167*, 715–722. [CrossRef] [PubMed]
29. Stone, G.W.; Maehara, A.; Lansky, A.J.; Bruyne B de Cristea, E.; Mintz, G.S.; Mehran, R.; McPherson, J.; Farhat, N.; Marso, S.P.; Parise, H.; et al. A Prospective Natural-History Study of Coronary Atherosclerosis. *N. Eng. J. Med.* **2011**, *364*, 226–235. [CrossRef]
30. Xing, L.; Higuma, T.; Wang, Z.; Aguirre, A.D.; Mizuno, K.; Takano, M.; Dauerman, H.L.; Park, S.-J.; Jang, Y.; Kim, C.-J.; et al. Clinical Significance of Lipid-Rich Plaque Detected by Optical Coherence Tomography: A 4-Year Follow-Up Study. *J. Am. Coll. Cardiol.* **2017**, *69*, 2502–2513. [CrossRef] [PubMed]
31. Alfonso, F.; Paulo, M.; Dutary, J. Endovascular Imaging of Angiographically Invisible Spontaneous Coronary Artery Dissection. *JACC Cardiovasc. Interv.* **2012**, *5*, 452–453. [CrossRef]
32. Reynolds, H.R.; Srichai, M.B.; Iqbal, S.N.; Slater, J.N.; Mancini, G.B.J.; Feit, F.; Pena-Sing, I.; Axel, L.; Attubato, M.J.; Yatskar, L.; et al. Mechanisms of myocardial infarction in women without angiographically obstructive coronary artery disease. *Circulation* **2011**, *124*, 1414–1425. [CrossRef] [PubMed]
33. Ouldzein, H.; Elbaz, M.; Roncalli, J.; Cagnac, R.; Carrié, D.; Puel, J.; Alibelli-Chemarin, M.-J. Plaque rupture and morphological characteristics of the culprit lesion in acute coronary syndromes without significant angiographic lesion: Analysis by intravascular ultrasound. *Ann. Cardiol. Angeiol.* **2012**, *61*, 20–26. [CrossRef] [PubMed]
34. Kranjec, I.; Mrevlje, B.; Legutko, J.; Dudek, D. Optical coherence tomography: Guided primary percutaneous coronary intervention in acute myocardial infarction. A bridge too far? *Kardiol. Pol.* **2015**, *73*, 309–316. [CrossRef] [PubMed]
35. Yabushita, H.; Bouma, B.E.; Houser, S.L.; Aretz, H.T.; Jang, I.-K.; Schlendorf, K.H.; Kauffman, C.R.; Shishkov, M.; Kang, D.-H.; Halpern, E.F.; et al. Characterization of human atherosclerosis by optical coherence tomography. *Circulation* **2002**, *106*, 1640–1645. [CrossRef]
36. Jang, I.-K.; Tearney, G.J.; MacNeill, B.; Takano, M.; Moselewski, F.; Iftima, N.; Shishkov, M.; Houser, S.; Aretz, H.T.; Halpern, E.F.; et al. In vivo characterization of coronary atherosclerotic plaque by use of optical coherence tomography. *Circulation* **2005**, *111*, 1551–1555. [CrossRef]
37. Oosterveer, T.T.M.; van der Meer, S.M.; Scherptong, R.W.C.; Jukema, J.W. Optical Coherence Tomography: Current Applications for the Assessment of Coronary Artery Disease and Guidance of Percutaneous Coronary Interventions. *Cardiol. Ther.* **2020**, *9*, 307–321. [CrossRef]
38. Tornvall, P.; Gerbaud, E.; Behaghel, A.; Chopard, R.; Collste, O.; Laraudogoitia, E.; Leurent, G.; Meneveau, N.; Montaudon, M.; Perez-David, E.; et al. Myocarditis or "true" infarction by cardiac magnetic resonance in patients with a clinical diagnosis of myocardial infarction without obstructive coronary disease: A meta-analysis of individual patient data. *Atherosclerosis* **2015**, *241*, 87–91. [CrossRef]
39. Dastidar, A.G.; Baritussio, A.; De Garate, E.; Drobni, Z.; Biglino, G.; Singhal, P.; Milano, E.G.; Angelini, G.D.; Dorman, S.; Strange, J.; et al. Prognostic Role of CMR and Conventional Risk Factors in Myocardial Infarction with Nonobstructed Coronary Arteries. *JACC Cardiovasc. Imaging* **2019**, *12*, 1973–1982. [CrossRef]

40. Yilmaz, A.; Mahrholdt, H.; Athanasiadis, A.; Vogelsberg, H.; Meinhardt, G.; Voehringer, M.; Kispert, E.-M.; Deluigi, C.; Baccouche, H.; Spodarev, E.; et al. Coronary vasospasm as the underlying cause for chest pain in patients with PVB19 myocarditis. *Heart* **2008**, *94*, 1456–1463. [CrossRef]
41. Pelliccia, F.; Kaski, J.C.; Crea, F.; Camici, P.G. Pathophysiology of Takotsubo Syndrome. *Circulation* **2017**, *135*, 2426–2441. [CrossRef]
42. Eitel, I.; Stiermaier, T.; Graf, T.; Möller, C.; Rommel, K.-P.; Eitel, C.; Schuler, G.; Thiele, H.; Desch, S. Optical Coherence Tomography to Evaluate Plaque Burden and Morphology in Patients with Takotsubo Syndrome. *J. Am. Heart Assoc.* **2016**, *5*, e004474. [CrossRef]
43. Sugiyama, T.; Yamamoto, E.; Fracassi, F.; Lee, H.; Yonetsu, T.; Kakuta, T.; Soeda, T.; Saito, Y.; Yan, B.P.; Kurihara, O.; et al. Calcified Plaques in Patients with Acute Coronary Syndromes. *JACC Cardiovasc. Interv.* **2019**, *12*, 531–540. [CrossRef]
44. Dai, J.; Xing, L.; Jia, H.; Zhu, Y.; Zhang, S.; Hu, S.; Lin, L.; Ma, L.; Liu, H.; Xu, M.; et al. In vivo predictors of plaque erosion in patients with ST-segment elevation myocardial infarction: A clinical, angiographical, and intravascular optical coherence tomography study. *Eur. Heart J.* **2018**, *39*, 2077–2085. [CrossRef] [PubMed]
45. Mrevlje, B.; Kleczyński, P.; Kranjec, I.; Jąkała, J.; Noc, M.; Rzeszutko, Ł.; Dziewierz, A.; Wizimirski, M.; Dudek, D.; Legutko, J. Optical coherence tomography versus intravascular ultrasound for culprit lesion assessment in patients with acute myocardial infarction. *Postepy Kardiol Interwencyjnej* **2020**, *16*, 145–152. [CrossRef] [PubMed]
46. Opolski, M.P.; Spiewak, M.; Marczak, M.; Debski, A.; Knaapen, P.; Schumacher, S.P.; Staruch, A.D.; Grodecki, K.; Chmielak, Z.; Lazarczyk, H.; et al. Mechanisms of Myocardial Infarction in Patients with Nonobstructive Coronary Artery Disease: Results From the Optical Coherence Tomography Study. *JACC Cardiovasc. Imaging* **2018**, *12*, 2210–2221. [CrossRef] [PubMed]
47. Fracassi, F.; Crea, F.; Sugiyama, T.; Yamamoto, E.; Uemura, S.; Vergallo, R.; Porto, I.; Lee, H.; Fujimoto, J.; Fuster, V.; et al. Healed Culprit Plaques in Patients With Acute Coronary Syndromes. *J. Am. Coll. Cardiol.* **2019**, *73*, 2253–2263. [CrossRef]
48. Mas-Lladó, C.; Maristany, J.; Gómez-Larab, J.; Pascual, M.; del Mar Alameda, M.; Gómez-Jaume, A.; Pozo-Contreras, R.D.; Peral-Disdier, V. Value of the optical coherence tomography in the diagnosis of unstable patients with non-significant coronary stenosis. *REC Interv. Cardiol.* **2020**, *2*, 272–279. [CrossRef]
49. Reynolds, H.R.; Maehara, A.; Kwong, R.Y.; Sedlak, T.; Saw, J.; Smilowitz, N.R.; Mahmud, E.; Wei, J.; Marzo, K.; Matsumura, M.; et al. Coronary Optical Coherence Tomography and Cardiac Magnetic Resonance Imaging to Determine Underlying Causes of MINOCA in Women. Available online: https://www.ahajournals.org/doi/10.1161/CIRCULATIONAHA.120.052008 (accessed on 11 February 2021).
50. Gerbaud, E.; Arabucki, F.; Nivet, H.; Barbey, C.; Cetran, L.; Chassaing, S.; Seguy, B.; Lesimple, A.; Cochet, H.; Montaudon, M.; et al. OCT and CMR for the Diagnosis of Patients Presenting With MINOCA and Suspected Epicardial Causes. *JACC Cardiovasc. Imaging* **2020**, *13*, 2619–2631. [CrossRef]
51. Russo, M.; Fracassi, F.; Kurihara, O.; Kim, H.O.; Thondapu, V.; Araki, M.; Shinohara, H.; Sugiyama, T.; Yamamoto, E.; Lee, H.; et al. Healed Plaques in Patients with Stable Angina Pectoris. *Arterioscler. Thromb. Vasc. Biol.* **2020**, *40*, 1587–1597. [CrossRef]
52. Buccheri, D.; Piraino, D.; Orrego, P.S.; Cortese, B. Is vasospasm overestimated in acute coronary syndromes presenting with non-obstructive coronary artery disease? The case for intravascular imaging. *Int. J. Cardiol.* **2016**, *203*, 1125–1126. [CrossRef] [PubMed]
53. Saw, J.; Mancini, G.B.J.; Humphries, K.; Fung, A.; Boone, R.; Starovoytov, A.; Aymong, E. Angiographic appearance of spontaneous coronary artery dissection with intramural hematoma proven on intracoronary imaging. *Catheter. Cardiovasc. Interv.* **2016**, *87*, E54–E61. [CrossRef]
54. Kaski, J.C.; Crea, F.; Meran, D.; Rodriguez, L.; Araujo, L.; Chierchia, S.; Davies, G.; Maseri, A. Local coronary supersensitivity to diverse vasoconstrictive stimuli in patients with variant angina. *Circulation* **1986**, *74*, 1255–1265. [CrossRef]
55. Pristipino, C.; Beltrame, J.F.; Finocchiaro, M.L.; Hattori, R.; Fujita, M.; Mongiardo, R.; Cianflone, D.; Sanna, T.; Sasayama, S.; Maseri, A. Major racial differences in coronary constrictor response between japanese and caucasians with recent myocardial infarction. *Circulation* **2000**, *101*, 1102–1108. [CrossRef] [PubMed]
56. Mohri, M.; Koyanagi, M.; Egashira, K.; Tagawa, H.; Ichiki, T.; Shimokawa, H.; Takeshita, A. Angina pectoris caused by coronary microvascular spasm. *Lancet* **1998**, *351*, 1165–1169. [CrossRef]
57. Shin, E.-S.; Ann, S.H.; Singh, G.B.; Lim, K.H.; Yoon, H.-J.; Hur, S.-H.; Her, A.-Y.; Koo, B.-K.; Akasaka, T. OCT-Defined Morphological Characteristics of Coronary Artery Spasm Sites in Vasospastic Angina. *JACC Cardiovasc. Imaging* **2015**, *8*, 1059–1067. [CrossRef]
58. Park, H.-C.; Shin, J.H.; Jeong, W.K.; Choi, S.I.; Kim, S.-G. Comparison of morphologic findings obtained by optical coherence tomography in acute coronary syndrome caused by vasospasm and chronic stable variant angina. *Int. J. Cardiovasc. Imaging* **2015**, *31*, 229–237. [CrossRef]
59. Tanaka, A.; Shimada, K.; Tearney, G.J.; Kitabata, H.; Taguchi, H.; Fukuda, S.; Kashiwagi, M.; Kubo, T.; Takarada, S.; Hirata, K.; et al. Conformational Change in Coronary Artery Structure Assessed by Optical Coherence Tomography in Patients With Vasospastic Angina. *J. Am. Coll. Cardiol.* **2011**, *58*, 1608–1613. [CrossRef] [PubMed]
60. Dastidar, A.G.; Rodrigues, J.C.L.; Johnson, T.W.; De Garate, E.; Singhal, P.; Baritussio, A.; Scatteia, A.; Strange, J.; Nightingale, A.K.; Angelini, G.D.; et al. Myocardial Infarction With Nonobstructed Coronary Arteries: Impact of CMR Early after Presentation. *JACC Cardiovasc. Imaging* **2017**, *10*, 1204–1206. [CrossRef] [PubMed]

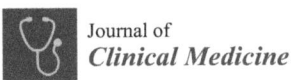 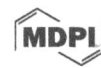

Article

# Management of High-Risk Atherosclerotic Patients by Statins May Be Supported by Logistic Model of Intima-Media Thickening

Dorota Formanowicz [1,*,†], Jacek B. Krawczyk [2,†], Bartłomiej Perek [3,†], Dawid Lipski [4,‡] and Andrzej Tykarski [4,‡]

1. Department of Medical Chemistry and Laboratory Medicine, Poznan University of Medical Sciences, 60-806 Poznan, Poland
2. School of Mathematics & Statistics, The University of Sydney, Sydney, NSW 2006, Australia; jacek.krawczyk@sydney.edu.au
3. Department of Cardiac Surgery and Transplantology, Poznan University of Medical Sciences, 61-001 Poznan, Poland; bperek@ump.edu.pl
4. Department of Hypertension, Angiology and Internal Disease, Poznan University of Medical Sciences, 61-001 Poznan, Poland; dlipski@ump.edu.pl (D.L.); tykarski@o2.pl (A.T.)
\* Correspondence: doforman@ump.edu.pl
† These authors contributed equally to this work.
‡ These authors conducted patient IMT measurements, which have been used in this work.

**Abstract:** While the use of statins in treating patients with atherosclerosis is an undisputed success, the questions regarding an optimal starting time for treatment and its strength remain open. We proposed in our earlier paper published in Int. J. Mol. Sci. (2019, 20) that the growth of intima-media thickness of the carotid artery follows an S-shape (i.e., logistic) curve. In our subsequent paper in PLoS ONE (2020, 15), we incorporated this feature into a logistic control-theoretic model of atherosclerosis progression and showed that some combinations of patient age and intima-media thickness are better suited than others to start treatment. In this study, we perform a new and comprehensive calibration of our logistic model using a recent clinical database. This allows us to propose a procedure for inferring an optimal age to start statin treatment for a particular group of patients. We argue that a decrease in the slope of the IMT logistic growth curve, induced by statin treatment, is most efficient where the curve is at its steepest, whereby the efficiency means lowering the future IMT levels. Using the procedure on an aggregate group of severely sick men, 38 years of age is observed to correlate with the steepest point of the logistic curve, and, thus, it is the preferred time to start statin treatment. We believe that detecting the logistic curve's steepest fragment and commencing statin administration on that fragment are courses of action that agree with clinician intuition and may support decision-making processes.

**Keywords:** atherosclerosis; statins; control-theoretic model; logistic growth

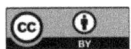

Citation: Formanowicz, D.; Krawczyk, J.B.; Perek, B.; Lipski, D.; Tykarski, A. Management of High-Risk Atherosclerotic Patients by Statins May Be Supported by Logistic Model of Intima-Media Thickening. J. Clin. Med. 2021, 10, 2876. https://doi.org/10.3390/jcm10132876

Academic Editor: Anna Kabłak-Ziembicka

Received: 18 May 2021
Accepted: 23 June 2021
Published: 29 June 2021

**Publisher's Note:** MDPI stays neutral with regard to jurisdictional claims in published maps and institutional affiliations.

**Copyright:** © 2021 by the authors. Licensee MDPI, Basel, Switzerland. This article is an open access article distributed under the terms and conditions of the Creative Commons Attribution (CC BY) license (https://creativecommons.org/licenses/by/4.0/).

## 1. Introduction

Knowledge of the intima-media (IMT) growth process is essential for decision making regarding statin therapy initiation and intensification. The purpose of our study is to assess whether the mathematical modeling of IMT growth, proposed in [1,2], can assist clinicians at crucial stages of the process.

Thickening of the intima-media complex, which is an undisputed symptom of atherosclerosis, is an inevitable consequence of the process of aging of the human vascular system. The age-related changes can be observed at both micro- and macro-levels. At the micro-level, cellular senescence manifests as reduced cell proliferation, an irreversible arrest of growth, apoptosis, DNA damage, etc. [3]. At the macro-level, atherosclerotic plaques with calcium deposits can be detected by imaging examinations applied routinely in clinical practice; see [4]. The deposits are of clinical significance, as they are the final stage of vascular degeneration.

Clearly, many factors contribute to atherosclerosis development; see e.g., [5]. In particular, there are some inherited predisposing factors and other factors that may be modified by our lifestyle, which include diet; physical activity; and adherence to recommendations of optimal management of many atherosclerosis-modifying diseases, such as arterial hypertension, diabetes, and hyperlipidemia—see [6].

According to our knowledge, it is very difficult, if at all possible, to regress atherosclerotic plaque development. However, in some cases, doctors are able to stabilize the plaque and, therefore, inhibit disease progression. This can happen if intensive treatment with high-dose statins is applied; see [7].

However, doubts surrounding the dosage of statins and the therapy timing remain. A few years ago, a cohort study [8] on the general UK population reported statin overuse in patients with low cardiovascular risk and underuse in patients with high cardiovascular risk. Furthermore, another study (see [9]) points to possible adverse events, such as muscle and liver injury, cognitive impairment, new-onset diabetes mellitus, and even hemorrhagic stroke, as a result of long-term statin therapy. Moreover, there is no strong clinical evidence that the elderly would benefit from statin therapy; see [10]. Statin therapy should be individualized and based on the patient's risk profile. This study uses a model that may alleviate the above concerns.

The measurement of the carotid artery IMT can be achieved by the simple and noninvasive technique of measuring atherosclerotic burden [11]. Consequently, IMT has been utilized as a reliable marker of drug efficiency and tested in clinical trials devoted to atherosclerosis treatment. Moreover, IMT is widely accepted as a screening tool that can be used together with the traditional risk factors assessment. The size and dynamics of IMT can help in determining optimal therapeutic interventions as well as in the application of other diagnostic tools; see [12]. Although there are studies that have presented a discrepancy between carotid IMT changes, prognosis, and the course of cardiovascular pathologies [13,14], the overwhelming clinical data (see [15–19]) strongly confirm that the IMT will continue to be used as a valuable tool in clinical research.

It was conjectured in [1] that the IMT growth process follows an S-shape (i.e., *logistic*) curve. An application of a mathematical model based on this proposition to atherosclerosis management by statins was developed in [2]. However, the number of observations in [1] of the logistic model being calibrated was low (27); therefore, the quantitative reasoning based on that model was mainly of conceptual value rather than being immediately applicable to management of atherosclerosis. The recent availability of the large Cardio Poznan Database (122 observations) [20] has created an opportunity for us to perform a new calibration of the logistic model from [1] and provide some managerial advice.

In the next section, we describe briefly the Cardio Poznan Database, the source of our new data. Then, Section 3 discusses the new data support for the S-shaped IMT growth. Subsequently, in Section 4, we propose a procedure for inferring an optimal age to start statin treatment for a particular group of patients. The paper ends with brief Concluding Remarks and an Appendix, which contains a few summary statistics concerning the observations gathered in the database.

**2. Cardio Poznan Data**

The data collection project, see [20], received a positive opinion (decision No. KB 341/21) of the Bioethics Committee of the Poznan University of Medical Sciences.

The data collection involved 122 consecutive patients: 78 males (63.9%) and 44 females (36.1%). Their mean age was 49.6 years, and the standard deviation was 15.6 years. These patients were treated in the Department of Hypertension and Angiology and Internal Medicine at the Poznan University of Medical Sciences in the first quarter of 2020. From this group, we selected the male subjects ($n = 31$) who had arterial hypertension-related cardiac disease, i.e., coronary artery disease (CAD) and/or vascular complications, such as peripheral vascular disease (PVD). This group of 31 *male* patients represents the observation sample for our study. These patients are referred to as *severely sick men*. They are split into two subgroups: (1) patients undergoing statin therapy, denoted as *statin(+)*, and (2) patients not treated with statins, denoted as *statin(-)*.

We provide a summary of the demographic and clinical data of the studied patients in Appendix A, Table A1. The findings of the laboratory tests and imaging examinations (carotid artery Doppler ultrasonography) are provided in Table A2.

## 3. Support for S-Shaped Growth of the Atherosclerotic Plaque

### 3.1. Importance of S-Shaped Growth for Atherosclerosis Treatment

Confirming both, the S-shape of the IMT growth process (see [1,2]) and its quantitative features is important for clinical reasons. Notably, knowledge of the S-shape model for the atherosclerosis process will enable us to indicate the patient age ranges of the disease's fast and slow growth. Specifically, we aim to identify when the atherosclerotic process is fast. In an attempt to prevent the IMT from thickening, the ideal place (here, the age range) to start statin treatment is when the curve is steep, i.e., before it eventually flattens at the patient's older age. Below, we present why we think this line of thought could help clinicians.

A slow IMT growth can occur when the patient is very young—too early to administer statins—or when the patient is very old (see [21])—too late to start treatment. Assuming statin treatment slows down the plaque growth by a certain amount, if this amount is subtracted from fast growth, the disease-slowing effect will be more substantial than if statins are administered when the disease progresses slowly. A mathematical explanation for this effect involves the model of nonlinearity. This emulates nonlinearity of the underlying medical process, as postulated in [1]. With the help of new data, we aim to confirm the logistic growth of IMT and establish the steepest fragment on an IMT growth model.

### 3.2. The S-Shape Conjecture

The S-shape of the atherosclerosis process was postulated in [1] (see also [2]). Regrettably, the number of data points available in [1] is low, and the proposed model's goodness-of-fit statistics are mixed. In an attempt to improve the statistical significance of the model, we now use a larger dataset [20] and carry out a new parameter identification procedure for the logistic model of atherosclerosis.

The starting point of our analysis of atherosclerosis in [1], continued in [2], is Figure 1 presented below (produced out of Figures A1 and A2 published in [1]). The figure panels show S-shaped curves calibrated ibidem using our previous data on IMT vs. age of severely sick men on dialysis.

The S-shaped curves in Figure 1 are of the following analytic form:

$$x(t) = \frac{cx_0 e^{at}}{c + x_0(e^{at} - 1)}. \qquad (1)$$

Each is a solution to the logistic differential equation $\frac{dx}{dt} = ax\left(1 - \frac{x}{c}\right), x(0) = x_0$ where

- $x_0$ is an initial condition;
- $c$ (called "carrying capacity" in population dynamics) is the terminal size of IMT toward which a patient's plaque size converges, given this patient's overall health level; presumably, a severely sick patient will have a large $c$ and if, eventually, IMT = $c$, the artery will not be able to handle this plaque thickness and the patient will pass away;
- $a$ determines the speed of plaque buildup.

The difference in the appearances of the S-shaped curves is attributed to the patients' medical conditions. Typically, patients whose medical conditions require dialysis will have a large $c$ that will grow more steeply. This is why the left panel curve grows faster and reaches higher values. The model coefficients for the severely sick men on dialysis (see the left panel) are provided in Table 1. (The model coefficients for the healthy patients' behavior are omitted, because healthy patients are not considered in this paper.)

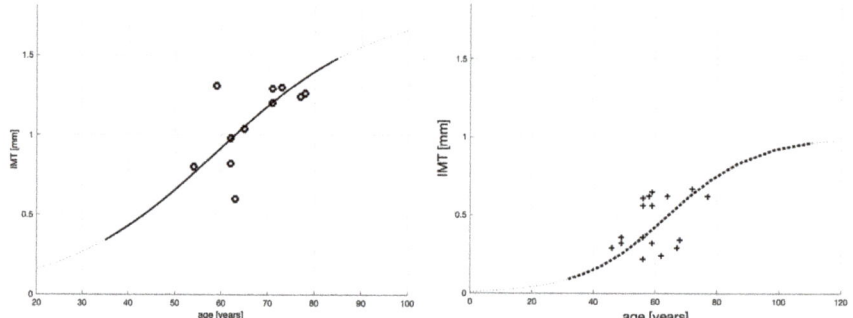

**Figure 1.** Fitting of the IMT time profile for severely sick patients (on dialysis)—**left panel** (11 observations), and fitting of the IMT time profile for healthy patients—**right panel** (16 observations).

**Table 1.** Parameters of the IMT time profile model for severely sick patients (on dialysis); see [1]. SSE is the sum of squared estimate of errors, and RMSE is the root mean square error. $R^2$ is the coefficient of determination.

| $x_0$ | $c$ | $a$ | SSE | RMSE | $R^2$ | Sample Size |
|---|---|---|---|---|---|---|
| 0.05 | 1.8 | 0.06 | 0.389 | 0.1881 | 0.36 | 11 |

The evidence provided by the curves, together with the existing clinical literature cited in [1], led us to propose ibidem that the atherosclerotic plaque's growth over a patient's life span has an S-shape and can be represented mathematically by a logistic function.

As mentioned above, the number of data points in Figure 1 is low, and the curves' goodness-of-fit statistics, reported in [1] and cited in Table 1, are mixed. For example, while the coefficient of determination $R^2 = 0.36$ for the case of severely sick patients might be considered satisfactory, the model-corresponding values of SSE = 0.389 and RMSE = 0.1881 are ordinary for such a small data sample of 11 observation points. Nevertheless, we conjectured ibidem that in aggregate, the above goodness-of-fit statistics provide support for a logistic process of IMT formation. However, given the low number of observations, they do not carry sufficient weight for the obtained model to be relied upon in clinical diagnostics and treatment, which are our ultimate goals of the model usage (see [2]).

## 4. New Data Support

### 4.1. Patient Aggregate

Figure 2 shows the new 62 IMT measurement points from [20] for the left and right arteries of severely sick men (see the legend for points marked L and R). The 11 black circles are the same as those in the left panel of Figure 1 and represent the 2008–2011 sample ([22]) of the severely sick men on dialysis. Their IMT values point to accelerated atherosclerosis.

The data from [1] did not distinguish between the left and right arteries; thus, it is likely that both were represented. Furthermore, both datasets are *aggregates* of sick patients who take statins (for different period lengths) and sick patients who do not take statins. Hence, from the point of view of gravity of the sickness, the old and new data may be compatible.

We used the new data to obtain the logistic curve in Figure 2. The identified parameters of this curve are provided in Table 2.

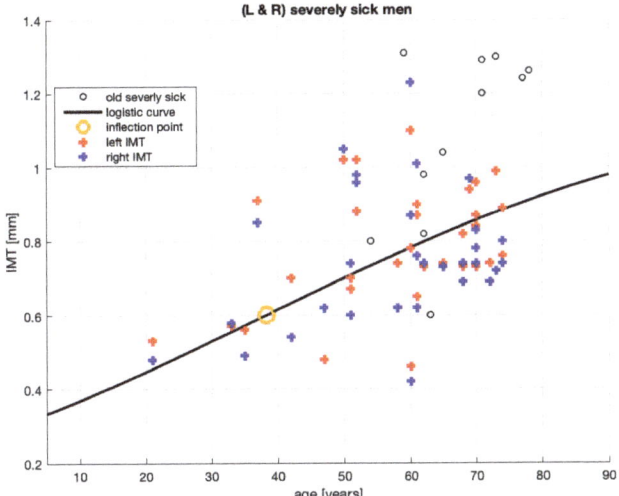

**Figure 2.** Fitting of the IMT time profile for severely sick men from [20].

**Table 2.** Parameters of the IMT growth model for severely sick men; see [20] (infl. point stands for the inflation point, and max slope indicates the fastest growth of IMT in mm/y for this group of patients).

| $x_0$ | $c$ | $a$ | SSE | RMSE | $R^2$ | Infl. Point | Max Slope | Sample Size |
|---|---|---|---|---|---|---|---|---|
| 0.3 | 1.2 | 0.02875 | 1.689 | 0.1664 | 0.0526 | [≈38, 0.6] | 0.008625 | 62 |

There are several comments to make concerning Figure 2.

1. The 2008–2011 population of sick men on dialysis (shown in Figure 1 left panel; see also the black empty circles in Figure 2) must indeed have been composed of sicker patients than those in the current sample. The black empty circles with a value of IMT over IMT ≥ 1.2 (mm), for example, constitute more than 50% of the whole sample; among the blue and red crosses (current sample), only 1 in 62 exceeds this value.
2. The old data spread of patient ages (horizontal axis) is much smaller (53–78 years old) than that of the new data (19–74 years old). This, combined with the fairly large spread of the old-sample IMT values (vertical axis), means that the old curve's steepness ( Figure 1) should be greater than that of the new one (Figure 2). Indeed, we computed the slope on this curve to be between 58 and 67 years old, and it is more than three times larger than the maximum slope reported in Table 2 (i.e., 0.0265 vs. 0.0086). This is consistent with the severity of *accelerated* atherosclerosis among the-old data patients.
3. We note that it should be easier to fit a 3-parameter (logistic) curve to 9 observations than to 62. Therefore, the distance between an observation point and its model should be shorter in the old model, but it is not. Remarkably, the RMSE of the new model is smaller than that of the old one. This indicates that the logistic model for the new data guarantees a smaller mean distance between an observation point and its logistic model's value. Therefore, in terms of these distances, the new logistic model is better aligned with the new data than the old model was with the old data.
4. The new model $R^2$ is smaller than that of the old model, which is an undesirable result. However, small or even negative values of $R^2$ may occur when fitting non-linear functions to data. Our model is non-linear. Therefore, $R^2$ alone cannot be used to judge how good, or bad, our model is.

**Proposition 1.** *We propose that, on balance, for small RMSE (good) versus small $R^2$ (bad), the logistic curve in Figure 2 supports the conjecture of the authors of [1] regarding the S-shaped process of the IMT growth.*

**Proposition 2.** *The steepest part of the logistic curve is around its inflection point ($\approx$38, 0.6; see Table 2 and the beige circle on the curve in Figure 2). Therefore, propose that for the group of sick men, starting patient medication at around 38 years old may be the most beneficial approach.*

The new dataset (from [20]), which we use in this study, concerns severely sick patients. However, this set is an aggregate of many patient types. The data are *inhomogeneous* in (at least) two aspects. First, they contain statin-medicated and statin-non-medicated patients. Second, the medicated patients take various doses of different statins (atorvastatin and rosuvastatin) for a varying number of months. Of course, model coefficients crucially depend on the sample patients' conditions. For example, the 2008–2011 data [22] of the severely sick men *on dialysis* generated a steeper S curve than that of the new data. Arguably, models built for a homogeneous patient group should be more reliable than a model built for a patient aggregate. In the next sections, we *disaggregate* the severely sick patient group into non-medicated and medicated patient subgroups and propose an IMT growth model for each subgroup.

*4.2. Non-Medicated, Severely Sick Men*

The group analyzed here is composed of patients who are severely sick but remain non-medicated. We refer to this subset of patients classified in the database [20] as *non-medicated*.

We now analyze the IMT growth process of the non-medicated patients.

Figure 3 shows 18 pairs (age and IMT) of the measurement points for severely sick, non-medicated men from [20]. Of course, these points are also represented in Figure 2. Now, they are analyzed alone.

The parameters of the logistic curve in Figure 3, which represents the IMT growth model, are provided in Table 3.

**Table 3.** Parameters of the IMT growth model for non-medicated, severely sick men from [20].

| $x_0$ | $c$ | $a$ | SSE | RMSE | $R^2$ | Infl. Point | Max Slope | Sample Size |
|---|---|---|---|---|---|---|---|---|
| 0.275 | 0.9 | 0.03962 | 0.2713 | 0.1263 | 0.0563 | [$\approx$21, 0.45] | 0.008915 | 18 |

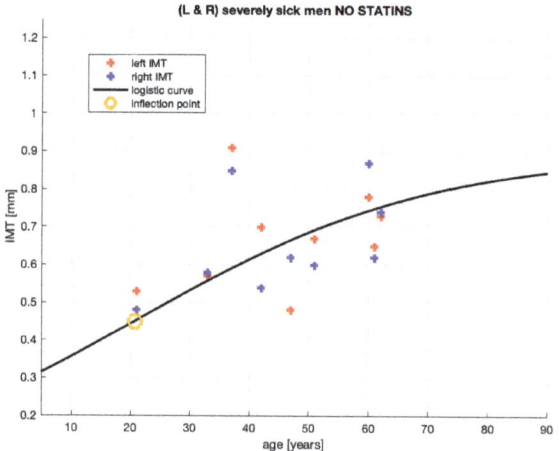

**Figure 3.** Fitting of the IMT time profile for non-medicated, severely sick men from [20].

Observing Figure 3, it can be noted that, in comparison to that of Figure 2, the logistic curve stabilizes here at a much lower IMT value. This may suggest that these patients' atherosclerotic plaque has been developing in a different manner to that of the other patient aggregate. This is discussed further in Section 4.1.

These patients are likely to have stable atherosclerotic plaque and be free from many of the clinical symptoms recorded in [20]. In particular, they may have developed collateral circulation, hence remaining in a clinically stable condition. Moreover, the IMT measurements, consequential for our study, are the IMT's thickness quantifications only. However, using the thickness measurement only, it is impossible to conclude the morphology of the atherosclerotic plaque. Nevertheless, it may be the morphology that is relevant to the classification of a patient as *severely sick*. For better insight into these statin-non-medicated patients, their characteristics, demographic data, and clinical and laboratory data are compared with those of severely sick but statin-medicated patients in Table A2.

While this group of non-statin-medicated patients might not profit from statin treatment, the observations of their IMT growth, as shown in Figure 3 and Table 3, assist in furthering the discussion of the growth's S-shape.

5. As per the goodness-of-fit statistics, the obtained model for the non-medicated, severely sick men is more reliable than that for the aggregate of the severely sick men. In particular, RMSE shrunk from 0.1664 mm for the aggregated patient group to 0.1263 mm for the non-medicated group. This means that the root mean square error (RMSE)—practically, the expected distance between an actual measurement and the corresponding model value— diminished by about 25%.
6. SSE and $R^2$ also improved (the latter only marginally).
7. The observations of [5,6] were expected. As previously mentioned, the non-medicated, severely sick men constitute a more homogeneous group than the severely sick aggregate of which they are a subset. Arguably, more uniformity in patient conditions will improve the goodness-of-fit statistics.

We draw the information on qualitative and quantitative properties of the IMT growth process in the non-medicated patients from Figure 3 and Table 3 as follows:

8. Patient age when the plaque growth is maximum (see the inflection points marked by the beige circles in each figure) differs between the groups. The maxima are 38 and 21 years old
9. The non-medicated patient model's $R^2$ is slightly larger than that of the aggregate group. We cannot though dwell on this improvement, however, since both models' determination coefficients are very small.

**Proposition 3.** *The above comments lead to the proposal that the model for the non-medicated, severely sick men (see Figure 3 and Table 3) supports the conjecture of the authors of [1] regarding the S-shaped process of the IMT growth.*

### 4.3. Statin-Medicated, Severely Sick Men

The complement to the non-medicated, severely sick men within the severely sick men aggregate in [20] is the group of severely sick men receiving statins or *statin-medicated* men. We now analyze the IMT growth process of these statin-medicated patients.

Figure 4 shows 44 pairs (age, IMT) of the measurement points for severely sick statin-medicated men from [20]. Of course, these points are also represented in Figure 2. Now, they are analyzed alone.

The parameters of the logistic curve in Figure 4, which represents the IMT growth model, are provided in Table 4.

**Table 4.** Parameters of the IMT growth model for statin-medicated, severely sick men; see [20].

| $x_0$ | $c$ | $a$ | SSE | RMSE | $R^2$ | Infl. Point | Max Slope | Sample Size |
|---|---|---|---|---|---|---|---|---|
| 0.325 | 1.25 | 0.02625 | 1.369 | 0.1784 | −0.13 | [≈40, 0.625] | 0.008203 | 44 |

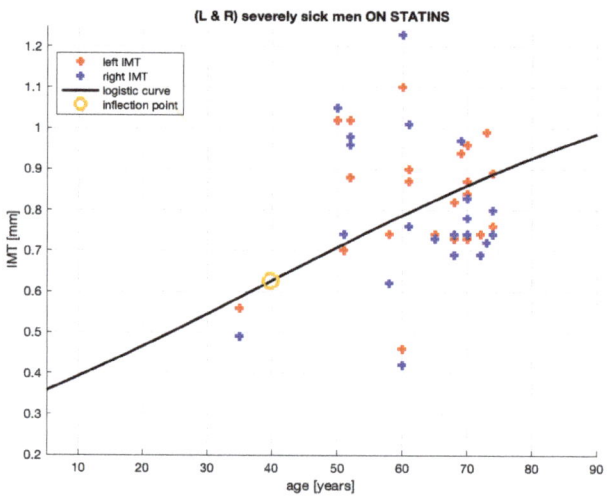

**Figure 4.** Fitting of the IMT time profile for statin-medicated, severely sick men from [20].

Below are our comments regarding the model for the statin-medicated, severely sick men.

10. The group analyzed here, while extracted from the severely sick men aggregate, is not necessarily composed of patients of much the same conditions. It is composed of patients who are severely sick and receive statins. Some patients in this group receive atorvastatin, some others—rosuvastatin, two not identical statin medications; the treatment periods vary between 2 and 36 months; the doses vary between 5 and 40 [mg]. This implies that—in this group—some patients may have suffered from an advanced stage of atherosclerosis mitigated by statins administered for short or for long periods. Undoubtedly, these inhomogeneities will complicate obtaining a reliable *quantitative* relationship between the age and plaque thickness formation.

11. Observing Figure 4, it can be noted that, generally, the logistic curve appears to be very similar to the curve obtained for the patient aggregate in Figure 2. This includes the suggested ages for starting statin treatment, which are 40 and 38.

12. The similarities are not unexpected given that, from the 64-patient measurements in Figure 2, only 18 were subtracted as non-medicated (see Figure 3). The parameters of the logistic curves are also similar.

13. Qualitatively, the model corresponds quite well to the intuition we may have about this patient group. To be medicated, their initial conditions $x_0$ should be worse than in the aggregate of the medicated and non-medicated patients. Indeed, the $x_0$ levels are 0.325 > 0.3, where the first number is for the statin-medicated group and the second is for the aggregate. Their $c$ levels 1.25 > 1.2 suggest that should these patients have remained non-medicated, the plaque would have grown larger in the medicated group than in the aggregate. The patients *are* being medicated and, as a result of that, the plaque grows at a slower pace for these patients than for the patient aggregate. See the coefficients $a$ and the maximum slopes document.

14. The slower plaque growth in the medicated patients is also observed in Figure 5: the dash-dotted (blue) line remains below the solid (black) line, where the latter corresponds to the patient aggregate.

15. The goodness-of-fit statistics of the statin-medicated patient model do not suggest that this model is better than the one proposed for the patient aggregate. Although SSE has improved (1.369 < 1.689), the expected distances between an actual measurement and the corresponding model's value (RMSE 0.1784 > 0.1664) and $R^2$ have worsened. We remind the reader that even $R^2 < 0$ should not alone disqualify a nonlinear model.

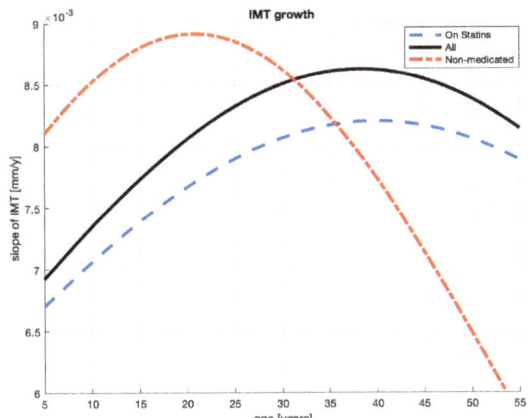

**Figure 5.** The slopes of the plaque formation processes for the severely sick men on statins, without statins, and their aggregate.

**Proposition 4.** *The logistic growth model (see Figure 4 and Table 4) for the statin-medicated, severely sick men has an explanatory value in that it helps to explain the IMT plaque formation process for this group of patients. However, the goodness-of-fit statistics for this model do not indicate that this model is an improvement on the patient aggregate's model referred to in Proposition 1.*

## 5. How to Infer an Optimal Age for Starting Statin Treatment

We have previously proposed that the optimal patient age for a specific group of patients to start statin treatment is when the curve is at its steepest. This seems the best locus on the S-curve to prevent it from rising or, in clinical terms, to prevent IMT from thickening. Figures 1–4 can help to find such loci for a specific group of patients.

The patterns of the speed of plaque formation differ between the aggregate of the severely sick patients and the non-medicated patients. We can see these speeds in Figure 5: the solid line represents the patient aggregate and the dash-dotted line the non-medicated patients. The dashed line indicates patients on statin; see the next section.

The maximum speed of the plaque formation for the non-medicated patients (a) is higher than the patients' aggregate i.e., 0.008915 > 0.008625 for the former and latter group and (b) occurs 17 years earlier for the former and latter groups.

We claimed in Proposition 2 that 38 years of age (see infl. point in Table 2) is the right age to start statin treatment in the aggregated group. Our argument is that a decrease—induced by treatment—in the slope of the IMT logistic curve is most efficient when the curve is at its steepest, whereby the efficiency concerns lowering the future IMT levels. Beginning treatment of non-medicated patients at the young age of 21 years old (see infl. point in Table 3) appears to be early. However, as judged by the logistic curve in Figure 3, these patients do not need medication. Arguably, their own bodies manage to considerably slow down plaque growth at this age. Just after the inflection point, we can see in Figure 5 that the dash-dotted (red) line quickly drops far below the other lines. The corresponding graph of the plaque formation in Figure 3 flattens as if these non-medicated patients were submitted to treatment. In fact, one could claim that it is their own bodies that generate this plaque formation pattern.

Briefly, an analysis of IMT slopes can help in making decisions regarding the best patient age for commencing statin treatment. The steepest slope can be learned from the slope's first derivative graph (see Figure 5). The steepest slope is where the derivative attains a maximum.

## 6. Limitations and Strength of This Study

An important limitation of our study is that it concerns male patients only. The reason for this is that the female population was less represented in [20]. Furthermore, the female patient population is less homogeneous than the male patient population in that their symptoms associated with cardiovascular pathologies are more variable and therefore more difficult to calibrate in the model than those of male patients.

Another limitation is related to the patient sample size in [20]. Although significantly larger than that in [1], our sample size is modest when compared with that of international studies; see e.g., the JUPITER trial [23]. With more patients in the database, perhaps augmented by a population-based study, we would be able to attempt to model IMT growth in female patients.

Notwithstanding these limitations, we strongly believe that the male patient sample size we used in this study was sufficient to validate the model proposed and explained in [1,2]. The results of the biostatistical data analyzed in this paper should assure clinicians regarding our model's usefulness.

## 7. Concluding Remarks

Our study showed that logistic models of IMT growth can support clinician decisions concerning the use of statins in the treatment of atherosclerosis. Specifically, we suggest that the steepest segment of the IMT-growth's S-shape curve, obtained for a specific group of patients, can be recommended as the appropriate disease phase to commence treatment. In numerical terms, we identified some statistical evidence that 38 years old may be an appropriate age to start treatment for the group of severely sick men in [20].

**Author Contributions:** Conceptualization: D.F., J.B.K., and B.P.; methodology: D.F., J.B.K., and B.P.; validation: D.F., J.B.K. and B.P.; formal analysis: D.F., J.B.K. and B.P.; investigation: D.F., J.B.K. and B.P.; writing—original draft preparation: D.F., J.B.K. and B.P.; writing—review and editing: D.F., J.B.K. and B.P.; data collection and furnishing: D.L. and A.T. All authors have read and agreed to the published version of the manuscript.

**Funding:** D.F., B.P., D.L. and A.T. were supported by Poznan University of Medical Sciences' statutory founds.

**Institutional Review Board Statement:** Bioethics Committee at Poznan University of Medical Sciences has confirmed in decision No. KB 341/21 that this study was not a medical experiment and therefore according to Polish law and the GCP regulations this research did not require approval of the Bioethics Committee.

**Informed Consent Statement:** The IMT assessment used in this study to validate our atherosclerotic plaque build-up model is a routine non-invasive diagnostic procedure performed using Doppler ultrasound. Anonymous use of the IMT results and the routinely performed laboratory parameters did not require any informed consent of the subjects.

**Data Availability Statement:** Data are available at https://www.researchgate.net/publication/351355752_CARDIO_POZNAN_DATA (accessed on 25 June 2021).

**Conflicts of Interest:** The authors declare no conflict of interest.

## Appendix A. CARDIO POZNAN DATA—Summary Statistics

We refer the reader to the Excel file at [20] for our field observations. Here, we present a few summary statistics concerning the observations.

Table A1. Summary of demographic and clinical CARDO POZNAN DATA severely sick male patients.

|  | All [n = 31] | Statin(−) [n = 9] | Statin(+) [n = 22] |
|---|---|---|---|
| Age [years] | 58.3 (13.4) | 47.4 (14.9) | 62.6 (10.2) |
| 70 years + | 8 (25.8) | 0 | 8 (36.4) |
| Height [m] | 1.77 (0.08) | 1.83 (0.08) | 1.75 (0.07) |
| Weight [kg] | 92.2 (16.7) | 106.4 (21.3) | 96.2 (13.9) |
| BMI [kg/m$^2$] | 32.3 (4.8) | 32.7 (6.5) | 32.2 (4.1) |
| Obesity (BMI > 30 kg/m$^2$) | 19 (61.3) | 5 (55.6) | 14 (63.6) |
| CAD | 18 (58.1) | 1 (11.1) | 17 (77.3) |
| ACS in history | 7 (22.6) | 0 | 7 (31.8) |
| PVD | 16 (51.6) | 2 (22.2) | 14 (63.6) |
| Cerebral * | 16 (51.6) | 2 (22.2) | 14 (63.6) |
| stroke | 2 (6.5) | 0 | 2 (9.1) |
| Lower extremities | 5 (16.1) | 0 | 5 (22.7) |
| CKD ** | 7 (22.6) | 3 (33.3) | 4 (18.2) |
| COPD | 3 (9.7) | 1 (11.1) | 2 (9.1) |
| Thyroid diseases | 2 (6.5) | 1 (11.1) | 1 (4.5) |
| GI disorders | 1 (3.2) | 1 (11.1) | 0 |
| Active smokers | 9 (29.0) | 3 (33.3) | 6 (27.3) |
| DM | 12 (38.7) | 2 (22.2) | 10 (45.5) |

Variables are presented as either means (standard deviation (SD)) for continuous data or numbers (%) for categorical data. * Included symptomatic (stroke/TIA) and asymptomatic with significant lesions (>80% of diameter) in the carotid artery (noted in Doppler ultrasound examination); ** Defined if eGFR calculated by means of simplified (short) MDRD formula was below 60 mL/min/1.73 m$^2$ BSA (body surface area). *Abbreviations*: ACS = acute coronary syndrome; CABG = coronary artery bypass grafting; CAD = coronary disease; CKD = chronic kidney disease; COPD = chronic obstructive; pulmonary disease; GI = gastrointestinal; PCI = percutaneous coronary intervention; PVD = peripheral vascular disease.

Table A2. Results of laboratory studies and Doppler ultrasonography of Poznan Cardio severely sick male patients.

|  | All [n = 31] | Statin(−) [n = 9] | Statin(+) [n = 22] |
|---|---|---|---|
| WBC [10 e9/L] | 8.02 (1.99) | 8.70 (2.10) | 7.74 (1.91) |
| Neutrophils | 5.14 (1.50) | 5.67 (1.88) | 4.92 (1.29) |
| Lymphocytes | 1.86 (0.66) | 1.95 (0.79) | 1.81 (0.62) |
| NLR | 3.15 (1.69) | 3.67 (2.79) | 2.93 (0.99) |
| RBC [10 e12/L] | 4.75 (0.30) | 4.78 (0.3) | 4.79 (0.31) |
| HGB [mM/L] | 9.14 (0.74) | 9.20 (1.05) | 9.11 (0.60) |
| Platelets [10 e9/L] | 250 (60) | 251 (43) | 250 (67) |
| PLR | 154.0 (75.1) | 157.5 (87.6) | 152.5 (71.7) |
| Total cholesterol [mM/L] | 4.49 (1.07) | 4.66 (1.07) | 4.42 (1.09) |
| LDL cholesterol | 2.86 (1.21) | 3.37 (1.12) | 2.65 (1.20) |
| HDL cholesterol | 1.12 (0.34) | 1.11 (0.17) | 1.12 (0.26) |
| Triglicerydes [mM/L] | 1.90 (1.43) | 1.64 (0.87) | 2.0 (1.61) |
| Creatinine [mg/dL] | 1.29 (0.80) | 1.65 (1.38) | 1.15 (0.32) |
| eGFR [mL/min/1.73 m$^2$] | 74.8 (26.7) | 76.7 (39.6) | 74.2 (20.5) |
| CRP [mg/L] | 10.3 (3.4) | 8.3 (4.2) | 11.3 (2.9) |
| IMT [mm] | 0.78 (0.16) | 0.70 (0.12) | 0.81 (0.16) |

Variables are presented as means (SD). *Abbreviations*: CRP = C-reactive protein; eGFR = estimated glomerular filtration rate; HDL = high-density lipids; HGB = hemoglobin concentration; IMT = intima-media thickness; NLR = neutrophil-to-lymphocyte ratio; PLR = platelet-to-lymphocyte ratio; RBC = red blood cell count; WBC = white blood cells count.

## Appendix B. Assessment of Carotid Intima-Media Thickness (IMT)

The carotid IMT measures were performed with the use of high-quality sonography (System EPIQ 5, Philips N.V., The Netherlands) using the linear 12–3 MHz transducer. IMT was measured bilaterally at the distal wall of carotid arteries in length (cm) starting 1 cm below the carotid bulb. At least five thickness measurements were performed on each site, and its average value was accepted as the outcome.

## Appendix C. Data Management and Statistical Analysis

Continuous variables were validated for normality by means of the Shapiro–Wilk W test. If they satisfied criteria of normal distribution, they were expressed as means (SD).

## References

1. Formanowicz, D.; Krawczyk, J.B.; Perek, B.; Formanowicz, P. A Control-Theoretic Model of Atherosclerosis. *Int. J. Mol. Sci.* **2019**, *20*, 785. [CrossRef] [PubMed]
2. Formanowicz, D.; Krawczyk, J.B. Controlling the thickness of the atherosclerotic plaque by statin medication. *PLoS ONE* **2020**, *15*, e0239953. [CrossRef] [PubMed]
3. Wang, J.; Bennett, M. Aging and Atherosclerosis: Mechanisms, Functional Consequences, and Potential Therapeutics for Cellular Senescence. *Circ. Res.* **2012**, *111*, 245–259. [CrossRef]
4. Biondi-Zoccai, G.; Mastrangeli, S.; Romagnoli, E.; Peruzzi, M.; Frati, G.; Roever, L.; Giordano, A. What We Have Learned from the Recent Meta-analyses on Diagnostic Methods for Atherosclerotic Plaque Regression. *Curr. Atheroscler. Rep.* **2018**, *20*, 2. [CrossRef]
5. Perrotta, I.; Aquila, S. The Role of Oxidative Stress and Autophagy in Atherosclerosis. *Oxidative Med. Cell. Longev.* **2015**, *2015*, 130315. [CrossRef]
6. Herrington, W.; Lacey, B.; Sherliker, P.; Armitage, J.; Lewington, S. Epidemiology of atherosclerosis and the potential to reduce the global burden of atherothrombotic disease. *Circ. Res.* **2016**, 1666–1665 doi:10.1161/CIRCRESAHA.115.307611. [CrossRef] [PubMed]
7. Nissen, S.; Nicholls, S.; Sipahi, I.; Libby, P.; Raichlen, J.; Ballantyne, C.; Davignon, J.; Erbel, R.; Fruchart, J.; Tardif, J.C.; et al. Effect of very high-intensity statin therapy on regression of coronary atherosclerosis: The ASTEROID trial. *JAMA* **2006**, 1556–1565. doi:10.1001/jama.295.13.jpc60002. [CrossRef]
8. van Staa, T.; Smeeth, L.; Ng, E.; Goldacre, B.; Gulliford, M. The efficiency of cardiovascular risk assessment: Do the right patients get statin treatment? *Heart* **2013**, *99*, 1597–1602. [CrossRef]
9. Adhyaru, B.; Jacobson, T. Safety and efficacy of statin therapy. *Nat. Rev. Cardiol.* **2018**, *15*, 757–769. [CrossRef]
10. Gitsels, L.; Bakbergenuly, I.; Steel, N.; Kulinskaya, E. Do statins reduce mortality in older people? Findings from a longitudinal study using primary care records. *Fam. Med. Community Health* **2021**, *9*, e000780. [CrossRef]
11. Nezu, T.; Hosomi, N.; Aoki, S.; Matsumoto, M. Carotid intima-media thickness for atherosclerosis. *J. Atheroscler. Thromb.* **2016**, 18–31. [CrossRef]
12. Centurión, O.A. Carotid intima-media thickness as a cardiovascular risk factor and imaging pathway of atherosclerosis. *Crit. Pathw. Cardiol.* **2016**, *15*, 152–160. [CrossRef]
13. Goff, D.C.; Lloyd-Jones, D.M.; Bennett, G.; Coady, S.; D'Agostino, R.B.; Gibbons, R.; Greenland, P.; Lackland, D.T.; Levy, D.; O'Donnell, C.J.; et al. 2013 ACC/AHA Guideline on the Assessment of Cardiovascular Risk. *Circulation* **2014**, *129*, S49–S73. [CrossRef]
14. Costanzo, P.; Perrone-Filardi, P.; Vassallo, E.; Paolillo, S.; Cesarano, P.; Brevetti, G.; Chiariello, M. Does Carotid Intima-Media Thickness Regression Predict Reduction of Cardiovascular Events?: A Meta-Analysis of 41 Randomized Trials. *J. Am. Coll. Cardiol.* **2010**, *56*, 2006–2020. [CrossRef]
15. Kablak-Ziembicka, A.; Tracz, W.; Przewlocki, T.; Pieniazek, P.; Sokolowski, A.; Konieczynska, M. Association of increased carotid intima-media thickness with the extent of coronary artery disease. *Heart* **2004**, *90*, 1286–1290. [CrossRef]
16. Zaidi, N.; Gilani, S.; Mehboob, R.; Waseem, H.; Hassan, A. A Diagnostic accuracy of carotid intima-media thickness by B-mode ultrasonography in coronary artery disease patients. *Arch. Med. Sci. Atheroscler. Dis.* **2020**, e79–e84. [CrossRef]
17. Liu, D.; Du, C.; Shao, W.; Ma, G. Diagnostic Role of Carotid Intima-Media Thickness for Coronary Artery Disease: A Meta-Analysis. *BioMed Res. Int.* **2020**, *5*. [CrossRef]
18. Simon, A.; Megnien, J.L.; Chironi, G. The Value of Carotid Intima-Media Thickness for Predicting Cardiovascular Risk. *Arterioscler. Thromb. Vasc. Biol.* **2010**, *30*, 182–185. [CrossRef] [PubMed]
19. Willeit, P.; Tschiderer, L.; Allara, E.; Reuber, K.; Seekircher, L.; Gao, L.; Liao, X.; Lonn, E.; Gerstein, H.C.; Yusuf, S.; et al. Carotid Intima-Media Thickness Progression as Surrogate Marker for Cardiovascular Risk. *Circulation* **2020**, *142*, 621–642. [CrossRef] [PubMed]
20. Data Base. Poznan Cardio Data. 2020. Available online: https://www.researchgate.net/publication/351355752_CARDIO_POZNAN_DATA (accessed on 25 June 2021).
21. Homma, S.; Hirose, N.; Ishida, H.; Ishii, T.; Araki, G. Carotid plaque and intima-media thickness assessed by B-mode ultrasonography in subjects ranging from young adults to centenarians. *Stroke* **2001**, *32*, 830–835. [CrossRef] [PubMed]

22. Formanowicz, D.; Wanic-Kossowska, M.; Pawliczak, E.; Radom, M.; Formanowicz, P. Usefulness of serum interleukin-18 in predicting cardiovascular mortality in patients with chronic kidney disease—Systems and clinical approach. *Sci. Rep.* **2015**, *5*. [CrossRef] [PubMed]
23. Ridker, P.M. The JUPITER Trial. *Circ. Cardiovasc. Qual. Outcomes* **2009**, *2*, 279–285. [CrossRef] [PubMed]

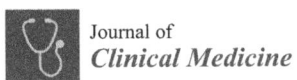

*Review*

# Fibrin Clot Properties in Atherosclerotic Vascular Disease: From Pathophysiology to Clinical Outcomes

Michał Ząbczyk [1,2,†], Joanna Natorska [1,2,†] and Anetta Undas [1,2,*]

1. John Paul II Hospital, 31-202 Kraków, Poland; michalzabczyk@op.pl (M.Z.); j.natorska@szpitaljp2.krakow.pl (J.N.)
2. Institute of Cardiology, Jagiellonian University Medical College, 31-202 Kraków, Poland
* Correspondence: mmundas@cyf-kr.edu.pl; Tel.: +48-126-143-004; Fax: +48-126-142-120
† Michał Ząbczyk and Joanna Natorska contributed equally.

**Abstract:** Fibrin is a major component of thrombi formed on the surface of atherosclerotic plaques. Fibrin accumulation as a consequence of local blood coagulation activation takes place inside atherosclerotic lesions and contributes to their growth. The imbalance between thrombin-mediated fibrin formation and fibrin degradation might enhance atherosclerosis in relation to inflammatory states reflected by increased fibrinogen concentrations, the key determinant of fibrin characteristics. There are large interindividual differences in fibrin clot structure and function measured in plasma-based assays and in purified fibrinogen-based systems. Several observational studies have demonstrated that subjects who tend to generate denser fibrin networks displaying impaired clot lysis are at an increased risk of developing advanced atherosclerosis and arterial thromboembolic events. Moreover, the majority of cardiovascular risk factors are also associated with unfavorably altered fibrin clot properties, with their improvement following effective therapy, in particular with aspirin, statins, and anticoagulant agents. The prothrombotic fibrin clot phenotype has been reported to have a predictive value in terms of myocardial infarction, ischemic stroke, and acute limb ischemia. This review article summarizes available data on the association of fibrin clot characteristics with atherosclerotic vascular disease and its potential practical implications.

**Keywords:** atherosclerosis; coronary artery disease; fibrin clot; fibrinolysis; thromboembolism

**Citation:** Ząbczyk, M.; Natorska, J.; Undas, A. Fibrin Clot Properties in Atherosclerotic Vascular Disease: From Pathophysiology to Clinical Outcomes. *J. Clin. Med.* **2021**, *10*, 2999. https://doi.org/10.3390/jcm10132999

Academic Editors: Anna Kabłak-Ziembicka and Gregory Y. H. Lip

Received: 18 June 2021
Accepted: 29 June 2021
Published: 5 July 2021

**Publisher's Note:** MDPI stays neutral with regard to jurisdictional claims in published maps and institutional affiliations.

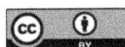

**Copyright:** © 2021 by the authors. Licensee MDPI, Basel, Switzerland. This article is an open access article distributed under the terms and conditions of the Creative Commons Attribution (CC BY) license (https://creativecommons.org/licenses/by/4.0/).

## 1. Introduction

Growing evidence indicates that the formation of denser fibrin networks, which are less susceptible to lysis, characterizes patients with atherosclerosis and arterial thromboembolic events. Several cardiovascular risk factors, such as hyperlipidemia, hypertension, smoking, or diabetes have also been shown to be associated with unfavorably altered fibrin clot properties in the general population. Low-dose aspirin, statins, better diabetes control, or smoking cessation have been shown to increase fibrin clot permeability and its susceptibility to lysis. Moreover, it has been shown that non-vitamin K antagonist oral anticoagulants (NOACs) are able to improve fibrin clot characteristics and contribute to the reduced risk of adverse clinical outcomes. The current review article summarizes available basic research and clinical papers deposited on PubMed over the last decade regarding associations between fibrin clot phenotype and atherosclerotic vascular disease, supported by the seminal papers from previous years. Moreover, data on novel therapeutic strategies, which can potentially influence fibrin clot characteristics, have been discussed.

## 2. Atherosclerotic Plaque Formation

Atherosclerosis is a major cause of cardiovascular disease that encompasses coronary artery disease, cerebrovascular disease, peripheral arterial disease, and aortic atherosclerosis. The current concept of the pathogenesis of atherosclerosis is based on chronic inflammation associated with modified lipid deposition and dysregulated immunity within the arterial wall [1–3]. The key driver of atherosclerosis is elevated low-density lipoprotein (LDL) prone to undergoing oxidative modification. Following endothelial cell injury with the subsequent influx of monocytes transformed into heterogeneous macrophages and other inflammatory cells, modified LDLs are extracellularly accumulated below the endothelium, leading to fatty streaks, an initial stage of plaque formation [2]. The formation of fibroatheroma and, finally, advanced atherosclerotic plaque is associated with the secretion of multiple chemoattractants and growth factors by leukocytes and arterial smooth muscle cells (SMCs) [2]. The proliferation of SMCs is associated with the production of large amounts of extracellular connective tissue matrix, including collagen, elastin, and proteoglycans [2,3]. Oxidized LDLs (oxLDLs) are taken up by immune cells within the atherosclerotic lesion with their subsequent transformation into foam cells, leading to plaque growth [4].

Neovascularization within the advanced plaque contributes to its gradual growth in part due to intraplaque hemorrhages. An increased density of microvessels has been found in ruptured atherosclerotic plaques [5], suggesting an important link between neovascularization and plaque instability [6]. Recent studies strongly suggest that plaque healing occurs in the natural course of atherosclerosis, with higher prevalence of healed plaques in patients with chronic manifestations of atherosclerotic vascular disease compared to those with recurrent acute coronary syndromes [7,8]. Unstable or vulnerable atherosclerotic plaques that show such characteristics as a thin fibrous cap, high macrophage content, high amounts of proinflammatory factors or a large necrotic core composed of foam cells and extracellular cholesterol [9] are prone to rupture, accompanied by occlusive thrombosis.

## 3. Blood Coagulation and Fibrin Formation in Atherosclerosis

The role of blood coagulation in the development and progression of atherosclerotic vascular disease reaches beyond thromboembolic complications. Macrophages can produce tissue factor (TF) [4], expressed also on microvesicles and its expression is regulated by inflammatory mediators, demonstrating the link between inflammation and thrombosis [10]. TF is the high-affinity receptor and cofactor for factor (F) VII/VIIa and the resultant TF-FVIIa complex activates FIX and FX [10]. A prothrombinase complex formed on activated platelets, including FXa, its cofactor FVa converts prothrombin to thrombin, the key enzyme of blood coagulation [11]. Pro-atherogenic actions of thrombin are associated with the activation of protease-activated receptors (PARs), leading to increased endothelial permeability, SMC migration and proliferation, and the activation of platelets and leukocytes, which promote vascular calcification and plaque development [11]. Activated platelets interact with leukocytes and stimulate them to release proinflammatory cytokines, reactive oxygen species, and provide the surface for the formation of tenase and prothrombinase complexes to generate thrombin from circulating prothrombin [10]. Fibrin formation occurs when minimal amounts of prothrombin have been activated (less than 5% of thrombin generation capacity) [8]. Fibrin accumulation within atherosclerotic plaque is involved in the disease progression, especially at the late stage of plaque formation [12]. Presence of fibrin within the necrotic core of damaged plaques supports its role in plaque growth and rupture [12,13]. Intraplaque fibrin has been shown to be more common in symptomatic than in asymptomatic atherosclerotic plaques [12]. Thrombin-activated FXIII, which covalently crosslinks fibrin fibers, also catalyzes the formation of intermolecular bonds between α2-antiplasmin, fibronectin, vitronectin, thrombospondin, and collagen, which in part explains fibrin accumulation with impaired fibrinolytic degradation within the lesions. Borissoff et al. [14] showed that ApoE-/-mice, which are prone to atherosclerosis, with genetically imposed 50% reduction in prothrombin were characterized by diminished atherosclerotic lesion formation and increased plaque stability, which suggests that coagulation activation is implicated in plaque development and progression and could be a potential therapeutic target. Thrombin promotes the accumulation of neutrophils and the production of reactive oxygen species, enhancing vascular inflammation. Of pivotal importance are observations made in 2010 suggesting that enhanced blood coagulation can be associated with plaque stability, given the fact that TF, FII, FX, and FXII activities are diminished along with plaque transformation to advanced stage [15]. Borissoff et al. [15] have also suggested that the loss of coagulation protein activity may contribute to the risk of plaque rupture.

Adventitial fibroblasts in normal arteries are able to express TF, while in atherosclerotic lesions, TF is also expressed by SMCs, foam cells, and macrophages, which can additionally release microparticle-derived TF [16]. TF was locally detected in 43% of patients with unstable coronary syndromes and in 12% of patients with stable coronary syndromes [17]. Moreover, about 40% higher blood levels of FVII have been reported in men with vulnerable atherosclerotic plaques in the coronary arteries, compared to those who had stable plaques [18]. The colocalization of several proteins involved in blood coagulation within the plaques, largely on macrophages, microvesicles, and SMCs [19], provides the rationale for the role of a local thrombin-mediated conversion of soluble fibrinogen into fibrin, the final product of blood coagulation, in the formation of atherosclerotic lesions.

Several studies have suggested that increased fibrinogen concentration, a key determinant of fibrin formation and its characteristics, is a risk factor for atherosclerotic vascular diseases, in particular coronary artery stenosis and myocardial infarction (MI) [20–22]. In the meta-analysis of 154,211 participants from 31 prospective studies, the hazard ratio (HR) for coronary heart disease and stroke was 1.78 (95% confidence interval [CI] 1.19–2.66) per 1 g/L increase in plasma fibrinogen concentrations [23]. The US National Health and Nutrition Examination Survey (NHANES) study showed that fibrinogen is associated with cardiovascular disease and about a 2.5-fold higher risk of all-cause and cardiovascular mortality during the 14 years of follow-up [24]. On the other hand, a Mendelian randomization study has shown no causal effect of fibrinogen on cardiovascular disease [25].

The localization of fibrin degradation products (i.e., D-dimer) within the human arterial wall suggests their potential atherogenic properties [26]. Higher D-dimer levels can be associated with atherosclerotic plaque remodeling or ongoing fibrinolysis [27]; however, both processes may trigger lipid deposition and modulate local inflammation within atherosclerotic plaques. Moreover, high levels of plasminogen activator inhibitor type 1 (PAI-1) have been identified both in the blood of coronary artery disease (CAD) patients and within unstable plaques [28]. Some genetically determined fibrinogen disorders, dysfibrinogenemias, have also been linked to atherosclerotic vascular disease and its thromboembolic manifestations, supporting the view that alterations to fibrin structure and function might be of greater importance than the fibrinogen concentration itself [29–31].

Fibrin acts as a scaffold for intravascular blood thrombi, enhancing platelet aggregation and thrombin generation, leading to a further increase in fibrin formation [29]. Fibrin(ogen) can interact with red blood cells through specific receptors, such as CD47, and with platelets (i.e., integrin αIIbβ3 or intercellular adhesion molecule 1) [29]. Cellular components embedded within the fibrin network after thrombus formation can modulate its properties. FXIII-dependent red blood cell retention in clots has been shown to impair the fibrin network structure, which delays thrombus degradation [32]. Scanning electron microscopic analysis of intracoronary thrombi obtained from patients with ST-segment elevation MI (STEMI) showed that fibrin content increased from about 30% to 80%, while red blood cell content decreased from 31% to 2% over time after the onset of chest pain [33,34]. It suggests that thrombus formation and its major component, fibrin, is a dynamic process [35,36]. Moreover, intravascular thrombi rich in red blood cells contain more neutrophils, reflecting a high thrombus burden, which has been shown to be associated with impaired reperfusion assessed at six months after the index event among patients with STEMI [35]. The presence of polyhedral erythrocytes, polyhedrocytes, has been linked with higher erythrocyte content, higher fibrinogen, and more significant stenosis in the culprit artery [36].

A contribution of blood components, in particular key coagulation factors to atherothrombosis along with potential therapeutic targets, which can modulate fibrin clot structure and function are summarized in Figure 1.

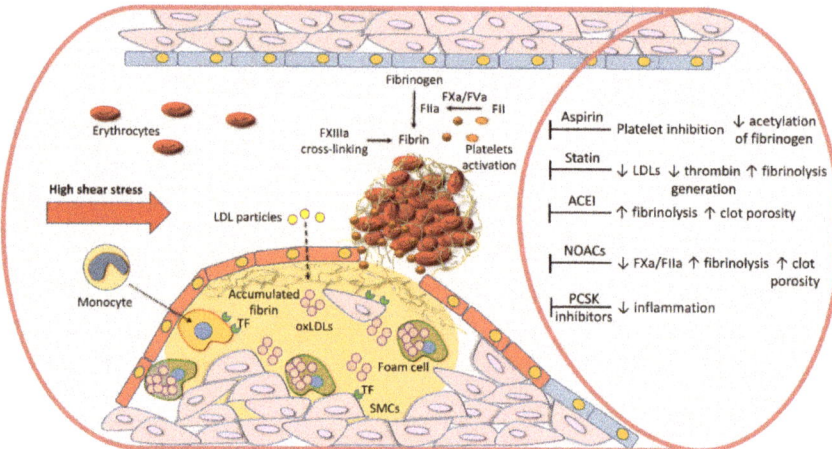

**Figure 1.** The initiation of an atherosclerotic lesion is associated with retention of low-density lipoproteins (LDL) and their oxidation (oxLDLs). oxLDLs stimulate recruitment of blood monocytes and their differentiation into macrophages. An uptake of oxLDLs by macrophages results in the formation of foam cells. Upon stimulation, vascular smooth muscle cells (SMCs) migrate and proliferate. Tissue factor (TF), expressed on macrophages and SMCs, is involved in coagulation activation, resulting in prothrombin (factor II, FII) conversion to thrombin (FIIa), which, in a prothrombinase complex with active FV (FVa), converts fibrinogen to fibrin. Several drugs, including aspirin, statins, angiotensin-converting enzyme inhibitors (ACEI), or non-vitamin K antagonist oral anticoagulants (NOACs) have been shown to modulate fibrin clot phenotype by different mechanisms. Proprotein convertase subtilisin kexin (PCSK) type 9 inhibitors are able to attenuate interplaque inflammation, but their effect on fibrin clot properties has not been reported yet. ↑—up-regulation, ↓—down-regulation.

## 4. Measures of Fibrin Clot Properties

Several parameters have been used in human subjects to assess fibrin clot properties. The structure of a fibrin clot generated from plasma (or purified fibrinogen) can be described using clot permeability ($K_s$ or Darcy's constant; reflecting volume of a buffer flowing through a fibrin gel during prespecified time) [37–39], turbidity (clot absorbance measured using a spectrophotometer at 405 or 340 nm) [40], or the direct measurement of fibrin fiber diameter, pore size, or fiber branching using microscopic techniques [41]. Fibrin clot susceptibility to lysis is measured by turbidimetry using several assays with either exogenous tissue plasminogen activator or plasmin added to clotted plasma [40,42,43]. A so-called prothrombotic fibrin clot phenotype encompasses reduced $K_s$ associated with typical changes in fibrin structure, such as lower fibrin fibers diameter, lower pore size area between particular fibers, and an increased number of branch points, along with faster fibrin formation and prolonged lysis time (Figure 2).

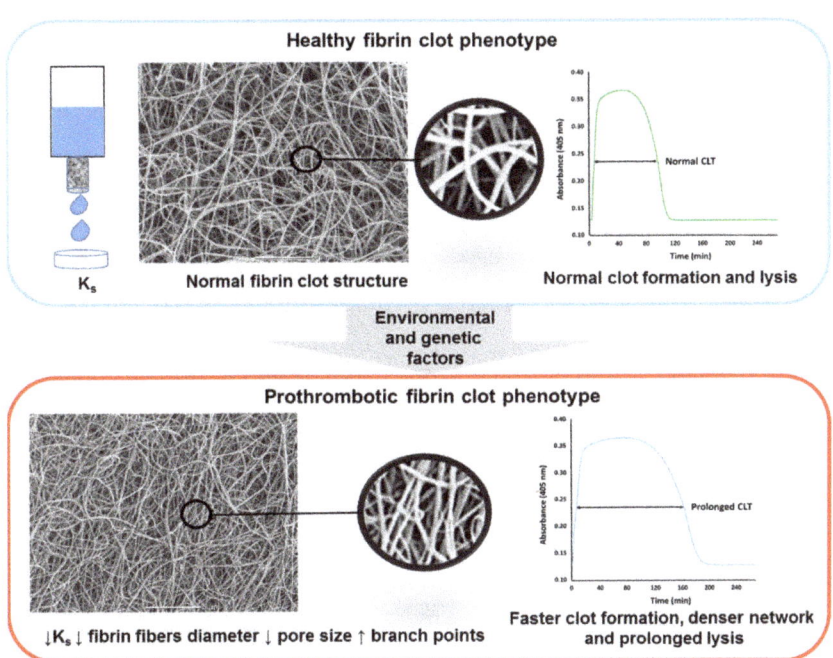

**Figure 2.** Fibrin clot structure differs between healthy persons and patients with atherosclerosis. A key measure describing plasma fibrin clot structure is its permeability. Reduced fibrin clot permeability ($K_s$) is a typical feature of the prothrombotic fibrin clot phenotype, which is associated with lower fibrin fiber diameter, lower pore size area, and increased number of fibrin branch points. Faster clot formation results in denser fibrin network (indicated by higher clot turbidity), which is relatively resistant to lysis (prolonged clot lysis time; CLT). ↑—up-regulation, ↓—down-regulation.

## 5. Cardiovascular Risk Factors

The majority of well-established cardiovascular risk factors which have been reported to be associated with prothrombotic fibrin clot properties are presented in Table 1 [44–54]. Of note, there is controversy around the association of unfavorably altered clot properties and hypercholesterolemia. Low HDL cholesterol has been reported to be associated with more prothrombotic clot features [55].

**Table 1.** Cardiovascular risk factors in association with fibrin clot properties.

| Cardiovascular Risk Factor | Study Design | No. of Subjects | Measure | Reference |
|---|---|---|---|---|
| Age | Case-control | 642 controls (and 421 MI patients) | No clear effect on CLT in controls | [44] |
|  | Cohort study | 80 healthy controls | ↑ CLT and Lys50 with increasing age | [45] |
|  | Cohort study | 2010 healthy controls | ↑ clot turbidity and CLT with increasing age | [46] |
|  | Cross-sectional study | 2000 healthy controls | No clear effect on CLT | [47] |
| Body-mass index (BMI) | Cohort study | 1288 healthy subjects | BMI positively associated with CLT in men and women | [48] |

Table 1. Cont.

| Cardiovascular Risk Factor | Study Design | No. of Subjects | Measure | Reference |
|---|---|---|---|---|
| Family history of coronary artery disease | Case-control | 100 healthy male relatives of patients with premature coronary artery disease and 100 healthy controls | ↓ $K_s$ and ↑ clot turbidity in relatives of patients | [39] |
| Current smoking | Case-control | 642 controls (and 421 MI patients) | No clear effect on CLT | [44] |
| | Cross-sectional study | 2000 healthy controls | No clear effect on CLT | [47] |
| | Case-control | 34 healthy male smokers and 34 nonsmokers | ↑ clot strength, ↑ clot turbidity, ↓ fibrin fiber diameter in smokers | [49] |
| | Case-control | 44 male cigarette smokers and 44 nonsmokers | ↓ $K_s$ and ↑ clot lysis time | [50] |
| | Cohort study | 30 healthy subjects | No clear effect on CLT | [51] |
| Lipid profile | Cohort study | 30 healthy subjects | Low-density lipoprotein cholesterol level positively associated with CLT | [51] |
| Diabetes | Case-control | 642 controls (and 421 MI patients) | No clear effect on CLT | [44] |
| | Case-control | 150 patients with type 2 diabetes and 50 controls | ↓ $K_s$ and ↑ clot turbidity associated with glycated hemoglobin levels | [52] |
| | Interventional study | 20 type 2 diabetes subjects | ↑ $K_s$ after achievement of glycemic control; $K_s$ associated with glycated hemoglobin levels | [53] |
| Arterial hypertension | Cohort study | 61 patients with essential arterial hypertension | ↑ $K_s$, ↓ clot lysis time, ↓ clot resistance to lysis at 6 months of antihypertensive treatment | [54] |

Myocardial infarction (MI), clot lysis time (CLT), fibrin clot permeability ($K_s$), ↑—up-regulation, ↓—down-regulation.

## 6. Coronary Artery Disease
### 6.1. Acute MI

Acute MI is a leading cause of mortality in high-income countries and is a major thrombotic manifestation of atherosclerotic lesions in coronary arteries [56]. Dense fibrin networks, as evidenced by reduced $K_s$ and impaired clot susceptibility to lysis, have been reported in patients with acute MI, at least in part associated with increased oxidative stress and the extent of inflammation [57]. Prolonged clot lysis time has been confirmed as a risk factor for MI in men and women in a case–control study performed on 800 acute MI patients and 1123 controls [58]. It has been hypothesized that unfavorably modified fibrin clot properties observed in acute MI are also driven by increased thrombin generation and platelet activation, expressed by a release of large amounts of proteins affecting clot features, for instance beta-thromboglobulin and platelet factor 4 [34]. In a cohort of 421 men with acute MI compared to 642 controls, hypofibrinolysis has been associated with the risk of a first MI in young men, but not in subjects aged ≥ 50 years, and CLT strongly correlated with body mass index [44]. As expected, patients with acute coronary events compared to stable coronary artery disease were characterized by a more prothrombotic fibrin clot phenotype, as reflected by lower $K_s$ and prolonged lysis time, related to a higher body mass index, higher blood pressure and higher C-reactive protein levels [57]. Platelet-derived factors, such as P-selectin of platelet-factor 4, exert a similar effect, promoting prothrombotic fibrin clot features [59]. Serum levels of P-selectin and soluble CD40 ligand were also positively associated with thrombus fibrin content [34].

It has been demonstrated that fibrin is the main constituent (60%) of intracoronary thrombi obtained during thrombectomy in acute STEMI (within 12 h since the symptom onset), with amounts increasing with time. Increased intracoronary fibrin content has also been found to be positively associated with denser plasma fibrin networks, reflected by reduced $K_s$ [36], which indicates that plasma clot characteristics have an impact on fibrin formed in intravascular thrombi. Recently, it has been suggested that intracoronary thrombi may have another type of fibrin on the surface. We have identified a thin layer of a fibrin biofilm on the surface of 15% intracoronary thrombi from acute MI patients, which was solely associated with higher plasma fibrinogen levels [60]. Heparin infusion during coronary angiography and thrombectomy probably reduces this proportion. This observation provided additional ex vivo evidence supporting the findings of Macrae and colleagues [61], who have shown that fibrin forms a film connected to the clot network and covers whole blood clots, which may protect against infiltration by bacteria or viruses, with potential impact on wound healing and thrombus fragmentation. Despite that there are no available reports describing the presence of fibrin biofilm on thrombi obtained from other locations. The relevance of the biofilm formation in human thrombosis requires further investigation.

It is unclear whether fibrin clot composition differs among patients with the same condition. Proteomics data has shown that clot-bound protein composition can influence fibrin properties [62]. A preliminary shotgun proteomic analysis performed on plasma clots from four patients during acute MI and two months later revealed time-dependent changes in the clot structure, which may influence clot stability and its susceptibility for lysis [63]. Differences in fibrinolysis proteins, such as increased amounts of $\alpha$2-antiplasmin, in acute MI may at least in part explain time-dependent changes in the clot structure following MI [63].

From a practical point of view, the issue of prognostication based on plasma fibrin clot characteristics appears to be of vital importance. Growing evidence indicates that the prothrombotic fibrin phenotype can predict cardiovascular events. A PLATO substudy performed on 4354 patients following acute MI has shown that a validated turbidimetric assay employed to assess plasma clot lysis time and clot maximum turbidity at hospital discharge, while on dual antiplatelet therapy, is able to predict adverse clinical outcomes during a 12 month follow-up period [64]. After adjustment for cardiovascular risk factors, each 50% increase in lysis time was associated with a 1.17-times higher risk of cardiovascular death or MI, and a 1.36-fold higher risk of cardiovascular death alone. A similar increase in plasma clot maximum turbidity was associated with a 1.24-fold increased risk of death (hazard ratio 1.24, 95% confidence interval 1.03–1.50) [64]. Fibrin clot density and resistance to lysis increased with higher levels of N-terminal pro B-type natriuretic peptide (NT-proBNP) and troponin T, which are known to be associated with a greater inflammatory response. The authors concluded that higher NT-proBNP levels can be associated with worse outcomes as a consequence of impaired fibrin clot features, which may lead to an increased risk of atherothrombosis [64]. Even after additional adjustment for leukocyte count, high-sensitivity C-reactive protein, high-sensitivity troponin T, cystatin C, NT-proBNP, and growth differentiation factor-15 levels, the association with death remained significant solely for lysis time [64]. It remains to be established whether clot density, or permeability, could have a similar prognostic value.

*6.2. Stable CAD*

Stable CAD, defined as angina pectoris, MI history, or presence of atherosclerotic plaques, has been associated with unfavorably modified fibrin clot properties [65]. Reduced fibrin clot lysability has been reported in asymptomatic women with present coronary plaque determined by computed tomography angiography, compared to both women without plaque and men, suggesting a sex-dependent link between coronary atherosclerosis and prolonged clot lysis time [66]. Patients with symptomatic CAD formed clots with more rigid structures and increased fibrin fiber mass-to-length ratio [67]. A history of MI in 33 young patients with documented CAD was associated with prothrombotic fibrin clot characteristics, including increased clot stiffness and a slower fibrinolysis rate, compared to healthy controls [68]. Increased lipoprotein(a) levels, a well-established risk factor for premature atherosclerosis, have been shown to alter fibrin clot properties and were associated with reduced $K_s$ and prolonged clot lysis time in patients with a history of MI [69]. Moreover, in advanced CAD patients, lipoprotein(a), a genetically determined risk factor for premature atherosclerosis, levels predicted $K_s$ but not lysis time [70]. Similarly, type 2 diabetes concomitant to CAD was associated with prolonged clot lysis time and a more compact fibrin clot structure compared to non-diabetic CAD patients [71]. The rs495828 risk allele within the ABO locus, which is known to be associated with an increased risk of MI in CAD patients, has also been shown to be associated with a more compact fibrin network structure, as evidenced by higher clot maximum absorbance, but not lysis time, among 773 stable CAD patients [72]. In a long-term follow-up study, the area under the curve of turbidimetrically monitored clot formation and lysis predicted future cardiovascular events in stable CAD (HR = 2.4, 95%CI 1.2–4.6) [73]. Altogether, CAD is associated with the prothrombotic clot phenotype governed by several largely environmental factors.

### 7. Peripheral Arterial Disease

Prothrombotic fibrin clot properties were observed for the first time in 2009 in patients with intermittent claudication, a typical manifestation of peripheral arterial disease (PAD) [74,75] which occurs in 18–20% in individuals over 70 years of age, including the most serious presentation, limb ischemia, affecting up to 3% of patients with PAD. [76]. The group from Leeds reported that unfavorably altered fibrin clot structure and function are detectable in apparently healthy close relatives of patients with claudication [74,75]. In 106 PAD patients, there was a reduction by 20% in $K_s$ when compared to controls, and it was associated with 31% prolonged CLT; the two alterations in fibrin properties predicted PAD progression during long-term follow-up [77]. Similarly, 13.4% reduced $K_s$ with no difference in CLT was found in patients with a history of acute lower limb ischemia compared to individuals without any history of such event [77]. Interestingly, premature PAD has also been identified as the clinical condition associated with a less favorable fibrin clot phenotype, in particular 30% lower clot permeability, compared to normal conditions, and no difference in the phenotype is observed in typical older PAD patients [78]. Moreover, in critical limb ischemia patients, who represent up to 3% of patients with PAD, restenosis detected within one year following endovascular therapy was associated with slightly reduced $K_s$ and prolonged CLT at baseline, accompanied by elevated thrombin generation and von Willebrand factor antigen; however, the fibrin clot variables cannot predict re-intervention, amputation, and death during further 3-year follow-up [79].

### 8. Aortic Aneurysm

Scott et al. [80] have shown that patients with abdominal aortic aneurysm (AAA) form denser fibrin clots with smaller pore sizes which are more resistant to lysis. Such prothrombotic clot phenotype was associated with the size of aneurysm and may play a role in its development. A further study performed on 169 AAA patients, including about 40% with a history of stable angina or MI, showed that plasma levels of D-dimer and thrombin-antithrombin (TAT) complexes were independent predictors of AAA growth rate [81]. An increase in D-dimer level by 500 ng/mL, or TAT level by 1 µg/mL was associated with enlargement of the aneurysm size by 0.21 and 0.24 mm per year, respectively. However, it is not known to date whether prothrombotic fibrin clot phenotype in patients with aneurysm may contribute to clinical outcomes in particular its rupture or rapid enlargement.

### 9. Pharmacological Treatment and Fibrin Clot Properties

*9.1. Cholesterol-Lowering Agents*

Statins (3-hydroxy-methylglutaryl coenzyme A reductase inhibitors) may exert several cholesterol-independent antithrombotic effects, including the down-regulation of TF expression and enhanced protein C activation via increased endothelial thrombomodulin expression [82]. Although data linking hypercholesterolemia with prothrombotic clot characteristics are limited and unconvincing, statins (simvastatin or atorvastatin at a dose of 40 mg/day for 4 weeks) used in patients with stable CAD to effectively reduce LDL cholesterol have been shown to reduce plasma clot density, reflected by higher $K_s$ and shortened

CLT, despite no impact on plasma fibrinogen levels [83]. Favorable effects of statins on fibrin clot structure and function were supported by the study in which a 3-month use of simvastatin (40 mg/d) led to a slight, though significant, increase in $K_s$ and a shortened clot lysis time in patients with LDL cholesterol < 3.4 mmol/L free of clinically evident CAD, like in the JUPITER trial with rosuvastatin [84]. This effect appeared to be associated with a decrease in CRP concentrations, suggesting links between the antithrombotic and anti-inflammatory effects of statins.

Novel therapeutic strategies to lower LDL cholesterol based on fully humanized monoclonal antibodies that bind free plasma proprotein convertase subtilisin/kexin type 9 (PCSK9) [85], different cholesteryl ester transfer protein (CETP) inhibitors [86], and antisense oligonucleotides targeting apolipoprotein(a) [87,88] are currently under investigation. To our knowledge, their potential effects on fibrin clot properties have not been investigated yet.

### 9.2. Aspirin

Aspirin was the first effective antiplatelet therapy for the prevention of ischemic events in patients with atherosclerotic vascular disease. Aspirin treatment has been shown to be associated with the formation of thicker fibrin fibers and improved clot susceptibility to lysis in stable CAD patients [89]. The mechanism of aspirin action on fibrin clot structure is unclear; however, fibrinogen acetylation [90,91] has been postulated as a major contributor despite controversies as to whether aspirin at therapeutic doses (75–150 mg/day) might exert such effects observed largely in vitro. Interestingly, low-dose aspirin (75 mg/day) has been shown to exert a stronger effect on fibrin clot properties than 320 mg/day [92,93]. In ten stable CAD patients treated with aspirin at a dose of 75 mg/day, aspirin withdrawal was associated with 32% reduced $K_s$ after one week and 41% reduced $K_s$ after two weeks when compared to values observed during treatment [94]. It is unclear to what extent fibrin-related mechanisms might add to the well-known antithrombotic effect caused by cyclooxygenase-1 inhibition and antiaggregatory effects on platelets.

### 9.3. Angiotensin-Converting Enzyme Inhibitors (ACEI)

Antihypertensive therapy with ACEI has been found to modulate fibrin clot properties in association with reduced complement component C3 levels [54]; however, similar effects were noted for other agents lowering blood pressure. In a double-blind study performed in men aged < 70 years with a history of MI or hospitalization for unstable angina, a four-week treatment with quinapril was associated with a $K_s$ increase by 13% and shortening of clot lysis time by 28% [83]. It has been suggested that the effect of ACEIs on increased fibrin clot porosity can be associated with reduced plasma fibrinogen levels [95].

### 9.4. NOACs

NOACs, including rivaroxaban and apixaban, which are selective and direct FXa inhibitors, and dabigatran as a direct thrombin inhibitor, are used to prevent and treat thromboembolic events [96]. Clots formed from normal plasma spiked with rivaroxaban (174 ng/mL) or apixaban (128 ng/mL) at therapeutic levels resulted in a less dense and more permeable clot structure with thicker fibers [97]. Varin et al. [98] have demonstrated more permeable fibrin networks composed of thicker fibrin fibers in plasma spiked with rivaroxaban at a concentration of 0.15 µg/mL, which was in line with the findings of Janion-Sadowska et al. [99] made in plasma-based assays in patients 2–6 h after rivaroxaban intake (20 mg/day). A seminal COMPASS trial has shown that rivaroxaban use at a dose of 2.5 mg twice daily combined with 100 mg of aspirin can prevent cardiovascular death in patients with advanced cardiovascular disease, mostly represented by those with stable CAD [100,101]. It has also been shown that pharmacological inhibition of FXa promotes the regression of advanced atherosclerotic plaques and enhances plaque stability in mice treated with rivaroxaban (1.2 mg/g) for 14 weeks [102], suggesting that the inhibition of FXa may be beneficial both in the prevention and regression of atherosclerotic vascular disease by down-regulated activation of PARs. The influence of low-dose rivaroxaban on fibrin clot phenotype still remains to be elucidated; however, based on the current knowledge, it can be assumed that rivaroxaban 2.5 mg bid might improve fibrin properties like rivaroxaban 20 mg/day, though to a smaller extent, and thus contributing to reduced risk of adverse clinical outcomes largely thromboembolic by nature.

## 10. Clinical Implications

The formation of dense fibrin networks which are relatively resistant to lysis has been observed in patients with atherosclerotic vascular disease, in particular CAD and PAD, along with those who experience arterial thromboembolism. The prothrombotic features of fibrin clots that are largely determined by environmental factors can be improved by the control of cardiovascular risk factors, in particular the normalization of glycemia and statin use. Growing evidence suggests that measures of clot characteristics, such as clot permeability and clot lysis time, may predict arterial thromboembolic events. Therefore, fibrin clot measures could serve as prognostic markers in patients at risk of arterial thromboembolism. However, there is a need for large studies to validate the available observations and standardization of the assays used to characterize the clot phenotype, though the first step initiated by the scientific subcommittee of the International Society on Thrombosis and Haemostasis has been made to implement the measurement of $K_s$ and CLT in clinical practice [43,103].

## 11. Conclusions

Taken together, several studies demonstrated that the formation of more compact fibrin networks displaying lower susceptibility to lysis are implicated in the progression of atherosclerosis and the occurrence of thromboembolic manifestations, in particular MI (see Table 2). The observations might support accumulating data on clinical benefits from the use of anticoagulant agents in the prevention of cardiovascular mortality. It remains to be established whether any specific modulators of fibrinolytic efficiency might be useful in the prevention of clinical outcomes in atherosclerotic vascular disease, still the major cause of morbidity and mortality worldwide.

**Table 2.** Table summarizing the recent data on plasma fibrin clot properties, including fibrin clot permeability ($K_s$) and clot lysis time (CLT) in atherosclerotic patients.

| Author (Year of Publication) | Study Type | Sample Size, Condition | Main Findings |
|---|---|---|---|
| Sadowski et al. (2014) [34] | Cohort study | 40 acute MI patients | Plasma levels of platelet activation markers correlated with thrombus fibrin content |
| Zalewski et al. (2015) [36] | Cohort study | 80 acute MI patients | Low $K_s$ was independently associated with high fibrin content within the intracoronary thrombi |
| Sumaya W et al. (2018) [64] | Cohort study | 4354 acute coronary syndrome patients | Prolonged lysis time was associated with cardiovascular death/MI |
| Ramanathan R et al. (2018) [66] | Cross-sectional study | 138 individuals without known cardiovascular disease | Women with coronary plaques had reduced fibrin clot lysability compared to women or men without coronary plaques |
| Neergaard-Petersen S et al. (2014) [71] | Cohort study | 581 CAD patients, including 148 subjects with type 2 diabetes | Type 2 diabetes in CAD patients was associated with prothrombotic fibrin clot compared to non-diabetic CAD patients |

Table 2. Cont.

| Author (Year of Publication) | Study Type | Sample Size, Condition | Main Findings |
|---|---|---|---|
| Winther-Larsen A et al. (2020) [72] | Cohort study | 773 patients with stable CAD | The *ABO* risk allele (rs495828) was associated with a more compact fibrin network in stable CAD patients |
| Neergaard-Petersen S et al. (2020) [73] | Cohort study | 786 patients with stable CAD | Increased area under the curve of clot formation and lysis predicted cardiovascular events |
| Karpińska I et al. (2020) [77] | Case-control study | 43 patients with a history of acute limb ischemia, 43 patients with cryptogenic stroke, 43 controls | Increased clot density and hypofibrinolysis characterized patients with acute limb ischemia compared to controls |
| Nowakowski et al. (2019) [79] | Case-control study | 85 patients with critical limb ischemia and restenosis and 47 PAD patients | Restenosis compared to PAD was associated with reduced $K_s$ and prolonged CLT |
| Scott DJ et al. (2011) [80] | Case-control study | 42 patients with large AAA, 40 patients with small AAA, and 49 controls | Patients with AAA compared to controls formed denser plasma clots, which were more resistant to lysis |

Myocardial infarction (MI), coronary artery disease (CAD), peripheral arterial disease (PAD), abdominal aortic aneurysm (AAA).

**Author Contributions:** Conceptualization, A.U.; methodology, M.Z. and J.N.; writing—original draft preparation, M.Z. and A.U.; writing—review and editing, A.U.; visualization, M.Z. and J.N.; supervision, A.U.; project administration, A.U.; funding acquisition, A.U. All authors have read and agreed to the published version of the manuscript.

**Funding:** This research was funded by the Jagiellonian University Medical College, grant number N41/DBS/000184.

**Conflicts of Interest:** The authors declare no conflict of interest.

## References

1. Libby, P.; Ridker, P.M.; Hansson, G.K. Progress and challenges in translating the biology of atherosclerosis. *Nature* **2011**, *473*, 317–325. [CrossRef]
2. Schaftenaar, F.; Frodermann, V.; Kuiper, J.; Lutgens, E. Atherosclerosis: The interplay between lipids and immune cells. *Curr. Opin. Lipidol.* **2016**, *27*, 209–215. [CrossRef] [PubMed]
3. Barrett, T.J. Macrophages in atherosclerosis regression. *Arterioscler. Thromb. Vasc. Biol.* **2020**, *40*, 20–33. [CrossRef] [PubMed]
4. Jaipersad, A.S.; Lip, G.Y.; Silverman, S.; Shantsila, E. The role of monocytes in angiogenesis and atherosclerosis. *J. Am. Coll. Cardiol.* **2014**, *63*, 1–11. [CrossRef]
5. Moreno, P.R.; Purushothaman, K.R.; Fuster, V.; Echeverri, D.; Truszczynska, H.; Sharma, S.K.; Badimon, J.J.; O'Connor, W.N. Plaque neovascularization is increased in ruptured atherosclerotic lesions of human aorta: Implications for plaque vulnerability. *Circulation* **2004**, *110*, 2032–2038. [CrossRef]
6. Vergallo, R.; Porto, I.; D'Amario, D.; Annibali, G.; Galli, M.; Benenati, S.; Bendandi, F.; Migliaro, S.; Fracassi, F.; Aurigemma, C.; et al. Coronary atherosclerotic phenotype and plaque healing in patients with recurrent acute coronary syndromes compared with patients with long-term clinical stability: An in vivo optical coherence tomography study. *JAMA Cardiol.* **2019**, *4*, 321–329. [CrossRef] [PubMed]
7. Fracassi, F.; Crea, F.; Sugiyama, T.; Yamamoto, E.; Uemura, S.; Vergallo, R.; Porto, I.; Lee, H.; Fujimoto, J.; Fuster, V.; et al. Healed culprit plaques in patients with acute coronary syndromes. *J. Am. Coll. Cardiol.* **2019**, *73*, 2253–2263. [CrossRef]
8. Mann, K.G.; Brummel, K.; Butenas, S. What is all that thrombin for? *J. Thromb. Haemost.* **2003**, *1*, 1504–1514. [CrossRef]
9. Brown, R.A.; Shantsila, E.; Varma, C.; Lip, G.Y. Current understanding of atherogenesis. *Am. J. Med.* **2017**, *130*, 268–282. [CrossRef] [PubMed]
10. Grover, S.P.; Mackman, N. Tissue factor: An essential mediator of hemostasis and trigger of thrombosis. *Arterioscler. Thromb. Vasc. Biol.* **2018**, *38*, 709–725. [CrossRef] [PubMed]
11. Borissoff, J.I.; Spronk, H.M.; Heeneman, S.; ten Cate, H. Is thrombin a key player in the 'coagulation-atherogenesis' maze? *Cardiovasc. Res.* **2009**, *82*, 392–403. [CrossRef] [PubMed]

12. Borissoff, J.I.; Spronk, H.M.; ten Cate, H. The hemostatic system as a modulator of atherosclerosis. *N. Engl. J. Med.* **2011**, *364*, 1746–1760. [CrossRef] [PubMed]
13. Finn, A.V.; Nakano, M.; Narula, J.; Kolodgie, F.D.; Virmani, R. Concept of vulnerable/unstable plaque. *Arterioscler. Thromb. Vasc. Biol.* **2010**, *30*, 1282–1292. [CrossRef]
14. Borissoff, J.I.; Otten, J.J.T.; Heeneman, S.; Leenders, P.; van Oerle, R.; Soehnlein, O.; Loubele, S.T.B.G.; Hamulyák, K.; Hackeng, T.M.; Daemen, M.J.A.P.; et al. Genetic and pharmacological modifications of thrombin formation in apolipoprotein e-deficient mice determine atherosclerosis severity and atherothrombosis onset in a neutrophil-dependent manner. *PLoS ONE* **2013**, *8*, e55784. [CrossRef]
15. Borissoff, J.I.; Heeneman, S.; Kilinç, E.; Kassák, P.; Van Oerle, R.; Winckers, K.; Govers-Riemslag, J.W.; Hamulyák, K.; Hackeng, T.M.; Daemen, M.J.; et al. Early atherosclerosis exhibits an enhanced procoagulant state. *Circulation* **2010**, *122*, 821–830. [CrossRef]
16. Grover, S.P.; Mackman, N. Tissue factor in atherosclerosis and atherothrombosis. *Atherosclerosis* **2020**, *307*, 80–86. [CrossRef]
17. Annex, B.H.; Denning, S.M.; Channon, K.M.; Sketch, M.H., Jr.; Stack, R.S.; Morrissey, J.H.; Peters, K.G. Differential expression of tissue factor protein in directional atherectomy specimens from patients with stable and unstable coronary syndromes. *Circulation* **1995**, *91*, 619–622. [CrossRef]
18. Ragino, Y.I.; Striukova, E.V.; Murashov, I.S.; Polonskaya, Y.V.; Volkov, A.M.; Kurguzov, A.V.; Chernjavskii, A.M.; Kashtanova, E.V. Association of some hemostasis and endothelial dysfunction factors with probability of presence of vulnerable atherosclerotic plaques in patients with coronary atherosclerosis. *BMC Res. Notes* **2019**, *12*, 336. [CrossRef] [PubMed]
19. Tavora, F.; Cresswell, N.; Li, L.; Ripple, M.; Burke, A. Immunolocalisation of fibrin in coronary atherosclerosis: Implications for necrotic core development. *Pathology* **2010**, *42*, 15–22. [CrossRef] [PubMed]
20. Dunn, E.J.; Ariëns, R.A.; de Lange, M.; Snieder, H.; Turney, J.H.; Spector, T.D.; Grant, P.J. Genetics of fibrin clot structure: A twin study. *Blood* **2004**, *103*, 1735–1740. [CrossRef]
21. Gao, X.Y.; Zhou, B.Y.; Zhang, M.Z.; Zhao, X.; Qing, P.; Zhu, C.G.; Wu, N.Q.; Guo, Y.L.; Gao, Y.; Li, X.L.; et al. Association between fibrinogen level and the severity of coronary stenosis in 418 male patients with myocardial infarction younger than 35 years old. *Oncotarget* **2017**, *8*, 81361–81368. [CrossRef]
22. Tatli, E.; Ozcelik, F.; Aktoz, M. Plasma fibrinogen level may predict critical coronary artery stenosis in young adults with myocardial infarction. *Cardiol. J.* **2009**, *16*, 317–320.
23. Fibrinogen Studies Collaboration; Danesh, J.; Lewington, S.; Thompson, S.G.; Lowe, G.D.; Collins, R.; Kostis, J.B.; Wilson, A.C.; Folsom, A.R.; Wu, K.; et al. Plasma fibrinogen level and the risk of major cardiovascular diseases and nonvascular mortality: An individual participant meta-analysis. *JAMA* **2005**, *294*, 1799–1809.
24. Pieters, M.; Ferreira, M.; de Maat, M.P.M.; Ricci, C. Biomarker association with cardiovascular disease and mortality—The role of fibrinogen. A report from the NHANES study. *Thromb. Res.* **2021**, *198*, 182–189. [CrossRef] [PubMed]
25. Ward-Caviness, C.K.; de Vries, P.S.; Wiggins, K.L.; Huffman, J.E.; Yanek, L.R.; Bielak, L.F.; Giulianini, F.; Guo, X.; Kleber, M.E.; Kacprowski, T.; et al. Mendelian randomization evaluation of causal effects of fibrinogen on incident coronary heart disease. *PLoS ONE* **2019**, *14*, e0216222. [CrossRef]
26. Smith, E.B.; Keen, G.A.; Grant, A.; Stirk, C. Fate of fibrinogen in human arterial intima. *Arteriosclerosis* **1990**, *10*, 263–275. [CrossRef] [PubMed]
27. Kleinegris, M.C.; ten Cate, H.; ten Cate-Hoek, A.J. D-dimer as a marker for cardiovascular and arterial thrombotic events in patients with peripheral arterial disease. A systematic review. *Thromb. Haemost.* **2013**, *110*, 233–243. [PubMed]
28. Kohler, H.P.; Grant, P.J. Mechanisms of disease: Plasminogen-activator inhibitor type 1 and coronary artery disease. *N. Engl. J. Med.* **2000**, *342*, 1792–1801.
29. Undas, A.; Casini, A. Congenital structural and functional fibrinogen disorders: A primer for internists. *Pol. Arch. Intern. Med.* **2019**, *129*, 913–920. [CrossRef] [PubMed]
30. Kryczka, K.E.; Płoski, R.; Księżycka, E.; Kruk, M.; Kostrzewa, G.; Kowalik, I.; Demkow, M.; Lubiszewska, B. The association between the insertion/deletion polymorphism of the angiotensin-converting enzyme gene and the plasma fibrinogen level in women and men with premature coronary artery atherosclerosis. *Pol. Arch. Intern. Med.* **2020**, *130*, 748–756. [CrossRef]
31. Treliński, J.; Witkowski, M.; Chojnowski, K.; Neerman-Arbez, M.; Wypasek, E.; Undas, A. Fibrinogen Łódź: A new cause of dysfibrinogenemia associated with recurrent thromboembolic arterial events. *Pol. Arch. Intern. Med.* **2019**, *129*, 934–935. [CrossRef]
32. Byrnes, J.R.; Duval, C.; Wang, Y.; Hansen, C.E.; Ahn, B.; Mooberry, M.J.; Clark, M.A.; Johnsen, J.M.; Lord, S.T.; Lam, W.A.; et al. Factor XIIIa-dependent retention of red blood cells in clots is mediated by fibrin α-chain crosslinking. *Blood* **2015**, *126*, 1940–1948. [CrossRef]
33. Cines, D.B.; Lebedeva, T.; Nagaswami, C.; Hayes, V.; Massefski, W.; Litvinov, R.I.; Rauova, L.; Lowery, T.J.; Weisel, J.W. Clot contraction: Compression of erythrocytes into tightly packed polyhedra and redistribution of platelets and fibrin. *Blood* **2014**, *123*, 1596–1603. [CrossRef] [PubMed]
34. Sadowski, M.; Ząbczyk, M.; Undas, A. Coronary thrombus composition: Links with inflammation, platelet and endothelial markers. *Atherosclerosis* **2014**, *237*, 555–561. [CrossRef]
35. Yunoki, K.; Naruko, T.; Sugioka, K.; Inaba, M.; Iwasa, Y.; Komatsu, R.; Itoh, A.; Haze, K.; Inoue, T.; Yoshiyama, M.; et al. Erythrocyte-rich thrombus aspirated from patients with ST-elevation myocardial infarction: Association with oxidative stress and its impact on myocardial reperfusion. *Eur. Heart. J.* **2012**, *33*, 1480–1490. [CrossRef] [PubMed]

36. Zalewski, J.; Bogaert, J.; Sadowski, M.; Woznicka, O.; Doulaptsis, K.; Ntoumpanaki, M.; Ząbczyk, M.; Nessler, J.; Undas, A. Plasma fibrin clot phenotype independently affects intracoronary thrombus ultrastructure in patients with acute myocardial infarction. *Thromb. Haemost.* **2015**, *113*, 1258–1269.
37. Carr, M.E.; Shen, L.L.; Hermans, J. Mass-length ratio of fibrin fibers from gel permeation and light scattering. *Biopolymers* **1977**, *16*, 1–15. [CrossRef] [PubMed]
38. Blombäck, B.; Okada, M. Fibrin gel structure and clotting time. *Thromb. Res.* **1982**, *25*, 51–70. [CrossRef]
39. Mills, J.D.; Ariëns, R.A.; Mansfield, M.W.; Grant, P.J. Altered fibrin clot structure in the healthy relatives of patients with premature coronary artery disease. *Circulation* **2002**, *106*, 1938–1942. [CrossRef] [PubMed]
40. Carter, A.M.; Cymbalista, C.M.; Spector, T.D.; Grant, P.J.; EuroCLOT Investigators. Heritability of clot formation, morphology, and lysis: The EuroCLOT study. *Arterioscler. Thromb. Vasc. Biol.* **2007**, *27*, 2783–2789. [CrossRef]
41. Collet, J.P.; Park, D.; Lesty, C.; Soria, J.; Soria, C.; Montalescot, G.; Weisel, J.W. Influence of fibrin network conformation and fibrin fiber diameter on fibrinolysis speed: Dynamic and structural approaches by confocal microscopy. *Arterioscler. Thromb. Vasc. Biol.* **2000**, *20*, 1354–1361. [CrossRef] [PubMed]
42. Smith, A.A.; Jacobson, L.J.; Miller, B.I.; Hathaway, W.E.; Manco-Johnson, M.J. A new euglobulin clot lysis assay for global fibrinolysis. *Thromb. Res.* **2003**, *112*, 329–337. [CrossRef] [PubMed]
43. Pieters, M.; Philippou, H.; Undas, A.; de Lange, Z.; Rijken, D.C.; Mutch, N.J.; Subcommittee on Factor XIII and Fibrinogen, and the Subcommittee on Fibrinolysis. An international study on the feasibility of a standardized combined plasma clot turbidity and lysis assay: Communication from the SSC of the ISTH. *J. Thromb. Haemost.* **2018**, *16*, 1007–1012. [CrossRef] [PubMed]
44. Meltzer, M.E.; Doggen, C.J.; de Groot, P.G.; Rosendaal, F.R.; Lisman, T. Reduced plasma fibrinolytic capacity as a potential risk factor for a first myocardial infarction in young men. *Br. J. Haematol.* **2009**, *145*, 121–127. [CrossRef] [PubMed]
45. Siudut, J.; Iwaniec, T.; Plens, K.; Pieters, M.; Undas, A. Determinants of plasma fibrin clot lysis measured using three different assays in healthy subjects. *Thromb. Res.* **2021**, *197*, 1–7. [CrossRef]
46. Swanepoel, A.C.; De Lange, Z.; Cockeran, M.; Pieters, M. Lifestyle influences changes in fibrin clot properties over a 10-year period on a population level. *Thromb. Haemost.* **2021**. [CrossRef]
47. de Lange, Z.; Pieters, M.; Jerling, J.C.; Kruger, A.; Rijken, D.C. Plasma clot lysis time and its association with cardiovascular risk factors in black Africans. *PLoS ONE* **2012**, *7*, e48881. [CrossRef] [PubMed]
48. Eksteen, P.; Pieters, M.; de Lange, Z.; Kruger, H.S. The association of clot lysis time with total obesity is partly independent from the association of PAI-1 with central obesity in African adults. *Thromb. Res.* **2015**, *136*, 415–421. [CrossRef]
49. Barua, R.S.; Sy, F.; Srikanth, S.; Huang, G.; Javed, U.; Buhari, C.; Margosan, D.; Ambrose, J.A. Effects of cigarette smoke exposure on clot dynamics and fibrin structure: An ex vivo investigation. *Arterioscler. Thromb. Vasc. Biol.* **2010**, *30*, 75–79. [CrossRef] [PubMed]
50. Undas, A.; Topór-Madry, R.; Tracz, W.; Pasowicz, M. Effect of cigarette smoking on plasma fibrin clot permeability and susceptibility to lysis. *Thromb. Haemost.* **2009**, *102*, 1289–1291.
51. Pieters, M.; Guthold, M.; Nunes, C.M.; de Lange, Z. Interpretation and validation of maximum absorbance data obtained from turbidimetry analysis of plasma clots. *Thromb. Haemost.* **2020**, *120*, 44–54. [CrossRef] [PubMed]
52. Dunn, E.J.; Ariëns, R.A.; Grant, P.J. The influence of type 2 diabetes on fibrin structure and function. *Diabetologia* **2005**, *48*, 1198–1206. [CrossRef] [PubMed]
53. Pieters, M.; Covic, N.; van der Westhuizen, F.H.; Nagaswami, C.; Baras, Y.; Toit Loots, D.; Jerling, J.C.; Elgar, D.; Edmondson, K.S.; van Zyl, D.G.; et al. Glycaemic control improves fibrin network characteristics in type 2 diabetes—A purified fibrinogen model. *Thromb. Haemost.* **2008**, *99*, 691–700.
54. Rajzer, M.; Wojciechowska, W.; Kawecka-Jaszcz, K.; Undas, A. Plasma fibrin clot properties in arterial hypertension and their modification by antihypertensive medication. *Thromb. Res.* **2012**, *130*, 99–103. [CrossRef]
55. Ząbczyk, M.; Hońdo, Ł.; Krzek, M.; Undas, A. High-density cholesterol and apolipoprotein AI as modifiers of plasma fibrin clot properties in apparently healthy individuals. *Blood Coagul. Fibrinolysis* **2013**, *24*, 50–54. [CrossRef] [PubMed]
56. Herrington, W.; Lacey, B.; Sherliker, P.; Armitage, J.; Lewington, S. Epidemiology of Atherosclerosis and the potential to reduce the global burden of atherothrombotic disease. *Circ. Res.* **2016**, *118*, 535–546. [CrossRef]
57. Undas, A.; Szułdrzynski, K.; Stepien, E.; Zalewski, J.; Godlewski, J.; Tracz, W.; Pasowicz, M.; Zmudka, K. Reduced clot permeability and susceptibility to lysis in patients with acute coronary syndrome: Effects of inflammation and oxidative stress. *Atherosclerosis* **2008**, *196*, 551–557. [CrossRef]
58. Leander, K.; Blombäck, M.; Wallén, H.; He, S. Impaired fibrinolytic capacity and increased fibrin formation associate with myocardial infarction. *Thromb. Haemost.* **2012**, *107*, 1092–1099. [CrossRef] [PubMed]
59. Gajos, G.; Siniarski, A.; Natorska, J.; Ząbczyk, M.; Siudut, J.; Malinowski, K.P.; Gołębiowska-Wiatrak, R.; Rostoff, P.; Undas, A. Polyhedrocytes in blood clots of type 2 diabetic patients with high cardiovascular risk: Association with glycemia, oxidative stress and platelet activation. *Cardiovasc. Diabetol.* **2018**, *17*, 146. [CrossRef]
60. Ząbczyk, M.; Natorska, J.; Zalewski, J.; Undas, A. Fibrin biofilm can be detected on intracoronary thrombi aspirated from patients with acute myocardial infarction. *Cardiovasc. Res.* **2019**, *115*, 1026–1028. [CrossRef]
61. Macrae, F.L.; Duval, C.; Papareddy, P.; Baker, S.R.; Yuldasheva, N.; Kearney, K.J.; McPherson, H.R.; Asquith, N.; Konings, J.; Casini, A.; et al. A fibrin biofilm covers blood clots and protects from microbial invasion. *J. Clin. Investig.* **2018**, *128*, 3356–3368. [CrossRef]

62. Ząbczyk, M.; Stachowicz, A.; Natorska, J.; Olszanecki, R.; Wiśniewski, J.R.; Undas, A. Plasma fibrin clot proteomics in healthy subjects: Relation to clot permeability and lysis time. *J. Proteom.* **2019**, *208*, 103487. [CrossRef]
63. Suski, M.; Siudut, J.; Ząbczyk, M.; Korbut, R.; Olszanecki, R.; Undas, A. Shotgun analysis of plasma fibrin clot-bound proteins in patients with acute myocardial infarction. *Thromb. Res.* **2015**, *135*, 754–759. [CrossRef]
64. Sumaya, W.; Wallentin, L.; James, S.K.; Siegbahn, A.; Gabrysch, K.; Bertilsson, M.; Himmelmann, A.; Ajjan, R.A.; Storey, R.F. Fibrin clot properties independently predict adverse clinical outcome following acute coronary syndrome: A PLATO substudy. *Eur. Heart J.* **2018**, *39*, 1078–1085. [CrossRef] [PubMed]
65. Undas, A. Fibrin clot properties and their modulation in thrombotic disorders. *Thromb. Haemost.* **2014**, *112*, 32–42. [CrossRef] [PubMed]
66. Ramanathan, R.; Gram, J.B.; Sidelmann, J.J.; Dey, D.; Kusk, M.W.; Nørgaard, B.L.; Sand, N.P.R. Sex difference in fibrin clot lysability: Association with coronary plaque composition. *Thromb. Res.* **2019**, *174*, 129–136. [CrossRef] [PubMed]
67. Greilich, P.E.; Carr, M.E.; Zekert, S.L.; Dent, R.M. Quantitative assessment of platelet function and clot structure in patients with severe coronary artery disease. *Am. J. Med. Sci.* **1994**, *307*, 15–20. [CrossRef] [PubMed]
68. Collet, J.P.; Allali, Y.; Lesty, C.; Tanguy, M.L.; Silvain, J.; Ankri, A.; Blanchet, B.; Dumaine, R.; Gianetti, J.; Payot, L.; et al. Altered fibrin architecture is associated with hypofibrinolysis and premature coronary atherothrombosis. *Arterioscler. Thromb. Vasc. Biol.* **2006**, *26*, 2567–2573. [CrossRef]
69. Undas, A.; Stepien, E.; Tracz, W.; Szczeklik, A. Lipoprotein(a) as a modifier of fibrin clot permeability and susceptibility to lysis. *J. Thromb. Haemost.* **2006**, *4*, 973–975. [CrossRef]
70. Undas, A.; Plicner, D.; Stepień, E.; Drwiła, R.; Sadowski, J. Altered fibrin clot structure in patients with advanced coronary artery disease: A role of C-reactive protein, lipoprotein(a) and homocysteine. *J. Thromb. Haemost.* **2007**, *5*, 1988–1990. [CrossRef]
71. Neergaard-Petersen, S.; Hvas, A.M.; Kristensen, S.D.; Grove, E.L.; Larsen, S.B.; Phoenix, F.; Kurdee, Z.; Grant, P.J.; Ajjan, R.A. The influence of type 2 diabetes on fibrin clot properties in patients with coronary artery disease. *Thromb. Haemost.* **2014**, *112*, 1142–1150. [CrossRef]
72. Winther-Larsen, A.; Christiansen, M.K.; Larsen, S.B.; Nyegaard, M.; Neergaard-Petersen, S.; Ajjan, R.A.; Würtz, M.; Grove, E.L.; Jensen, H.K.; Kristensen, S.D.; et al. The ABO locus is associated with increased fibrin network formation in patients with stable coronary artery disease. *Thromb. Haemost.* **2020**, *120*, 1248–1256. [CrossRef] [PubMed]
73. Neergaard-Petersen, S.; Larsen, S.B.; Grove, E.L.; Kristensen, S.D.; Ajjan, R.A.; Hvas, A.M. Imbalance between fibrin clot formation and fibrinolysis predicts cardiovascular events in patients with stable coronary artery disease. *Thromb. Haemost.* **2020**, *120*, 75–82. [CrossRef]
74. Bhasin, N.; Parry, D.J.; Scott, D.J.; Ariëns, R.A.; Grant, P.J.; West, R.M. Regarding "Altered fibrin clot structure and function in individuals with intermittent claudication". *J. Vasc. Surg.* **2009**, *49*, 1088–1089. [CrossRef] [PubMed]
75. Bhasin, N.; Ariëns, R.A.; West, R.M.; Parry, D.J.; Grant, P.J.; Scott, D.J. Altered fibrin clot structure and function in the healthy first-degree relatives of subjects with intermittent claudication. *J. Vasc. Surg.* **2008**, *48*, 1497–1503. [CrossRef]
76. Olinic, D.M.; Stanek, A.; Tătaru, D.A.; Homorodean, C.; Olinic, M. Acute limb ischemia: An update on diagnosis and management. *J. Clin. Med.* **2019**, *8*, 1215. [CrossRef]
77. Karpińska, I.A.; Nowakowski, T.; Wypasek, E.; Plens, K.; Undas, A. A prothrombotic state and denser clot formation in patients following acute limb ischemia of unknown cause. *Thromb. Res.* **2020**, *187*, 32–38. [CrossRef] [PubMed]
78. Okraska-Bylica, A.; Wilkosz, T.; Słowik, L.; Bazanek, M.; Konieczyńska, M.; Undas, A. Altered fibrin clot properties in patients with premature peripheral artery disease. *Pol. Arch. Med. Wewn.* **2012**, *122*, 608–615. [CrossRef]
79. Nowakowski, T.; Malinowski, K.P.; Niżankowski, R.; Iwaniec, T.; Undas, A. Restenosis is associated with prothrombotic plasma fibrin clot characteristics in endovascularly treated patients with critical limb ischemia. *J. Thromb. Thrombolysis* **2019**, *47*, 540–549. [CrossRef]
80. Scott, D.J.; Prasad, P.; Philippou, H.; Rashid, S.T.; Sohrabi, S.; Whalley, D.; Kordowicz, A.; Tang, Q.; West, R.M.; Johnson, A.; et al. Clot architecture is altered in abdominal aortic aneurysms and correlates with aneurysm size. *Arterioscler. Thromb. Vasc. Biol.* **2011**, *31*, 3004–3010. [CrossRef] [PubMed]
81. Sundermann, A.C.; Saum, K.; Conrad, K.A.; Russell, H.M.; Edwards, T.L.; Mani, K.; Björck, M.; Wanhainen, A.; Owens, A.P. Prognostic value of D-dimer and markers of coagulation for stratification of abdominal aortic aneurysm growth. *Blood Adv.* **2018**, *2*, 3088–3096. [CrossRef] [PubMed]
82. Undas, A.; Brummel-Ziedins, K.E.; Mann, K.G. Anticoagulant effects of statins and their clinical implications. *Thromb. Haemost.* **2014**, *111*, 392–400.
83. Undas, A.; Celinska-Löwenhoff, M.; Löwenhoff, T.; Szczeklik, A. Statins, fenofibrate, and quinapril increase clot permeability and enhance fibrinolysis in patients with coronary artery disease. *J. Thromb. Haemost.* **2006**, *4*, 1029–1036. [CrossRef] [PubMed]
84. Undas, A.; Topór-Madry, R.; Tracz, W. Simvastatin increases clot permeability and susceptibility to lysis in patients with LDL cholesterol below 3.4 mmol/l. *Pol. Arch. Med. Wewn.* **2009**, *119*, 354–359. [CrossRef] [PubMed]
85. Stein, E.A.; Mellis, S.; Yancopoulos, G.D.; Stahl, N.; Logan, D.; Smith, W.B.; Lisbon, E.; Gutierrez, M.; Webb, C.; Wu, R.; et al. Effect of a monoclonal antibody to PCSK9 on LDL cholesterol. *N. Engl. J. Med.* **2012**, *366*, 1108–1118. [CrossRef] [PubMed]
86. Hovingh, G.K.; Kastelein, J.J.; van Deventer, S.J.; Round, P.; Ford, J.; Saleheen, D.; Rader, D.J.; Brewer, H.B.; Barter, P.J. Cholesterol ester transfer protein inhibition by TA-8995 in patients with mild dyslipidaemia (TULIP): A randomised, double-blind, placebo-controlled phase 2 trial. *Lancet* **2015**, *386*, 452–460. [CrossRef]

87. Tsimikas, S.; Viney, N.J.; Hughes, S.G.; Singleton, W.; Graham, M.J.; Baker, B.F.; Burkey, J.L.; Yang, Q.; Marcovina, S.M.; Geary, R.S.; et al. Antisense therapy targeting apolipoprotein(a): A randomised, double-blind, placebo-controlled phase 1 study. *Lancet* **2015**, *386*, 1472–1483. [CrossRef]
88. Viney, N.J.; van Capelleveen, J.C.; Geary, R.S.; Xia, S.; Tami, J.A.; Yu, R.Z.; Marcovina, S.M.; Hughes, S.G.; Graham, M.J.; Crooke, R.M.; et al. Antisense oligonucleotides targeting apolipoprotein(a) in people with raised lipoprotein(a): Two randomised, double-blind, placebo-controlled, dose-ranging trials. *Lancet* **2016**, *388*, 2239–2253. [CrossRef]
89. Williams, S.; Fatah, K.; Ivert, T.; Blombäck, M. The effect of acetyl salicylic acid on fibrin gel lysis by tissue plasminogen activator. *Blood Coagul. Fibrinolysis* **1995**, *6*, 718–725. [CrossRef]
90. Ajjan, R.A.; Standeven, K.F.; Khanbhai, M.; Phoenix, F.; Gersh, K.C.; Weisel, J.W.; Kearney, M.T.; Ariëns, R.A.; Grant, P.J. Effects of aspirin on clot structure and fibrinolysis using a novel in vitro cellular system. *Arterioscler. Thromb. Vasc. Biol.* **2009**, *29*, 712–717. [CrossRef]
91. Svensson, J.; Bergman, A.C.; Adamson, U.; Blombäck, M.; Wallén, H.; Jörneskog, G. Acetylation and glycation of fibrinogen in vitro occur at specific lysine residues in a concentration dependent manner: A mass spectrometric and isotope labeling study. *Biochem. Biophys. Res. Commun.* **2012**, *421*, 335–342. [CrossRef]
92. Williams, S.; Fatah, K.; Hjemdahl, P.; Blombäck, M. Better increase in fibrin gel porosity by low dose than intermediate dose acetylsalicylic acid. *Eur. Heart J.* **1998**, *19*, 1666–1672. [CrossRef]
93. He, S.; Bark, N.; Wang, H.; Svensson, J.; Blombäck, M. Effects of acetylsalicylic acid on increase of fibrin network porosity and the consequent upregulation of fibrinolysis. *J. Cardiovasc. Pharmacol.* **2009**, *53*, 24–29. [CrossRef] [PubMed]
94. Fatah, K.; Beving, H.; Albåge, A.; Ivert, T.; Blombäck, M. Acetylsalicylic acid may protect the patient by increasing fibrin gel porosity. Is withdrawing of treatment harmful to the patient? *Eur. Heart J.* **1996**, *17*, 1362–1366. [CrossRef]
95. Scott, E.M.; Ariëns, R.A.S.; Grant, P.J. Genetic and environmental determinants of fibrin structure and function. Relevance to clinical disease. *Arterioscler. Thromb. Vasc. Biol.* **2004**, *24*, 1558–1566. [CrossRef]
96. Franchini, M.; Mannucci, P.M. Direct oral anticoagulants and venous thromboembolism. *Eur. Respir. Rev.* **2016**, *25*, 295–302. [CrossRef]
97. Gauer, J.S.; Riva, N.; Page, E.M.; Philippou, H.; Makris, M.; Gatt, A.; Ariëns, R.A.S. Effect of anticoagulants on fibrin clot structure: A comparison between vitamin K antagonists and factor Xa inhibitors. *Res. Pract. Thromb. Haemost.* **2020**, *4*, 1269–1281. [CrossRef] [PubMed]
98. Varin, R.; Mirshahi, S.; Mirshahi, P.; Klein, C.; Jamshedov, J.; Chidiac, J.; Perzborn, E.; Mirshahi, M.; Soria, C.; Soria, J. Whole blood clots are more resistant to lysis than plasma clots—Greater efficacy of rivaroxaban. *Thromb. Res.* **2013**, *131*, e100–e109. [CrossRef] [PubMed]
99. Janion-Sadowska, A.; Natorska, J.; Siudut, J.; Ząbczyk, M.; Stanisz, A.; Undas, A. Plasma fibrin clot properties in the G20210A prothrombin mutation carriers following venous thromboembolism: The effect of rivaroxaban. *Thromb. Haemost.* **2017**, *117*, 1739–1749. [CrossRef]
100. Connolly, S.J.; Eikelboom, J.W.; Bosch, J.; Dagenais, G.; Dyal, L.; Lanas, F.; Metsarinne, K.; O'Donnell, M.; Dans, A.L.; Ha, J.W.; et al. Rivaroxaban with or without aspirin in patients with stable coronary artery disease: An international, randomised, double-blind, placebo-controlled trial. *Lancet* **2018**, *391*, 205–218. [CrossRef]
101. Desperak, P.; Hudzik, B.; Gąsior, M. Assessment of patients with coronary artery disease who may benefit from the use of rivaroxaban in the real world: Implementation of the COMPASS trial criteria in the TERCET registry population. *Pol. Arch. Intern. Med.* **2019**, *129*, 460–468. [CrossRef] [PubMed]
102. Posthuma, J.J.; Posma, J.J.N.; van Oerle, R.; Leenders, P.; van Gorp, R.H.; Jaminon, A.M.G.; Mackman, N.; Heitmeier, S.; Schurgers, L.J.; Ten Cate, H.; et al. Targeting Coagulation factor Xa promotes regression of advanced atherosclerosis in apolipoprotein-E deficient mice. *Sci. Rep.* **2019**, *9*, 3909. [CrossRef] [PubMed]
103. Pieters, M.; Undas, A.; Marchi, R.; De Maat, M.P.; Weisel, J.; Ariëns, R.A.; Factor XIII and Fibrinogen Subcommittee of the Scientific and Standardisation Committee of the International Society for Thrombosis and Haemostasis. An international study on the standardization of fibrin clot permeability measurement: Methodological considerations and implications for healthy control values. *J. Thromb. Haemost.* **2012**, *10*, 2179–2181. [CrossRef] [PubMed]

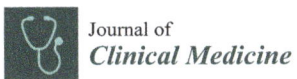 

*Review*

# Clinical Significance of Carotid Intima-Media Complex and Carotid Plaque Assessment by Ultrasound for the Prediction of Adverse Cardiovascular Events in Primary and Secondary Care Patients

Anna Kabłak-Ziembicka [1,2,*] and Tadeusz Przewłocki [3,4]

1. Department of Interventional Cardiology, Institute of Cardiology, Jagiellonian University Medical College, 31-202 Krakow, Poland
2. Noninvasive Cardiovascular Laboratory, John Paul II Hospital, Prądnicka 80, 31-202 Krakow, Poland
3. Department of Cardiac and Vascular Diseases, Institute of Cardiology, Jagiellonian University Medical College, John Paul II Hospital, 31-202 Krakow, Poland; tadeuszprzewlocki@op.pl
4. Department of Interventional Cardiology, John Paul II Hospital, Prądnicka 80, 31-202 Krakow, Poland
* Correspondence: kablakziembicka@op.pl

**Abstract:** Recently published recommendations from the American Society of Echocardiography on 'Carotid Arterial Plaque Assessment by Ultrasound for the Characterization of Atherosclerosis and Evaluation of Cardiovascular Risk' provoked discussion once more on the potential clinical applications of carotid intima-media complex thickness (CIMT) and carotid plaque assessment in the context of cardiovascular risk in both primary and secondary care patients. This review paper addresses key issues and milestones regarding indications, assessment, technical aspects, recommendations, and interpretations of CIMT and carotid plaque findings. We discuss lacks of evidence, limitations, and possible future directions.

**Keywords:** cardiovascular risk; carotid intima-media complex; carotid plaque; major adverse cardiac and cerebral events; prevention; scores

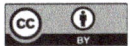

## 1. Introduction

Cardiovascular disease (CVD) is a leading global problem [1]. An estimated 17.9 million people died from CVDs in 2019, representing 32% of all global deaths [1]. Of these deaths, 85% were due to major adverse cardiac and cerebral events (MACCE) [1]. Atherosclerosis and its complications, i.e., MACCE, heart failure, disability, vascular dementia, renal failure, lower limb ischemia, etc. are responsible for more than 50% of all deaths in westernized societies [2]. According to the WHO targets, it is important to detect CVD as early as possible so that management with counseling and medicine can begin [1].

As atherosclerosis is a generalized disease affecting many arterial beds at the same time, assessment of carotid arteries theoretically creates a unique opportunity to mirror and track atherosclerotic disease [2–7].

Recently published recommendations from the American Society of Echocardiography on 'Carotid Arterial Plaque Assessment by Ultrasound for the Characterization of Atherosclerosis and Evaluation of Cardiovascular Risk' [8], once more opened discussion on the potential clinical applications of carotid intima-media complex thickness (CIMT) and carotid plaque assessments in the context of cardiovascular (CV) risk in both primary and secondary care patients.

CIMT assessment, with or without carotid plaque inclusion, was considered a surrogate measure of atherosclerosis to provide information on the CV outcome in asymptomatic patients with CV risk factors and patients with known atherosclerotic disease, or to measure the effect of medical therapy [8–42].

In epidemiological studies in asymptomatic individuals, increased CIMT values indicate higher risk of stroke, myocardial infarction (MI), or CV mortality [10]. The identification of carotid plaque even enhances this risk [8,11]. Carotid plaque presence, its number and size, volume, surface, echogenicity, or vascularization are all possible measures of MACCE [12–20]. Additionally, in secondary prevention for high-risk patients who already suffered from MI or stroke, the carotid atherosclerosis burden may have a role in the prediction of recurrent MACCE [21–25].

Despite so many advantages, the main flaw of CIMT and carotid plaque assessments is the heterogeneous techniques used for taking measurements, data reproducibility, and the limitations on the plaque composition judgements.

Therefore, this review paper addresses key issues and milestones regarding the indications, assessment, technical aspects, and interpretation of CIMT and carotid plaque findings. We discuss lacks of evidence, limitations, and possible future directions.

## 2. Historical Rationale for CIMT Assessment

The conception of CIMT and carotid plaque assessment dates back to the late years of the 20th century [43,44]. Its introduction was closely related to the development of high-resolution ultrasound techniques that allowed for the imaging of a double-layer carotid wall structure (intima-media and adventitia) [43,44].

The first report showed a difference in CIMT values between patients with hyperlipidemia as compared to healthy age-matched individuals [44]. In result, ultrasound images of the carotid artery at the level of the common carotid (CIMT-CCA), the carotid bifurcation (CIMT-CB), or the proximal segment of internal carotid artery (CIMT-ICA) were quickly adopted as a surrogate measure for atherosclerosis by epidemiological studies, i.e., the Kuopio Heart Study, the Atherosclerosis Risk in Communities Study, and the Cardiovascular Health Study [45–47].

Later, CIMT was recognized as the equivalent of "subclinical" CVD in asymptomatic patients before an individual develops symptoms such as angina, ischemic stroke (IS), or limb ischemia and was validated to predict CV outcomes [12–20].

## 3. Normal vs. Abnormal CIMT Value: Carotid Plaque Definitions

CIMT values are age and sex specific, and males have higher CIMT on average compared to females [48–52]. Therefore, normative absolute CIMT values are obsolete, and previous normative CIMT cut-off values such as the 0.9 mm mentioned in the European Society of Cardiology guideline should not be used [53]. Several studies have investigated normal CIMT value ranges, and they are summarized in Table 1.

Table 1. Normative values for CIMT. An overview of studies.

| Study | Population | Number of Participants | Site of CIMT Assessment | CIMT Cut-Off | CIMT Determinant | CIMT Cut-Off |
|---|---|---|---|---|---|---|
| Lim, T.K., et al. 2008 [48] | Healthy individuals: no CVD, no hypertension, no diabetes, BMI < 30 kg/m$^2$, and total cholesterol < 6 mmol/L. | 137 women and men | Bilaterally, far wall of CCA and CB | Over 97.5th percentile of the distribution | CCA and age: 35–39 y.o. | 0.60 mm |
| | | | | | 40–49 y.o. | 0.64 mm |
| | | | | | 50–59 y.o. | 0.71 mm |
| | | | | | over 60 y.o. | 0.81 mm |
| | | | | | CB and age: 30–39 y.o. | 0.83 mm |
| | | | | | 40–49 y.o. | 0.77 mm |
| | | | | | 50–59 y.o. | 0.85 mm |
| | | | | | over 60 y.o. | 1.05 mm |
| Estibaliz, J., et al. 2010 [49] | Healthy individuals with a BMI < 30 kg/m$^2$, blood pressure < 160/90 mmHg, LDL-C < 160 mg/dL, HDL-C > 30 mg/dL, TG < 200 mg/dL, glycaemia < 125 mg/dL, creatinine < 2 mg/dL, or thyrotropin < 6 µU/mL. | 74 women 64 men | Bilaterally, the average CIMT of the CCA, CB, and ICA | Over 75th percentile of the distribution | Female and age: <25 y.o. | 0.52 mm |
| | | | | | 25–34 y.o. | 0.58 mm |
| | | | | | 35–44 y.o. | 0.65 mm |
| | | | | | 45–54 y.o. | 0.70 mm |
| | | | | | 55–64 y.o. | 0.80 mm |
| | | | | | >64 y.o. | 0.93 mm |
| | | | | | Male and age: <25 y.o. | 0.59 mm |
| | | | | | 25–34 y.o. | 0.67 mm |
| | | | | | 35–44 y.o. | 0.66 mm |
| | | | | | 45–54 y.o. | 0.72 mm |
| | | | | | 55–64 y.o. | 0.81 mm |
| | | | | | >64 y.o. | 0.95 mm |

Table 1. Cont.

| Study | Population | Number of Participants | Site of CIMT Assessment | CIMT Cut-Off | CIMT Determinant | CIMT Cut-Off |
|---|---|---|---|---|---|---|
| Diaz, A., et al. 2018 [50] | Healthy individuals: BP < 140/90 mmHg in adults and < 90th percentile in younger subjects; no history of CVD, pulmonary, or renal disease; not taking antihyperlipidemic, blood lowering, or antidiabetic drugs; glycaemia < 110 mg/dL; total cholesterol <200 mg/dL; TG < 150 mg/dL and < 130 mg/dL for adults and subjects between 10 to 17 years, respectively. | 391 women 621 men | Bilaterally, averaged far wall of the CCA | Over 75th percentile of the distribution | Female and age: <20 y.o. 25; 35 y.o. 40; 50 y.o. 55; 65 y.o. ≥70 y.o. Male and age: <20 y.o. 25; 35 y.o. 40; 50 y.o. 55; 65 y.o. ≥70 y.o. | 0.47 mm 0.49; 0.55 mm 0.58; 0.67 mm 0.72; 0.83 mm 0.89 mm 0.49 mm 0.51; 0.56 mm 0.60; 0.68 mm 0.72; 0.83 mm 0.89 mm |
| Engelen, L., et al. 2013 [51] | 24 research centers worldwide. Individuals without CVD or CV risk factors (BP < 140/90 mmHg), no current smoking, glucose < 7.0 and/or post-load plasma glucose < 11.0 mmol/L, total cholesterol < 6.2 mmol/L, HDL-C > 1.17 mmol/L (for men) and > 1.30 mmol/L (for women), BMI < 30 kg/m², and no BP-, lipid-, and/or glucose-lowering medication | 2241 women 1993 men | Bilaterally, averaged far wall of the CCA | Over 75th percentile of the distribution | Female and age: <20 y.o. 25; 35 y.o. 40; 50 y.o. 55; 65 y.o. 70; 80 y.o. ≥85 y.o. Male and age: <20 y.o. 25; 35 y.o. 40; 50 y.o. 55; 65 y.o. 70; 80 y.o. ≥85 y.o. | 0.47 mm 0.50; 0.55 mm 0.58; 0.64 mm 0.66; 0.72 mm 0.75; 0.80 mm 0.83 mm 0.48 mm 0.51; 0.57 mm 0.59; 0.65 mm 0.68; 0.74 mm 0.80; 0.83 mm 0.86 mm |
| Randrianarisoa, E., et al. 2015 [52] | Healthy individuals: no CVD, no classic CV risk factors, and exclusion of metabolic syndrome, subclinical inflammation, insulin resistance, abnormal the body fat distribution, and prediabetes | 428 women 373 men | Bilaterally, far wall of the CCA | Over 90% limits of the distribution | Female and age: 18–29 y.o. 30–39 y.o. 40–49 y.o. 50–59 y.o. Male and age: 18–29 y.o. 30–39 y.o. 40–49 y.o. 50–59 y.o. | 0.47 mm 0.59 mm 0.67 mm 0.70 mm 0.47 mm 0.62 mm 0.72 mm 0.80 mm |

BMI, body mass index; BP, blood pressure; CB, carotid bulb; CCA, common carotid artery; CIMT, carotid intima-media thickness; CV, cardiovascular; CVD, cardiovascular disease; HDL-C, high-density lipoprotein cholesterol; ICA, internal carotid artery; LDL-C, low-density lipoprotein cholesterol; TG, triglycerides.

A CIMT value over the 75th percentile, according to American Society of Echocardiography (ASE), should be considered abnormal [54]. In 2002, the National Cholesterol Education Program (NCEP) Adult Treatment Panel III stated that an elevated CIMT (above 75th percentile for age and sex) could elevate a person with multiple risk factors at higher risk category [55].

In a research study enrolling 24 medical centers, the 75th percentile of the CIMT-CCA distribution was established at 0.5 and 0.51 mm in female and male below 25 years of age, while it was established at 0.80 and 0.83 mm in healthy individuals over 80 years of age, respectively (Table 1) [51]. Later, Randrianarisoa et al. performed an update on normal values for CIMT, including traditional as well as novel cardiovascular risk factors of atherosclerosis progression, like the body fat distribution, metabolic syndrome, subclinical inflammation, insulin resistance, and disturbances in glucose metabolism [52].

## 4. Techniques for CIMT and Carotid Plaque Assessment: Strengths and Weaknesses

B-mode high-resolution ultrasound is a noninvasive technique that provides one of the best methods for the detection of early stages of atherosclerotic disease [10]. Many studies have successfully applied CIMT as a technique to monitor arterial wall alterations based upon its association with CV risk factors, the incident CVD, and the outcome [9–20]. CIMT and carotid plaque measurements including mean-maximal or mean-mean CIMT, plaque thickness, area and volume, and plaque score were all used as imaging outcomes [9–20,56–59].

Unfortunately, diverse approaches for measuring CIMT and plaque as well as different cut-offs and acquisition techniques have caused confusion for the interpretation of CIMT and plaque findings [9–20]. Thus, technique, the number of segments of the carotid artery tree, the near or far wall, and the use of contrast-enhanced agents are all points for discussion [56].

Another, but not less important issue, is whether measurements can be manual, (semi)-automated, or if computer-assisted analysis software should be used to automatically track the intima-media layer [10,54,59]. Semi-automated edge detection is more often applied in the setting where only the CCA is examined, while manual edge detection is usually applied in the setting where the CB and the ICA are also measured [58].

For example, in the Carotid Atherosclerosis Progression Study (CAPS), CIMT was expressed as the mean CCA at the far wall and in the Cardiovascular Health Study (CHS) as the mean of the maximum at the near and far CCA and ICA, while in the Malmö Diet and Cancer Study (MDCS) and the Kuopio Ischemic Heart Disease Study (KIHD), it was expressed as the maximum CIMT-CCA at the far wall [12–16]. The Rotterdam study presented results as the maximum value from the near and far CCA [17], while the Atherosclerosis Risk in Communities Study (ARIC) measured CIMT as the mean of means at the right and left CCA, CB, and ICA [18,19].

The lack of methodological standardization of CIMT resulted in contraindication (Class III) for CIMT assessment as CV risk modifier from the 2021 ESC Guidelines on CVD prevention in clinical practice [60].

Thus, to overcome methodological flaws, guidelines for obtaining CIMT and carotid plaque measurements were published with the intention to reduce measurement variability, a key parameter for a high-quality study, statistical power, and sample size determination (Table 2, Figure 1).

Table 2. An overview on CIMT and carotid plaque definitions and acquisition techniques.

| Study | CIMT Assessment — Definition, Acquisition Technique | Carotid Plaque — Acquisition Technique, Definition |
|---|---|---|
| Mannheim IMT Consensus, 2012 [59] | Definition: CIMT is a double-line pattern visualized by ultrasound on both walls of the CCA in a longitudinal image, which consist of the leading edges of two anatomical boundaries: the lumen-intima and media-adventitia interfaces (Figure 1). Acquisition: High-resolution B-mode system with linear transducers at frequencies > 7 MHz, log gain compensation of app. 60 dB. Gain settings adjusted to obtain a symmetrical brightness on the near and far wall to eliminate artifacts in a longitudinal view lateral position. A long 10 mm length of a straight arterial segment is required for reproducible serial measurements. CIMT measurement within a region free of plaque with a clearly identified double-line pattern, preferably on the far wall of the CCA at least 5 mm below its end. CIMT can be measured at the CB or ICA in a region free of plaque, on a shorter length, taking caution of the large interindividual variability. These values must be recorded separately. CIMT measurements options include the mean, maximum, composite measures from both sides, and different arterial sites. Mean CIMT values averaged across the entire distance are less susceptible to outliers. The maximal CIMT may reflect more advanced stages with focal thickening or plaque formation. | Definition: Plaques are focal structures encroaching into the arterial lumen of at least 0.5 mm or 50% of the surrounding CIMT, or demonstrating a thickness of >1.5 mm as measured from the intima-lumen interface to the media-adventitia interface (Figure 1). Acquisition technique: Plaque location, thickness, area, and number scanned in longitudinal and cross-sections must be recorded. For plaque, a maximal thickness requires demonstration from 2 different angles of insonation, in longitudinal and cross-sectional views. The incremental value of recording texture (density, echogenicity, shadow) remains uncertain pending more research. |
| American Society of Echocardiography, 2008 [54] and 2020 [8] | Definition: not given Acquisition technique: B-mode imaging preferred over M-mode. Ultrasound system with a linear-array transducer at frequencies > 7 MHz. CIMT imaging (3–5 beat cine-loop and optimized R-wave gated still frames at each angle).Distal 1 cm of each CCA. Use of a semiautomated border detection program with validated accuracy. Scanning protocols from observational studies with published nomograms may be used if they are more germane to the age, sex, and race/ethnicity of the clinical population being investigated; however, the clinical laboratory must have sufficient expertise to perform them accurately and reproducibly. Use of values from clinically referred populations are discouraged, because of the high likelihood of referral bias and inaccurate risk estimates. Limiting CIMT measurements to the far wall of the CCA is the preferred strategy. Interpretation of carotid ultrasound studies for CVD risk assessment: Mean CIMT values from the far wall of the right and left CCAs (mean-mean) should be reported. Use of additional segments or maximum values is an alternative if there is local expertise and normative values with published associations to CVD risk are reported. Mean-mean values are more reproducible because multiple points along the traced segment are averaged, but are less sensitive to change. Mean-maximum values are more sensitive to change, but less reproducible. Evaluating for the presence or absence of plaque in conjunction with measuring CIMT-CCA offers a better representation of subclinical vascular disease and CVD risk than only measuring CIMT. | Definition: Carotid arterial plaque visualized with or without use of an ultrasound enhancing agent is defined as: (1) any focal thickening thought to be atherosclerotic in origin and encroaching into the lumen of any segment of the carotid artery (protuberant-type plaque), or (2) in the case of diffuse vessel wall atherosclerosis, when CIMT measures ≥ 1.5 mm in any segment of the carotid artery (diffuse-type plaque). Carotid plaque grading: Grade 0: no carotid plaque; Grade I: focal protuberant thickening of vessel wall < 1.5 mm; Grade II: focal protuberant plaque between 1.5 and 2.4 mm height, or diffuse thickening of the vessel wall between 1.5 and 2.4 mm; Grade III: either protuberant or diffuse thickening above 2.4 mm. Repeat measurements are not recommended unless the Grade and CIMT meets criteria for diffuse-type plaque (Grades II or III, and CIMT ≥ 1.5 mm) in which case it is a plaque equivalent. Acquisition technique: 2D techniques for quantifying plaque as initial approach with giving maximum plaque thickness. It should be measured from the side in which a plaque lesion is detected (unilateral) or from both the right and left carotid arterial segments (bilateral) using a caliper placed at the adventitial plane and extending into the center of the lumen at right angles to the vessel wall. For standardization, this measurement should be taken from segments of the long and short axis. 2D plaque area: the measurement should begin from medial-adventitial plane for the purposes of standardization. The quantification of plaque volume for an individual plaque lesion is recommended when required (e.g., morphologic assessment, serial assessment, or pre-operative consideration), using either the stacked-contour method or specialized semi-automated tools. 3D plaque volume: the quantification of right and/or left carotid plaque volume using 3D ultrasound for cardiovascular risk stratification with a single-plaque or single-region report, or a full-vessel protocol report. |

2D, 2-dimentional; 3D, 3-dimensional.

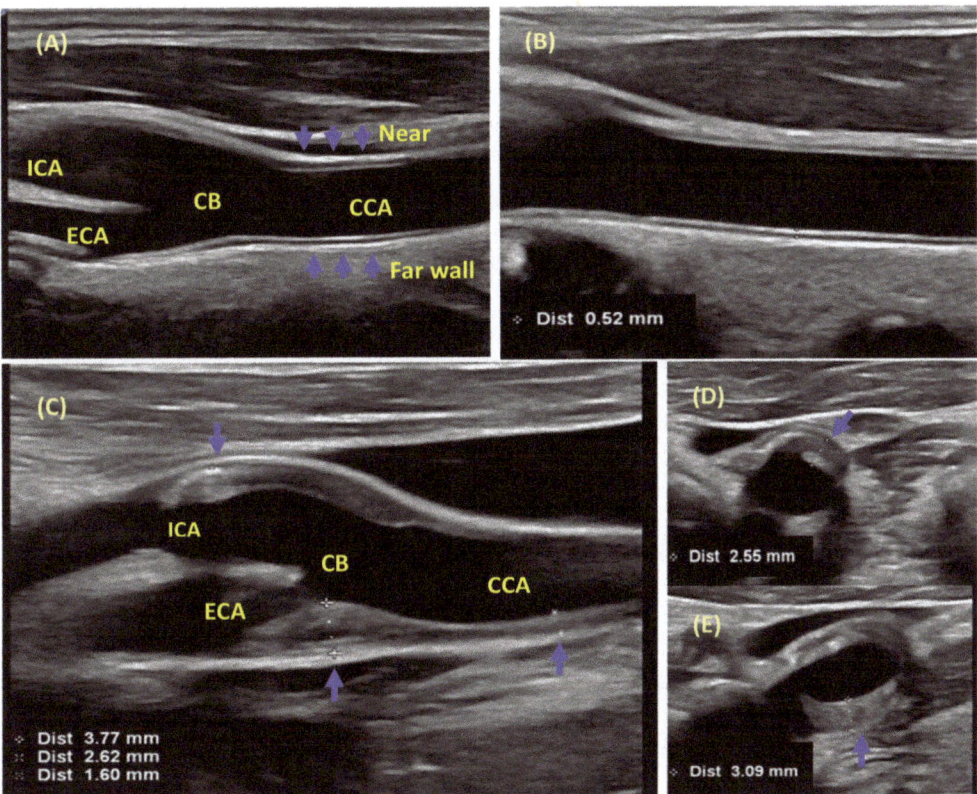

**Figure 1.** CIMT and carotid plaque assessment. (**A**) CIMT is a double-line pattern on both walls of the common carotid artery (CCA), the carotid bulb (CB), the internal carotid artery (ICA), and the external carotid artery (ECA) in a B-Mode 2D longitudinal image. Two parallel lines are the lumen-intima and media-adventitia interfaces. (**B**) According to the Mannheim IMT consensus [59], CIMT should be measured within a region free of plaque with a clearly identified double-line pattern, preferably on the far wall of the CCA at least 5 mm below its end. If the CIMT-CB and the CIMT-ICA are measured, the results should be reported separately from CIMT-CCA. According to the Mannheim [59], limiting CIMT measurements to the far wall of the CCA and distal 1 cm of each CCA is the preferred strategy. (**C**) Diffuse-type plaques (Grades II or III, and CIMT $\geq$ 1.5 mm). (**C–E**) In line with the ASE consensus, the maximal plaque height should be measured from the side in which a plaque is detected (unilateral) or from the right and left carotid arterial segments (bilateral), using a caliper placed at the adventitial plane and extending into the center of the lumen to the vessel wall. For the purposes of standardization, this measurement should be taken from the long (**C**) and short axis (**D,E**) of the carotid artery. Arrows indicate regions of taking CIMT, plaque measurements.

The 2008 ASE consensus statement for CIMT is based on the concept of identifying asymptomatic patients at high risk who might be candidates for more intensive, evidence-based medical interventions that reduce CVD risk (Table 2) [54]. The 2008 ASE guidelines recommend measuring CIMT and identifying carotid plaque by ultrasound for refining CVD risk assessment in patients at intermediate CVD risk (FRS 6%–20%) without established coronary heart disease (CHD), peripheral arterial disease (PAD), cerebrovascular disease, diabetes, or abdominal aortic aneurysm. Patients with the following clinical circumstances also might be considered for CIMT and carotid plaque measurement: (1) family history of premature CVD in a first degree relative (men < 55 years old, women <

65 years old); (2) individuals younger than 60 years old with severe abnormalities in a single risk factor (e.g., genetic dyslipidemia) who otherwise would not be candidates for pharmacotherapy; or (3) women younger than 60 years old with at least two CV risk factors.

The Mannheim IMT Consensus [59] recommended CIMT assessment for the initial detection of CHD risk in (1) asymptomatic patients at intermediate risk, (2) in the setting of two or more NCEP risk factors, (3) with metabolic syndrome, (4) with a family history of premature CHD, or (5) with a known coronary artery calcium (CAC) score of zero and FRS 11%–20%. According to Mannheim IMT consensus, measurements may include the CCA, the ICA, or the CB segments. Whereas nearly all patients have their CIMT-CCA imaged, successful imaging of the CIMT-ICA and of the CIMT-CB depends both upon the anatomical topography of the patient and on sonographer's expertise. Thus, the Mannheim IMT consensus advises rather for CIMT-CCA at far wall measurements than from the whole carotid artery tree. The overview of the Mannheim recommendations is presented in Table 2. The Mannheim definition of plaque was adopted by the 2021 ESC Guidelines on CVD prevention in clinical practice as possible CV risk modifier (Class II-b) [60].

The 2020 ASE recommendations for carotid plaque ultrasound suggested a stepwise approach to CV risk stratification using plaque grading via a focused carotid vascular ultrasound and subsequent 2D or 3D plaque quantification in the assessment of asymptomatic patients at risk (Table 2). In patients presented with symptoms suggestive of CHD but normal non-invasive tests (e.g., stress electrocardiogram, stress echocardiography, stress MRI, and nuclear imaging), patients with atherosclerotic plaques in the carotid artery may benefit from more aggressive medical treatment. In contrast, patients without plaque have an excellent CV prognosis [8]. The 2020 ASE consensus did not focus on CIMT, referring to 2008 ASE recommendations for CIMT assessment [8,54].

## 5. Simultaneity of Atherosclerotic Burden across Arterial Beds

Multi-site steno-occlusive arterial disease is invariably associated with worse clinical outcomes [4], accounting for 51% MACCE incidence rate in patients with arterial disease (at least 50% lumen reduction) in either coronary, carotid, and renal and lower extremity arterial territories as compared to 27%, 18%, and 9% in patients with 3-site, 2-site, and 1-site arterial disease at 4 years follow-up, respectively [4]. Furthermore, studies are ongoing about which patients with multi-site atherosclerotic occlusive disease would have decreased risk of MACCE following revascularization, and who would benefit more from medical treatment [61].

In the general population of individuals aged 30–79 years, the global prevalence of increased CIMT and carotid plaque is estimated to be 27.6% (16.9% to 41.3%) and 21.1% (13.2% to 31.5%), respectively [62,63]. Multisite arterial disease is common in patients with atherosclerotic involvement in one vascular bed, ranging from 10% to 15% in patients with CAD to 60% to 70% in patients with severe carotid stenosis or PAD [64,65].

At large, screening for asymptomatic disease in additional vascular sites has not been proved to improve prognosis. Nevertheless, the mean-max CIMT values from the CCA, the CB, and the ICA with a cut-off value of 1.30 mm nicely distinguish patients with no steno-occlusive arterial disease or stenosis limited to one arterial territory from individuals with larger arterial territory involvements (odds ratio, OR, 35.9, 95% Confidence Interval, 95% CI, 20 to 65) with a sensitivity of 81.6%, specificity of 88.8%, and positive and negative predictive value of 85.1% and 86.3%, respectively [66].

A variety of studies evaluated the relationship between CIMT and presence of atherosclerotic abnormalities in the other territories of the arterial system [67–77]. Most studies demonstrated associations between increasing CIMT value and presence and severity of a significant arterial disease (defined as at least 50% or more lumen reduction): CAD, renal artery stenosis, lower and upper extremity athero-oclussive disease, or the abdominal aorta [67–77]. However, correlations between CIMT with incidence and severity of lesions in the other arterial sites are modest, especially when only CIMT-CCA is reported [78–80].

Rohani et al. demonstrated a correlation between the extent of CAD and the mean CIMT-CCA of r = 0.44; Adams et al. demonstrated a correlation between 0.23 and 0.29, while Azarkish et al. demonstrated a correlation between 0.36 and 0.47 [78–80]. Interestingly, CIMT can rule out significant CAD in women and patients with degenerative aortic stenosis, e.g., a mean-maximum CIMT value of greater than 1.2 mm was predictive (sensitivity, 73.5%; specificity, 72.7%) of concomitant CAD in patients with aortic stenosis [70,73].

A recent meta-analysis of 89 studies showed moderate correlation between CIMT and severity of CAD (r = 0.60, $p < 0.001$) and the number of diseased vessels (r = 0.49, $p < 0.001$) [67]. Additionally, carotid plaque presence and calcification were less, and lipid-rich necrotic core was highly prevalent in nonsignificant versus significant CAD ($p < 0.001$, $p = 0.03$, $p < 0.001$, respectively) [67]. In another large meta-analysis, including 22 studies, the diagnostic sensitivity and specificity of CIMT for CAD were 0.68 and 0.70, respectively [81].

## 6. CIMT and Carotid Plaque in the Context of Cardiovascular Risk Factors

Various risk factors influence CIMT and carotid plaque, including age, gender, diabetes, dyslipidemia, hypertension, cigarette smoking, genetics, and inflammation [82–84]. Song et al. performed a systematic review and meta-analysis of the 75 articles on CIMT, carotid plaque, and carotid stenosis [62]. The influence of CV risk factors for increased CIMT and carotid plaque were 2.71 and 1.79 for age per 10-year increase, 0.49 and 0.55 for female sex, 1.76 and 1.70 for current smoking, 2.23 and 1.45 for diabetes, and 1.55 and 1.75 for hypertension, respectively (Table 3) [62]. Another meta-analysis by Ji et al. of 76 cross-sectional studies that evaluated 11 risk factors showed a pooled OR and 95% CI for the probability of the carotid plaque incidence (the Mannheim definition) to be associated with hypertension, diabetes, dyslipidemia, current smoking, hypertriglyceridemia, LDL-C, hypertriglyceridemia, hyperuricemia, hyperhomocysteinemia, and metabolic syndrome (Table 3) [85].

**Table 3.** Meta-analyses on the increased CIMT and carotid plaque incidence with cardiovascular risk factors.

| Risk Factor | Song et al. 2020 [62] Pooled Data OR (95% CI) | Ji et al. 2019 [85] Pooled Data OR (95% CI) |
|---|---|---|
| Increased CIMT (>1.0 mm) | | |
| Age | 2.71 (2.07–3.55) | N/A |
| Female sex | 0.49 (0.38–0.64) | N/A |
| Current smoking | 1.76 (1.34–2.30) | N/A |
| Diabetes | 2.23 (1.48–3.36) | N/A |
| Hypertension | 1.55 (1.03–2.34) | 2.60 (1.33–5.08) |
| Dyslipidemia | 0.90 (0.65–1.25) | N/A |
| Carotid plaque | | |
| Age | 1.79 (0.93–3.43) | - |
| Female sex | 0.55 (0.33–0.94) | - |
| Current smoking | 1.70 (1.41–2.04) | 1.41 (1.08–1.87) |
| Diabetes | 1.45 (1.12–1.90) | 1.31 (1.13–1.53) |
| Hypertension | 1.75 (1.44–2.13) | 1.81 (1.55–2.13) |
| Dyslipidemia | - | 1.20 (0.80–1.82) |
| HDL-C | 0.46 (0.21–0.99) | 1.28 (0.99–1.67) |
| LDL-C | - | 1.11 (1.08–1.13) |
| Hypertriglyceridemia | - | 1.33 (1.14–1.55) |
| Hyperuricemia | - | 1.57 (1.11–2.22) |
| Hyperhomocysteinemia | - | 1.88 (1.19–2.95) |
| Metabolic syndrome | - | 1.71 (1.10–2.66) |

In the NOMAS study that assessed 2D carotid plaque area in 1730 primary care individuals above 39 years old, the associations between carotid plaque and age, smoking, systolic blood pressure, diabetes, LDL-C:HDL-C ratio, and homocysteine levels were found, with respective contributions of 13.5%, 2.8%, 1.1%, 0.8%, 0.7%, and 0.7% [86].

There is much confusion with regard to lipoproteins and CIMT. Single-center studies indicate the relationship between higher CIMT and higher levels of total cholesterol (TC), LDL-C, lipoprotein (a), and non-HDL-cholesterol, as well as inverse associations with HDL-C; however, meta-analyses fail to show associations [62,85–89]. For example, in a study by Stamler et al. in a group of men aged 18 to 39 years, those with TC levels $\geq$ 6.21 mmol/L had a greater risk of CHD (2.15 to 3.63 times) and CV mortality (2.10 to 2.87 times) in comparison to individuals with TC < 5.17 mmol/L [90]. In this study, LDL-C, which is a classical atherogenic lipid, had a lower predictive value for the presence of carotid plaque than TC. The problem of lipids and atherosclerosis is much more complex, as there are many different fractions of lipoproteins that are atherogenic (i.e., very low-density lipoprotein cholesterol, intermediate-density lipoprotein cholesterol, or lipoprotein (a)) [90].

Of note, the accumulation of many various risk factors impacts overall CIMT and plaque parameters [91]. Many systemic inflammatory and thrombotic biomarkers are associated with increased CIMT and asymptomatic and symptomatic plaque incidence. Associations were proven for CIMT and interleukin-6 (IL-6), vascular cell adhesion molecule-1 (VCAM-1), Apolipoprotein E (ApoE), white blood cell (WBC) count, T lymphocytes, fibrin, and adiponectin [21,90]. Carotid plaque presence was associated with intercellular adhesion molecule 1 (ICAM-1), L-selectin, E-selectin, IL-1$\beta$, tumor necrosis factor $\alpha$ (TNF-$\alpha$), lipoprotein phospholipase A2 (Lp-PLA2), WBC count, and mi-RNAs [90]. While transformation of asymptomatic into symptomatic carotid plaque was associated with levels of high-sensitivity C-reactive protein (hs-CRP), serum amyloid-A Protein (SAA), TNF-$\alpha$, plasma-soluble urokinase plasminogen activator receptor (suPAR), matrix metalloproteinases (MPO-1, -2, -7, -9), tissue inhibitors of metalloproteinase (TIMP), ApoE, ApoA-I, Lp-PLA2, and miRNAs [92].

## 7. Additive Value of CIMT and Carotid Plaque to the Traditional Cardiovascular Risk Scoring Systems

As CIMT and carotid plaque are measures of atherosclerosis, it seems reasonable to combine established traditional risk scores with carotid imaging [93,94]. In a study by Elaid et al., 127 (37.8%) out of 336 initially 'low-risk' primary care patients (FRS event risk < 5% in 10 years) were re-classified as higher risk (>5%) when high CIMT (CIMT $\geq$ 75th percentile adjusted for age, gender, race, and presence of plaque) was found on ultrasound [95]. Plaque exceeding 1.5 mm was present in 17.3% of low-risk patients [95].

The risk calculators may integrate CIMT measurement with CV risk factors [86,93–102]. The ARIC study published an adjusted FRS calculator incorporating mean-maximum CIMT from six carotid segments and plaque assessment to determine the probability of MI or death from CHD within 10 years [96]. In that study including 13,145 individuals, approximately 23% were reclassified by adding CIMT and plaque information [96]. The addition of CIMT and plaque together to the traditional risk factors improved the prediction model from 0.742 for traditional risk factors to 0.755 for the CV risk factors, CIMT and plaque [96].

Recently, STRATEGY study assessed three scoring systems: the FRS, the Prospective Cardiovascular Münster Study Score (PROCAM), and the European Society of Cardiology SCORE in the context of possible additive CIMT value [85,92,95,96]. All scores correlated significantly with CIMT, but this correlation was only moderate [87]. The FRS correlated most strongly and predicted 27% of the CIMT variance in men and 20% in women [87].

The IMPROVE study, in a group of 3703 primary care patients aged 54–79 years with at least three CV risk factors, but free of any CV events prior to enrolment, evaluated the independence of carotid plaque thickness and the mean CIMT (measured in plaque-free areas bilaterally in the CCA, the CB, and the ICA) in CV risk stratification at 3 years follow-up [99]. In this study, both plaque and CIMT occurred as independent predictors of MACCE, with values of 1.98 (1.47 to 2.67) and 1.68 (1.23 to 2.29), respectively, as well as cerebrovascular events. However, only plaque was an independent predictor of coronary events like MI, sudden cardiac death (SCD), angina pectoris, and coronary revascularization [99]. The authors concluded that in reclassification analyses, CIMT and plaque significantly add to the FRS score [99]. In line, in the study by Gaibazzi et al., carotid plaques (not CIMT) and echocardiographic cardiac calcium were significant predictors of angiographic CAD in patients without prior CHD but with signs or symptoms suspect of CAD, again incrementally correlated to FRS [102].

Mitu et al. found a relationship between CIMT and arterial stiffness with SCORE, FRS, QRISK, and PROCAM in an asymptomatic population [100,101]. The SCORE risk correlated better with CIMT, while the FRS and QRISK seemed more specific for increased arterial stiffness parameters [100]. Of note, arterial stiffness proved its clinical value for MACCE in various clinical scenarios, e.g., in patients with aortic valve stenosis [103].

## 8. Primary and Secondary Care Population and MACCE

There is much evidence that higher CIMT corresponds to higher likelihood of MACCE. At least six primary care large-cohort prospective studies examined the predictive value of CIMT (without plaque) on MACCE (Table 4). In general, CIMT values in the highest range are associated with a 1.4- to 3.2-fold risk increase for MI, a 1.4- to 3.5-fold risk increase for IS, a 2.3- to 2.9-fold risk increase for CV death, and a 1.75-fold risk increase for SCD (Table 4) [11,12,15–19,104–108]. This was evidenced regardless of method used for CIMT calculation (mean-mean, mean-maximum, the CCA only, or combined CCA-CB-ICA) [12,13,15,104]. Importantly, in most studies, the ability of CIMT to predict future MACCE was independent of traditional risk factors [11,12,15–19,104–108].

There is much evidence that plaque presence is stronger predictor of MACCE than CIMT alone (Table 4) [11,59,94,108–120]. In a study comparing results of ARIC and CHS studies, the presence of plaque was associated with over 30% increased risk of SCD: 1.37 in the ARIC and 1.32 in the CHS [105]. In the Manhattan Study, carotid plaque thickness exceeding 1.9 mm was associated with a MACCE incidence risk of 2.8 (2.03 to 3.84), as compared to individuals with no plaque at all [110].

Further improvement in risk estimation may be gained by considering not only the largest identified plaque, but also the total plaque burden, plaque area, plaque score (a sum of all plaques heights), or a number of segments containing plaque in both carotid arteries (Table 4) [109,111–118,121]. According to some authors, the average of all the CIMTmax observed in each carotid segment (CIMTmean-max), is the variable that best describes the total plaque profile, and which has the best predictive power [21,118]. Additionally, carotid plaque burden measured by 3D ultrasound is highly correlated with CAC scores and predictive of MACCE (CV death, MI, and stroke) [111]. The High-Risk Plaque BioImage Study compared CIMT, carotid plaque burden, and maximum carotid plaque thickness in nearly 6000 individuals [111]. Both carotid plaque burden and carotid plaque thickness were predictive of primary and secondary MACCE, whereas CIMT was not [111].

Table 4. Overview of studies on the relationship between CIMT, carotid plaque, and MACCE in primary and secondary cardiovascular risk prevention individuals.

| Study | CIMT Measure | Interpretation | Participants Number, Type | Follow-Up (Years) | Outcome | HR (95% CI) |
|---|---|---|---|---|---|---|
| **Primary Cardiovascular Risk Prevention** | | | | | | |
| CIMT studies CAPS [12] | Mean-CCA | 4th vs. 1st quartile<br>4th vs. 1st quartile<br>4th vs. 1st quartile | 5052, PC<br>5052, PC<br>5052, PC | 4.2<br>4.2<br>4.2 | MI<br>IS<br>CV death | 2.3 (0.9–6.3)<br>2.3 (1.4–3.8)<br>3.2 (2.0–5.1) |
| CHS [13] | Max-CCA | 5th vs. 1st quartile<br>5th vs. 1st quartile<br>4th vs. 1st quartile | 4476, PC<br>4476, PC<br>5555, PC | 6.2<br>6.2<br>13.1 | MI<br>IS<br>SCD | 3.2 (2.0–5.1)<br>2.8 (1.8–4.2)<br>1.75 (1.25–2.51) |
| MDCS [15] | Mean-CCA | 3rd vs. 1st tertile<br>3rd vs. 1st tertile | 5163, PC<br>5163, PC | 7.0<br>7.0 | MI<br>IS | 2.1 (1.2–3.4)<br>3.0 (1.6–5.7) |
| KIDH [16] | Max-CCA | ≥1 mm vs. < 1.0 mm | 1275, PC | 1.0 | MI | 2.2 (0.7–6.7) |
| Rotterdam [17] | Mean-CCA | Per 0.16 mm, 1SD<br>Per 0.16 mm, 1SD | 1566, PC<br>1566, PC | 2.7<br>2.7 | MI<br>IS | 1.4 (1.2–1.8)<br>1.4 (1.3–1.8) |
| LILAC [104] | Mean-CCA, CB, ICA | Per 0.3 mm | 298, PC | 3.1 | CV death | 2.9 (1.0–6.8) |
| Carotid plaque studies CHS [105] | Plaque presence | Plaque vs. no plaque | 5555, PC | 13.1 | SCD | 1.32 (1.04–1.67) |
| ARIC [18,19] | Mean-CCA-CB-ICA+plaque | >1 mm<br>>1 mm<br>>1 mm<br>>1 mm | 10841, PC<br>10841, PC<br>14214, PC<br>14214, PC | 5.2<br>5.2<br>7.2<br>7.2 | MI<br>MI<br>IS<br>IS | M: 1.8 (1.3–2.7)<br>F: 5.1 (3.1–8.4)<br>M: 2.0 (1.2–3.1)<br>F: 3.3 (1.9–5.8) |
| ARIC [105] | Plaque (>1.5 mm)<br>Mean-CCA-CB-ICA+plaque | Plaque vs. no plaque<br>4th vs. 1st quartile | 15307, PC<br>15307, PC | 23.5<br>23.5 | SCD<br>SCD | 1.37 (1.13–1.67)<br>1.64 (1.15–2.63) |
| Ali J.S. et al. [107] | Mean-CCA-CB-ICA+plaque | 4th vs. 1st quartile | 706, PC | 4.78 | MI, IS, TIA, revascularization | 5.8 (1.3–26.60) |
| TROMSO [107,108] | Plaque area | 4th quartile of plaque area vs. no plaque | 3240 M, PC<br>3344 F, PC<br>2989 M, PC<br>3237 F, PC | 10<br>10<br>5.4<br>5.4 | IS<br>IS<br>MI<br>MI | 1.73 (1.19–2.52)<br>1.62 (1.04–2.53)<br>1.56 (1.04–2.36)<br>3.95 (2.16–7.19) |
| Manhattan Study [110] | Max. plaque thickness | Plaque > 1.9 mm vs. no plaque | 2189, PC | 6.9 | MI, IS, CV death | 2.80 (2.04–3.84) |
| BioImage Study [111] | 3D Plaque max thickness | 3rd tertile vs. no plaque | 5808, PC | 2.7 | MI, IS, CV death | 2.36 (1.13–4.92) |
| Xie et al. [112] | Sum of segments with plaque | ≥ 3 segments with plaque(s) | 3258, PC | 5 | CHD, IS | 2.43 (1.20–4.93) |
| Stork et al. [113] | Sum of all plaques areas | By number of plaques: < 2; 2 to 4; > 4 | 403, PC | 4 | CV death | 1.85 (1.14–3.01) |
| ARCO study [109] | Total plaque area | 3rd tertile of plaque area vs. no plaque | 2842, PC | 5.9 | MI, IS, CV death | 21.4 (2.8–163) |
| MESA study [114] | Total plaque score | Plaque score per 1 SD | 6814, PC | 11.3 | CV disease<br>CHD<br>IS | 1.27 (1.16–1.40)<br>1.35 (1.21–1.51)<br>1.15 (0.98–1.35) |
| Yang, C.W.; et al. [120] | Mean-max CIMT-CCA, CB, ICA plus plaque | CIMT/plaque >2 mm vs. <1 mm<br>CIMT >1 mm vs. <1 mm | 2956, PC<br>2956, PC | 9.41<br>9.41 | All-cause death<br>All-cause death | 1.79 (1.07–3.00)<br>1.65 (1.21–2.32) |

Table 4. Cont.

| Study | CIMT Measure | Interpretation | Participants Number, Type | Follow-Up (Years) | Outcome | HR (95% CI) |
|---|---|---|---|---|---|---|
| **Secondary cardiovascular risk prevention** | | | | | | |
| *CIMT studies* | | | | | | |
| Yoon et al. [23] | mean CCA | mean | 479, AIS | 9 | MI, IS, CLI, CV death | 2.21 (0.80–6.09) |
| Tada et al. [122] | mean-max CCA | mean | 2035, ASCVD | 4 | All-cause death CV death, MI, stroke, HF, revascularization | 0.89 (0.52–1.49) |
| *Carotid plaque studies* | | | | | | |
| Kolkenbeck-Ruh et al. [22] | Plaque thickness | CIMT plus plaque | 473, CLI or IS 479, controls | n/a | IS vs. controls CLI vs. controls | <60 years, HR 20.8 to 28.4 (7.24–111) >50 years, HR 5.61 to 8.85 (1.77–25.4) |
| Kabłak-Ziembicka et al. [4] | Mean-max CIMT-CCA, CB, ICA plus maximum plaque thickness | Mean CIMT/plaque ≥ 1.25 mm (3,4 vs. 1,2 quartile) | 652, Confirmed CHD 125, PC | 5 | MI, IS, CLI, CV death | 2.52 (1.50–4.24) |
| Yoon et al. [23] | Plaque presence (Mannheim definition) | Any vs. no plaque | 479, AIS | 9 | MI, IS, CLI, CV death | 1.70 (1.14–2.53) |
| Tada et al. [122] | Carotid plaque score | top quintile vs. bottom quintile | 2035, ASCVD | 4 | All-cause death, CV death, MI, IS, HF, revascularization | 3.38 (1.82–6.27) |

AIS, acute ischemic stroke; ASCVD, atherosclerotic cardiovascular disease; CLI, critical limb ischemia; CV, cardiovascular; F, female gender; HF, heart failure; IS, ischemic stroke; M, male gender; MI, myocardial infarction; PC, primary care subjects; SCD, sudden cardiac death; SSSS, symptomatic subclavian steal syndrome.

The estimated added predictive value of carotid plaque thickness in comparison to traditional risk factors accounts respectively for 0.73 vs. 0.72 in the CHS study [116], 0.72 vs. 0.67 in Stork et al.'s study [113], and 0.90 vs. 0.88 in Prati et al.'s study [115], as well as 0.75 vs. 0.74 in the Tromso, ARIC, and Xie et al. studies [105,108,112]. The addition of the carotid plaque score to the established risk factors can significantly improve risk discrimination (C-index 0.746 vs. 0.726; $p = 0.017$) [114].

Importantly, plaque echogenicity, surface, angiogenesis, and size (volume and area) are all among risk factors for both cerebrovascular and cardiac events [121,123–127]. There is strong association between an increased risk of IS and plaques that are low echogenic (echolucent), ulcerated, with neovascularization, or containing mobile fragments with estimated respective risk of IS (HR, 95% CI): 3.99 (3.06 to 5.19), 3.58 (1.66 to 7.71), 9.68 (3.14 to 123.2), and 1.57 (1.02 to 2.41), respectively [125].

In contrast to primary prevention studies, there are only few studies that address role of CIMT/plaque assessment to calculate risk of MACCE recurrence. Although the issue is clinically relevant, the assessment of CV risk in patients with already known atherooclussive disease at any arterial site (coronary, carotid, or other), or after index CV event (primary MI, IS, critical limb ischemia (CLI)) is not supported by the guidelines [55,125]. This attitude seems justified with regard to CIMT assessment (with exclusion of plaque parameters) and evidenced by studies of Yoon et al. and Tada et al. (Table 4) [23,122]. In contrast, in the study of Yoon et al. performed in 479 patients with index acute IS, carotid plaque (not mean CIMT-CCA) was associated with risk of secondary CV event (Table 4) [23].

In the study including 652 patients with angiographic stenosis ≥ 50% in at least one arterial territory (coronary, supra-aortic, renal, and/or lower extremity), who underwent a revascularization procedure for index lesion, a mean-max CIMT (plaque included) exceeding ≥ 1.25 mm (HR, 2.52; 95% CI, 1.5 to 4.24; $p$ = 0.001) was associated with increased risk of MACCE, abdominal aortic aneurysm rupture, or development of new symptomatic lesions requiring revascularization [4]. In this study, inclusion of CIMT and plaque into the stratification model significantly improved the prediction of CV event risk [4]. Incremental value of mean-max CIMT plus plaque, TNF-α, and hs-CRP to traditional risk factors in risk stratification was also found in another study of patients with confirmed atherosclerosis [21]. Yet, the study by Tada et al. showed a combined risk for all-cause death, CV death, MI, IS, revascularization, heart failure of 3.38 (95% CI, 1.82 to 6.27) among 2035 patients diagnosed with atherosclerotic CVD [122].

## 9. Follow-Up of Changes in CIMT and Carotid Plaque Thickness with Multiple Assessments—Is It Worth It?

Serial assessment of CIMT change over time is considered a good method to monitor the natural progression of atherosclerosis in epidemiological studies and/or to assess the average response to treatment in clinical trials [27,40,41,44,116,121,122,128–131]. A major advantage of measuring carotid plaque burden is that progression/regression of plaque can be measured in clinically relevant time frames. The spatial resolution of carotid ultrasound is approximately 0.3 mm, and on average, CIMT changes by only 0.015 mm/year [128]. It is therefore not possible to reliably measure change in CIMT within an individual over short period of time. The consensus sample size for studies of effects of therapy on CIMT is 200 to 300 patients per group, followed for 2 years [27]. Thus, an appropriate time span is required between individual CIMT and plaque size assessments.

In the Malmo Diet and Cancer Study (MDCS) including 3426 primary care middle-aged Swedish patients, there was a cumulative relationship between traditional CV risk factors and CIMT progression rates during the 16-year follow-up period. The ORs of a high CIMT-CCA progression rate (>75th percentile) were 1.0 (reference), 1.4 (95% CI: 1.1 to 1.7), 1.7 (95% CI: 1.3 to 2.2), and 2.1 (95% CI: 1.4 to 3.1), respectively, for individuals with none, one, two, and three risk factors [44]. Favorable changes in systolic blood pressure, LDL-C, and HDL-C during over 15 years of follow-up decreased the CIMT progression rate in the CCA [44]. Interestingly, averaged CIMT progression rates were lower in the CCA (0.011 mm/year for men and 0.010 mm/year for women) but greater in the CB (0.036 mm/year for men and 0.030 mm/year for women) [44].

In a prospective study of a primary care population in the Cholesterol-Lowering Atherosclerosis Study trial, during an 8.8-year observation, Hodis et al. showed that the risk of coronary events was increased with the rate of CIMT progression (Table 5). The researchers observed ORs of coronary events of 1.0 (reference), 1.6, 2.3, and 2.8 for CIMT progression rates of less than 0.011, 0.011 to 0.017, 0.018 to 0.033, and greater than 0.033 mm/year, respectively [40]. In another study, CIMT progression predicted CV events in patients with type 2 diabetes [41].

Table 5. The relationship between CIMT or carotid plaque progression over time and MACCE.

| Study | CIMT Measure | Interpretation Progression Rate, mm/Year | Participants Number, Type | Follow-Up (Years) | Outcome | HR (95% CI) |
|---|---|---|---|---|---|---|
| **Primary cardiovascular risk prevention** | | | | | | |
| CIMT studies Hodis, et al. [40] | Mean-CCA | < 0.011, 0.011 to 0.017, 0.018 to 0.033, > 0.033 | 188, PC | 8.8 | Coronary events | Ref. 1.0 1.6 (0.9–6.3) 2.3 (1.4–3.8) 2.8 (1.8–4.2) |
| IMPROVE study [118] | CIMT-CCA, BC, ICA | Fastest CIMT change > 0.026 mm/year | 3482, CRF ≥ 3 | 1.3 | MI, SCD, CV death, stroke, TIA | 1.98 (1.47–2.67) |
| Okayama, et al. [41] | CIMT-CCA at baseline and at least 2 more times | Median CIMT change > 0.011 mm/year | 342, diabetes | 7.6 | CV death, MI, IS | 2.24 (1.25–4.03) |
| Willeit et al. [132] Meta-analysis of 119 clinical trials with medical agents | CIMT-CCA, mean or max | CIMT regression of: 0.01 mm/year 0.02 mm/year 0.03 mm/year 0.04 mm/year | 100667, CRF | n/a | MI, stroke, CV death, revascularization | 0.84 (0.75–0.93) 0.76 (0.67–0.85) 0.69 (0.59–0.79) 0.63 (0.52–0.74) |
| Carotid plaque studies Wannarong, T., et al. [128] | CIMT, TPA, TPV at baseline and after 1 year | By tertiles of change | 349, PC | 3.17 | Death, stroke, TIA, MI | CIMT: $P = 0.455$ TPA: $P = 0.143$ TPV: $P < 0.001$ |
| **Secondary cardiovascular risk prevention** | | | | | | |
| Carotid plaque studies Wrotniak et al. [24] | Mean-max CIMT-CCA, CB, ICA plus plaque thickness, 2nd exam at M36-42 | > 0.060 mm/year | 108, SSSS | 4.8 | CV death, MI, IS, revascularization | 1.22 (1.02–1.46) |
| Gacof, J et al. [130] | Mean-max CIMT-CCA, CB, ICA plus plaque thickness, exams at yearly intervals | CIMT progression rate > 0.003 mm/year | 215, ACS | 4.4 | MI, IS, CV death, new onset angina revascularization | 3.0 (1.5–6.02) |
| Hirano et al. [133] | Max carotid plaqu eat baseline, 2nd exam after 6M | Per 0.1 mm increase over 6 months | 240, CHD | 3 | Cardiac death, MI, UA with revascularization | 1.21 (1.10–1.33) |
| Gacof, J et al. [134] | Mean-max CIMT CCA, CB, ICA plus plaque thickness, 2nd exam between M12-24, 3rd exam between M24-36 | Mean CIMT/plaque ≥ 0.056 mm/year Any CIMT/plaque regression | 466, ASCVD 466, ASCVD | 3.5 3.5 | MI, IS, CV death MI, IS, CV death | 1.22 (1.03–1.44) 0.25 (0.14–0.32) |

ACS, acute coronary syndrome; ASCVD, atherosclerotic cardiovascular disease, defined as lesions in at least one major arterial territory including coronary, carotid, renal, or lower extremity arteries exceeding 50% lumen reduction; CRF, cardiovascular risk factors; IS, ischemic stroke; M, month; MI, myocardial infarction; TPA, total plaque area; TPV, total plaque volume; UA, unstable angina.

A novel approach was recently proposed by the IMPROVE study to assess carotid CIMT progression [118]. In this study, the greatest value among the progressions of CIMTmax observed in the whole carotid tree identified focal increases of CIMT and was associated with cardiovascular risk (Table 5) [118].

In a secondary prevention population of 108 patients who had stent-supported angioplasty for symptomatic subclavian steal syndrome, followed for a mean of 4.8 years, Wrotniak et al. found CIMT progression of 0.060 mm/year to increase risk of MACCE and lesion progression by 22% (OR, 1.22; 95% CI, 1.02 to 1.46; $p = 0.033$) with a sensitivity of 75.0% and specificity of 61.8% [24]. In this study, despite medical treatment adhering to guidelines, atherosclerosis progression was found in 53 (49%), no change in 10 (9.3%), and regression in 45 (41.7%) patients [24].

Gacoń et al. demonstrated in a group of 215 patients admitted with acute coronary event, that patients with MACCE at follow-up, compared to MACCE-free subjects, had a greater annual CIMT progression rate either at first ($0.024 \pm 0.12$ vs. $0.009 \pm 0.16$ mm/year; $p < 0.001$) or at subsequent follow-up ultrasound visits ($0.050 \pm 0.1$ vs. $0.001 \pm 0.1$ mm/year; $p < 0.001$) [130]. Of note, initial CIMT values were similar in MACCE vs. MACCE-free patients ($1.43 \pm 0.40$ vs. $1.45 \pm 0.44$ mm; $p = 0.486$) [130].

In Hirano et al.'s study including 240 patients with CHD confirmed on angiography, the average number of carotid plaques ($\geq 1.1$ mm of CIMTmax) at baseline was $2.5 \pm 1.8$ in a patient [128]. The change in plaque-IMTmax over 6 months ranged from $-0.85$ to $0.97$ mm (mean, $-0.006 \pm 0.319$ mm). The study showed that progression of carotid plaque-IMTmax over 6 months despite anti-atherosclerotic therapy was an independent predictor of future coronary events in CHD patients (Table 5) [133].

It is extremely important to understand that CIMT and plaque progression rate is non-linear [42,130]. Among that innumerous studies that were published, a study by Olmastroni et al. deserves particular attention as it is a large primary care cohort (1175 participants), with participants initially at low and intermediate CV risk with a prospective follow-up of 12 years, with the use of individual CIMT growth curve modeling [42]. Participants completed four visits with ultrasound examination, which proved that the rate of change in CIMT over time is a sign of the development of atherosclerosis, with periods of rapid and attenuated CIMT growth, which cannot be a priori assumed as linear [42]. In that study, the fastest mean and max CIMT growth was observed in patients between 50 and 70 years old. Of 966 subjects free from carotid atherosclerosis at baseline, 31.8% developed multifocal carotid atherosclerosis and 11.8% developed focal carotid atherosclerosis [42].

The non-linear response of atherosclerosis to so-called optimal medical treatment was also reported by study of Gacoń et al., including 466 secondary care patients [134]. In this study, regression of the mean-max CIMT (with inclusion of plaque thickness when present) was observed in 37.1% of the study group at the first ultrasound re-examination between month 12 and 24, and it went down to 26.6% at the second re-examination between month 24 and 36 [134]. The attenuated CIMT/plaque progression was independently associated with a reduced risk of MACCE (HR, 0.25; 95% CI, 0.15 to 0.42), MI (HR, 0.32; 95% CI, 0.20 to 0.51), IS (HR, 0.29; 95% CI, 0.18 to 0.45), and CV death (HR, 0.24; 95% CI, 0.15 to 0.40) [134]. In contrast, a carotid atherosclerosis progression of >0.056 mm/year was associated with increased risk of MACCE, however, with only moderate sensitivity and specificity of 53.2% and 72.2%, respectively (Table 5). Thus, achieving regression in CIMT and plaque thickness may constitute a better measure of treatment efficacy.

## 10. CIMT and Carotid Plaque Changes in Response to Medical Treatment

CIMT was used in randomized clinical trials (RCT) to measure the effect of medical intervention, targeted at CV risk factor control, and the carotid atherosclerosis progression or regression, as possible modifiers of adverse CV outcomes [12,26–36]. Positive response to the medical intervention was defined as a measurable decrease in CIMT and carotid plaque values of the treated group compared to patients' group, with treatment failure defined as CIMT or carotid plaque increase despite treatment in the context of future MACCE [37–42].

As effective interventions targeting pre-existing CVD, lifestyle and diet may reduce the risk of carotid atherosclerosis [85]. Huang et al. suggested that antihypertensive medication use may be the strongest modifiable predictor of slowing CIMT progression over time, especially when measurements are taken at the CB [135]. Overall, 8 out of 10 analyzed statin RCTs showed that conventional statins therapy are efficient and safe to decrease the rate of carotid atherosclerosis progression in the long term, and aggressive statins may provide superior efficacy for carotid atherosclerosis regression [34]. According to Wannanong et al., for assessment of response to anti-atherosclerotic therapy, measurement of total plaque volume is superior to both CIMT and total plaque area measurements [128]. This finding is in line with meta-analysis of seven studies including 361 patients receiving statin therapy, in which there was significant decrease in lipid-rich necrotic-core volume at >12 months ($-9.9$ mm$^3$, 95% CI $-8.9$, $-2.3$); however, no significant reduction in carotid wall volume was seen on high-resolution carotid plaque MRI [136].

Conversely, according to the SAIP research group, the scientific bases for monitoring changes in single individuals are still not convincing [137]. First, Goldberger suggested caution in using CIMT as a surrogate endpoint of outcome in trials with statins, focused on CIMT progression/regression and MACCE incidence, although a smaller rate of change in CIMT was associated with a reduced MI incidence 0.82 (95% CI, 0.69 to 0.96; $p = 0.018$) [35]. Alas, there was no significant relationship between mean change in CIMT and nonfatal MI in RCTs [35]. Another large meta-analysis of 16 prospective studies performed by the PROG-IMT collaboration revealed a positive association between the mean CIMT-CCA and a 16% increase in CV risk, but no association between CIMT progression and CV events [132]. However, in this meta-analysis, the reproducibility between first and the second CIMT measurement was surprisingly low (correlation coefficient < 0.10), resulting in huge bias for data interpretation [138]. As consequence, the conclusion from meta-analyses of RCTs was that CIMT changes (regression or progression) did not correlate with changes in the incidence of MACCE induced by several drug treatments in different categories of subjects at intermediate to high CV risk [29].

This lack of associations between CIMT changes and clinical outcomes is surprising, as active medical treatment with either statins, calcium channel blockers, angiotensin-converting enzymes, or sartans was associated both with MACCE rate reduction as well as CIMT decrease in comparison to placebo groups [12,26–38].

To overcome existing confusion, a meta-analysis of 119 clinical trials involving 100,667 patients done by Willeit et al. shed some light on this puzzle [132]. Data from individual RCTs were systematized (Table 5). CIMT was assessed as the mean value at the CCA; if unavailable, the maximum value at the CCA or other CIMT measures were utilized. The primary outcome was a combined CVD endpoint defined as MI, stroke, revascularization procedures, or CV death. Authors estimated intervention effects on CIMT progression and incident CVD for each trial, before relating the two using a Bayesian meta-regression approach. This meticulous work resulted in conclusion that medical interventions reducing CIMT progression by only 0.01, 0.02, 0.03, or 0.04 mm/year would decrease the relative risks for CVD of 0.84 (95% CI, 0.75 to 0.93), 0.76 (95% CI, 0.67 to 0.85), 0.69 (95% CI, 0.59 to 0.79), or 0.63 (95% CI, 0.52 to 0.74), respectively [132].

## 11. Important Limitation for Comprehensive Data Analysis and Results Interpretation

Based on the experience in previous large-scale trials, there is a number of aspects that one may consider in designing a trial with CIMT as primary outcome parameter. For example, a major flaw in CIMT and carotid plaque measurements is the inter-observer and intra-observer reproducibility of measures. Although many recent studies demonstrated good agreements between intra-observer (between 91% and 97%) and inter-observer (between 88% and 91%) reliability of CIMT [120,122,139], data reproducibility must be assured.

An important limitation for comprehensive data analysis and results interpretation is the different methodology of CIMT and plaque measurements used in individual studies. That issue was clarified in the dedicated ASE and Mannheim recommendations [8,54,59].

Information on plaque changes in time carries useful information on treatment efficacy. Patients who are responders to medical treatment in terms of attenuation of carotid atherosclerosis growth have a decreased risk of MACCE. Therefore, last but not least, it is important to perform serial repeated carotid atherosclerotic burden measurements with appropriate period intervals between measurements, as atherosclerosis changes can fluctuate with periods of rapid and slow growth or regression. The single re-assessment of CIMT and plaque is a shortcoming.

## 12. Perspectives for CIMT and Carotid Plaque on Ultrasound

The 2020 ASE recommendations for carotid plaque ultrasound suggested a stepwise approach to CV risk stratification adopted from Greenland et al. [140] and Piepoli et al. [124]. At baseline, carotid vascular ultrasound and subsequent 2D or 3D plaque quantification would be performed in the assessment of asymptomatic patients at low or intermediate risk according to an FRS and European SCORE. Patients with no plaque or carotid plaque thickness less than 1.5 mm would be considered as low risk. Patients with plaques thickness (CIMT) between 1.5 and 2.4 mm would be allocated to the intermediate risk class, while whose with plaques exceeding 2.4 mm would be considered in the high CV risk class with subsequent assessment of patient and plaque vulnerability (neovascularization and echolucency) [8].

In conclusion, CIMT and carotid plaque reflects atherosclerosis burden in the whole arterial tree. Incidence and severity of CV risk factors (both traditional and non-traditional) have an impact on CIMT thickness and plaque burden, and more importantly, they are responsible for the rate of carotid atherosclerosis progression. CIMT and carotid plaque may play an additive role in scoring systems evaluating CV risk. Thus, it appears reasonable to combine established risk scores with CIMT and plaque imaging. Both in the primary and the secondary care populations of patients, baseline parameters of CIMT and plaque thickness are associated with risk of future CV events. Aggressive medical treatment focused on CV risk factors' elimination is associated with lesser progression of carotid atherosclerosis. However, whether medical interventions have an impact on the decreased risk of CV events through the reduction of CIMT and carotid plaque burden remains a matter of debate and needs further studies.

The authors of this review believe that averaged value of maximum CIMT with inclusion of maximum plaque thickness (when applicable) assessed at both the CCA, the CB, and the ICA is the best way to display atherosclerosis burden, and it well stratifies the CV risk and adverse events incidence both as baseline values and as a serial assessment. However, its clinical appliance should be matter of further investigations.

**Author Contributions:** Conceptualization, A.K.-Z.; methodology, A.K.-Z. and T.P.; writing—original draft preparation, A.K.-Z. and T.P.; writing—review and editing, A.K.-Z.; visualization, A.K.-Z. and T.P.; supervision, T.P.; project administration, A.K.-Z.; funding acquisition, A.K.-Z. All authors have read and agreed to the published version of the manuscript.

**Funding:** This research was funded by the Jagiellonian University Medical College, grant number N41/DBS/000752. This article was supported by the science fund of the John Paul II Hospital, Cracow, Poland (no. FN/22/2021 to A.K.-Z.).

**Institutional Review Board Statement:** Not applicable.

**Informed Consent Statement:** Not applicable.

**Data Availability Statement:** The data presented in this study are available on request from the corresponding author. The data are not publicly available due to privacy.

**Conflicts of Interest:** The authors declare no conflict of interest.

## References

1. World Health Organization. Cardiovascular diseases (CVDs) Fact Sheet. 2021. Available online: https://www.who.int/news-room/fact-sheets/detail/cardiovascular-diseases-(cvds) (accessed on 5 September 2021).
2. Pahwa, R.; Jialal, I. Atherosclerosis. Updated 2021 Aug 11. In *StatPearls [Internet]*; StatPearls Publishing: Treasure Island, FL, USA, 2021.
3. Libby, P.; Ridker, P.M.; Maseri, A. Inflammation and atherosclerosis. *Circulation* **2002**, *105*, 1135–1143. [CrossRef]
4. Kablak-Ziembicka, A.; Przewlocki, T.; Pieniazek, P.; Musialek, P.; Sokolowski, A.; Drwila, R.; Sadowski, J.; Zmudka, K.; Tracz, W. The role of carotid intima-media thickness assessment in cardiovascular risk evaluation in patients with polyvascular atherosclerosis. *Atherosclerosis* **2010**, *209*, 125–130. [CrossRef]
5. Kim, H.; Kim, S.; Han, S.; Rane, P.P.; Fox, K.M.; Qian, Y.; Suh, H.S. Prevalence and incidence of atherosclerotic cardiovascular disease and its risk factors in Korea: A nationwide population-based study. *BMC Public Health* **2019**, *19*, 1112. [CrossRef] [PubMed]
6. Lahoza, C.; Mostazaa, J. M. Atherosclerosis as a Systemic Disease. *Rev. Esp. Cardiol.* **2007**, *60*, 184–195. [CrossRef]
7. De Carlo, M. Chapter: Multisite Artery Disease. In *ESC CardioMed*, 3rd ed.; Camm, A.J., Lüscher, T.F., Maurer, G., Serruys, P.W., Eds.; Oxford University Press: Oxford, UK, 2018; ISBN 9780198784906. [CrossRef]
8. Johri, A.M.; Nambi, V.; Naqvi, T.Z.; Feinstein, S.B.; Kim, E.S.H.; Park, M.M.; Becher, H.; Sillesen, H. Recommendations for the Assessment of Carotid Arterial Plaque by Ultrasound for the Characterization of Atherosclerosis and Evaluation of Cardiovascular Risk: From the American Society of Echocardiography. *J. Am. Soc. Echocardiogr.* **2020**, *33*, 917–933. [CrossRef]
9. Polak, J.F.; O'Leary, D.H.; Kronmal, R.A.; Wolfson, S.K.; Bond, M.G.; Tracy, R.P.; Gardin, J.M.; Kittner, S.J.; Price, T.R.; Savage, P.J. Sonographic evaluation of carotid artery atherosclerosis in the elderly: Relationship of disease severity to stroke and transient ischemic attack. *Radiology* **1993**, *188*, 363–370. [CrossRef] [PubMed]
10. Bots, M.L.; Evans, G.W.; Tegeler, C.H.; Meijer, R. Carotid Intima-media Thickness Measurements: Relations with Atherosclerosis, Risk of Cardiovascular Disease and Application in Randomized Controlled Trials. *Chin. Med. J.* **2016**, *129*, 215–226. [CrossRef] [PubMed]
11. Inaba, Y.; Chen, J.A.; Bergmann, S.R. Carotid plaque, compared with carotid intima-media thickness, more accurately predicts coronary artery disease events: A meta-analysis. *Atherosclerosis* **2012**, *220*, 128–133. [CrossRef] [PubMed]
12. Lorenz, M.W.; von Kegler, S.; Steinmetz, H.; Markus, H.S.; Sitzer, M. Carotid intima-media thickening indicates a higher vascular risk across a wide age range: Prospective data from the Carotid Atherosclerosis Progression Study (CAPS). *Stroke* **2006**, *37*, 87–92. [CrossRef]
13. O'Leary, D.H.; Polak, J.F.; Kronmal, R.A.; Manolio, T.A.; Burke, G.L.; Wolfson, S.K., Jr. Carotid-artery intima and media thickness as a risk factor for myocardial infarction and stroke in older adults: Cardiovascular Health Study Collaborative Research Group. *N. Engl. J. Med.* **1999**, *340*, 14–22. [CrossRef]
14. Salonen, J.T.; Salonen, R. Ultrasound B-mode imaging in observational studies of atherosclerotic progression. *Circulation* **1993**, *87*, II56–II65. [PubMed]
15. Rosvall, M.; Janzon, L.; Berglund, G.; Engstrom, G.; Hedblad, B. Incident coronary events and case fatality in relation to common carotid intima-media thickness. *J. Intern. Med.* **2005**, *257*, 430–437. [CrossRef]
16. Kitamura, A.; Iso, H.; Imano, H.; Ohira, T.; Okada, T.; Sato, S.; Kiyama, M.; Tanigawa, T.; Yamagishi, K.; Shimamoto, T. Carotid intima-media thickness and plaque characteristics as a risk factor for stroke in Japanese elderly men. *Stroke* **2004**, *35*, 2788–2794. [CrossRef] [PubMed]
17. Van der Meer, I.; Bots, M.L.; Hofman, A.; del Sol, A.I.; van der Kuip, D.A.; Witteman, J.C. Predictive value of noninvasive measures of atherosclerosis for incident myocardial infarction: The Rotterdam study. *Circulation* **2004**, *109*, 1089–1094. [CrossRef]
18. Chambless, L.E.; Folsom, A.R.; Clegg, L.X.; Sharrett, A.R.; Shahar, E.; Nieto, F.J.; Rosamond, W.D.; Evans, G. Carotid wall thickness is predictive of incident clinical stroke: The Atherosclerosis Risk in Communities (ARIC) study. *Am. J. Epidemiol.* **2000**, *151*, 478–487. [CrossRef] [PubMed]
19. Chambless, L.E.; Heiss, G.; Folsom, A.R.; Rosamond, W.; Szklo, M.; Sharrett, A.R.; Clegg, L.X. Association of coronary heart disease incidence with carotid arterial wall thickness and major risk factors: The Atherosclerosis Risk in Communities ARIC) study, 1987–1993. *Am. J. Epidemiol.* **1997**, *146*, 483–494. [CrossRef] [PubMed]
20. Bild, D.E.; Bluemke, D.A.; Burke, G.L.; Detrano, R.; Diez Roux, A.V.; Folsom, A.R.; Greenland, P.; Jacob, D.R., Jr.; Kronmal, R.; Liu, K.; et al. Multi-Ethnic Study of Atherosclerosis: Objectives and design. *Am. J. Epidemiol.* **2002**, *156*, 871–881. [CrossRef]
21. Kabłak-Ziembicka, A.; Przewłocki, T.; Sokołowski, A.; Tracz, W.; Podolec, P. Carotid intima-media thickness, hs-CRP and TNF-alpha are independently associated with cardiovascular event risk in patients with atherosclerotic occlusive disease. *Atherosclerosis* **2011**, *214*, 185–190. [CrossRef]
22. Kolkenbeck-Ruh, A.; Woodiwiss, A.J.; Monareng, T.; Sadiq, E.; Mabena, P.; Robinson, C.; Motau, T.H.; Stevens, B.; Manyatsi, N.; Tiedt, S.; et al. Complementary impact of carotid intima-media thickness with plaque in associations with noncardiac arterial vascular events. *Angiology* **2019**, *71*, 122–130. [CrossRef]
23. Yoon, H.J.; Kim, K.H.; Park, H.; Cho, J.Y.; Hong, Y.J.; Park, H.W.; Kim, J.H.; Ahn, Y.; Jeong, M.H.; Cho, S.G.; et al. Carotid plaque rather than intima-media thickness as a predictor of recurrent vascular events in patients with acute ischemic stroke. *Cardiovasc. Ultrasound* **2017**, *15*, 19. [CrossRef]

24. Wrotniak, L.; Kabłak-Ziembicka, A.; Karch, I.; Pieniazek, P.; Rosławiecka, A.; Mleczko, S.; Tekieli, L.; Zmudka, K.; Przewłocki, T. Multiterritory Atherosclerosis and Carotid Intima-Media Thickness as Cardiovascular Risk Predictors After Percutaneous Angioplasty of Symptomatic Subclavian Artery Stenosis. *J. Ultrasound Med.* **2016**, *35*, 1977–1984. [CrossRef]
25. Zielinski, T.; Dzielinska, Z.; Januszewicz, A.; Rynkun, D.; Makowiecka Ciesla, M.; Tyczynski, P.; Prejbisz, A.; Demkow, M.; Kadziela, J.; Naruszewicz, M.; et al. Carotid Intima-Media Thickness as a Marker of Cardiovascular Risk in Hypertensive Patients with Coronary Artery Disease. *Am. J. Hyperten.* **2007**, *20*, 1058–1064. [CrossRef]
26. De Groot, E.; Jukema, J.W.; van Boven, A.J.; Reiber, J.H.; Zwinderman, A.H.; Lie, K.I.; Ackerstaff, R.A.; Bruschke, A.V. Effect of pravastatin on progression and regression of coronary atherosclerosis and vessel wall changes in carotid and femoral arteries: A report from the Regression Growth Evaluation Statin Study. *Am. J. Cardiol.* **1995**, *76*, 40C–46C. [CrossRef]
27. Bots, M.L.; Evans, G.W.; Riley, W.A.; Grobbee, D.E. Carotid intima-media thickness measurements in intervention studies: Design options, progression rates, and sample size considerations: A point of view. *Stroke* **2003**, *34*, 2985–2994. [CrossRef]
28. Taylor, A.J.; Kent, S.M.; Flaherty, P.J.; Coyle, L.C.; Markwood, T.T.; Vernalis, M.N. Arterial Biology for the Investigation of the Treatment Effects of Reducing Cholesterol: A randomized trial comparing the effects of atorvastatin and pravastatin on carotid intima medial thickness. *Circulation* **2002**, *106*, 2055–2060. [CrossRef]
29. Costanzo, P.; Perrone-Filardi, P.; Vassallo, E.; Paolillo, S.; Cesarano, P.; Brevetti, G.; Chiariello, M. Does carotid intima-media thickness regression predict reduction of cardiovascular events? A meta-analysis of 41 randomized trials. *J. Am. Coll. Cardiol.* **2010**, *56*, 2006–2020. [CrossRef] [PubMed]
30. Peters, S.A.; Palmer, M.K.; Grobbee, D.E.; Crouse, J.R., 3rd; Evans, G.W.; Raichlen, J.S.; Bots, M.L.; METEOR Study Group. Effect of number of ultrasound examinations on the assessment of carotid intima-media thickness changes over time: The example of the METEOR study. *J. Hypertens.* **2011**, *29*, 1145–1154. [CrossRef] [PubMed]
31. Furberg, C.D.; Adams, H.P., Jr.; Applegate, W.B.; Byington, R.P.; Espeland, M.A.; Hartwell, T.; Hunninghake, D.B.; Lefkowitz, D.S.; Probstfield, J.; Riley, W.A. Effect of lovastatin on early carotid atherosclerosis and cardiovascular events. Asymptomatic Carotid Artery Progression Study (ACAPS) Research Group. *Circulation* **1994**, *90*, 1679–1687. [CrossRef] [PubMed]
32. Kastelein, J.J.; van Leuven, S.I.; Burgess, L.; Evans, G.W.; Kuivenhoven, J.A.; Barter, P.J.; Revkin, J.H.; Grobbee, D.E.; Riley, W.A.; Shear, C.L.; et al. Designs of RADIANCE 1 and 2: Carotid ultrasound studies comparing the effects of torcetrapib/atorvastatin with atorvastatin alone on atherosclerosis. *Curr. Med. Res. Opin.* **2007**, *23*, 885–894. [CrossRef] [PubMed]
33. Li, H.; Xu, X.; Lu, L.; Sun, R.; Guo, Q.; Chen, Q.; Wang, J.; He, Z.; Zhang, Y. The comparative impact among different intensive statins and combination therapies with niacin/ezetimibe on carotid intima-media thickness: A systematic review, traditional meta-analysis, and network meta-analysis of randomized controlled trials. *Eur. J. Clin. Pharmacol.* **2021**, *77*, 1133–1145. [CrossRef]
34. Kang, S.; Wu, Y.; Li, X. Effects of statin therapy on the progression of carotid atherosclerosis: A systematic review and meta-analysis. *Atherosclerosis* **2004**, *177*, 433–442. [CrossRef] [PubMed]
35. Goldberger, Z.D.; Valle, J.A.; Dandekar, V.K.; Chan, P.S.; Ko, D.T.; Nallamothu, B.K. Are changes in carotid intima-media thickness related to risk of nonfatal myocardial infarction? A critical review and meta-regression analysis. *Am. Heart J.* **2010**, *160*, 701–714. [CrossRef] [PubMed]
36. Lorenz, M.W.; Markus, H.S.; Bots, M.L.; Rosvall, M.; Sitzer, M. Prediction of clinical cardiovascular events with carotid intima-media thickness: A systematic review and meta-analysis. *Circulation* **2007**, *115*, 459–467. [CrossRef] [PubMed]
37. Hodis, H.N.; Mack, W.J.; LaBree, L.; Selzer, R.H.; Liu, C.R.; Liu, C.H.; Azen, S.P. The role of carotid intima-media thickness in predicting clinical coronary events. *Ann. Intern Med.* **1998**, *128*, 262–269. [CrossRef]
38. Okayama, K.I.; Mita, T.; Gosho, M.; Yamamoto, R.; Yoshida, M.; Kanazawa, A.; Kawamori, R.; Fujitani, Y.; Watada, H. Carotid intima-media thickness progression predicts cardiovascular events in Japanese patients with type 2 diabetes. *Diabetes Res. Clin. Pract.* **2013**, *101*, 286–292. [CrossRef]
39. Johnson, H.M.; Douglas, P.S.; Srinivasan, S.R.; Bond, M.G.; Tang, R.; Li, S.; Chen, W.; Berenson, G.S.; Stein, J.H. Predictors of carotid intima-media thickness progression in young adults: The Bogalusa Heart Study. *Stroke* **2007**, *38*, 900–905. [CrossRef]
40. Haberka, M.; Bałys, M.; Matla, M.; Kubicius, A.; Maciejewski, Ł.; Gąsior, Z. Carotid artery stenosis and ultrasound vascular indexes predict the coronary revascularization in patients with high cardiovascular risk scheduled for coronary angiography. *Kardiol. Pol.* **2019**, *77*, 1028–1033. [CrossRef]
41. Rosvall, M.; Persson, M.; Ostling, G.; Nilsson, P.M.; Melander, O.; Hedblad, B.; Engstrom, G. Risk factors for the progression of carotid intima-media thickness over a 16-year follow-up period: The Malmö Diet and Cancer Study. *Atherosclerosis* **2015**, *239*, 615–621. [CrossRef]
42. Olmastroni, E.; Baragetti, A.; Casula, M.; Grigore, L.; Pellegatta, F.; Pirillo, A.; Tragni, E.; Catapano, A.L. Multilevel Models to Estimate Carotid Intima-Media Thickness Curves for Individual Cardiovascular Risk Evaluation. *Stroke* **2019**, *50*, 1758–1765. [CrossRef]
43. Pignoli, P.; Tremoli, E.; Poli, A.; Oreste, P.; Paoletti, R. Intimal plus medial thickness of the arterial wall: A direct measurement with ultrasound imaging. *Circulation* **1986**, *74*, 1399–1406. [CrossRef]
44. Poli, A.; Tremoli, E.; Colombo, A.; Sirtori, M.; Pignoli, P.; Paoletti, R. Ultrasonographic measurement of the common carotid artery wall thickness in hypercholesterolemic patients. A new model for the quantitation and follow-up of preclinical atherosclerosis in living human subjects. *Atherosclerosis* **1988**, *70*, 253–261. [CrossRef]
45. Salonen, J.T.; Seppanen, K.; Rauramaa, R.; Salonen, R. Risk factors for carotid atherosclerosis: The Kuopio Ischaemic Heart Disease Risk Factor Study. *Ann. Med.* **1989**, *21*, 227–229. [CrossRef]

46. Heiss, G.; Sharrett, A.R.; Barnes, R.; Chambless, L.E.; Szklo, M.; Alzola, C. Carotid atherosclerosis measured by B-mode ultrasound in populations: Associations with cardiovascular risk factors in the ARIC study. *Am. J. Epidemiol.* **1991**, *134*, 250–256. [CrossRef]
47. O'Leary, D.H.; Polak, J.F.; Wolfson, S.K., Jr.; Bond, M.G.; Bommer, W.; Sheth, S.; Psaty, B.M.; Sharrett, A.R.; Manolio, T.A. Use of sonography to evaluate carotid atherosclerosis in the elderly. The Cardiovascular Health Study. CHS Collaborative Research Group. *Stroke* **1991**, *22*, 1155–1163. [CrossRef]
48. Lim, T.K.; Lim, E.; Dwivedi, G.; Kooner, J.; Senior, R. Normal value of carotid intima-media thickness–a surrogate marker of atherosclerosis: Quantitative assessment by B-mode carotid ultrasound. *J. Am. Soc. Echocardiogr.* **2008**, *21*, 112–116. [CrossRef] [PubMed]
49. Estíbaliz, J.; Mateo-Gallego, R.; Bea, A.; Burillo, E.; Calmarza, P.; Civeiraa, F. Carotid Intima-Media Thickness in Subjects with No Cardiovascular Risk Factors. *Rev. Esp. Cardiol.* **2010**, *63*, 97–102.
50. Diaz, A.; Bia, D.; Zócalo, Y.; Manterola, H.; Larrabide, I.; Vercio, L.L.; Del Fresno, M.; Fischer, E.F. Carotid Intima Media Thickness Reference Intervals for a Healthy Argentinean Population Aged 11–81 Years. *Int. J. Hypertens.* **2018**, *2018*, 8086714. [CrossRef] [PubMed]
51. Engelen, L.; Ferreira, I.; Stehouwer, C.D.; Boutouyrie, P.; Laurent, S.; on behalf of the Reference Values for Arterial Measurements Collaboration. Reference intervals for common carotid intima-media thickness measured with echotracking: Relation with risk factors. *Eur. Heart J.* **2013**, *34*, 2368–2380. [CrossRef] [PubMed]
52. Randrianarisoa, E.; Rietig, R.; Jacob, S.; Blumenstock, G.; Haering, H.U.; Rittig, K.; Balletshofer, B. Normal values for intima-media thickness of the common carotid artery—An update following a novel risk factor profiling. *Vasa* **2015**, *44*, 444–450. [CrossRef]
53. Piepoli, M.F.; Hoes, A.W.; Agewall, S.; Albus, C.; Brotons, C.; Catapano, A.L.; Cooney, M.T.; Corrà, U.; Cosyns, B.; Deaton, C.; et al. 2016 European Guidelines on cardiovascular disease prevention in clinical practice: The Sixth Joint Task Force of the European Society of Cardiology and Other Societies on Cardiovascular Disease Prevention in Clinical Practice (constituted by representatives of 10 societies and by invited experts): Developed with the special contribution of the European Association for Cardiovascular Prevention & Rehabilitation (EACPR). *Eur. J. Prev. Cardiol.* **2016**, *23*, NP1–NP96.
54. Stein, J.H.; Korcarz, C.E.; Hurst, R.T.; Lonn, E.; Kendall, C.B.; Mohler, E.R.; Najjar, S.S.; Rembold, C.M.; Post, W.S.; American Society of Echocardiography Carotid Intima-Media Thickness Task Force. Use of carotid ultrasound to identify subclinical vascular disease and evaluate cardiovascular disease risk: A consensus statement from the American Society of Echocardiography carotid intima-media thickness task force. Endorsed by the Society for Vascular Medicine. *J. Am. Soc. Echocardiogr.* **2008**, *21*, 93–111.
55. National Cholesterol Education Program (NCEP) Expert Panel (ATP III). Third report of the National Cholesterol Education Program (NCEP) Expert Panel on Detection, Evaluation, and Treatment of High Blood Cholesterol in Adults (Adult Treatment Panel III) final report. *Circulation* **2002**, *106*, 3143–3421. [CrossRef]
56. Peters, S.A.; Den Ruijter, H.M.; Bots, M.L.; Moons, K.G. Improvements in risk stratification for the occurrence of cardiovascular disease by imaging subclinical atherosclerosis: A systematic review. *Heart* **2012**, *98*, 177–184. [CrossRef]
57. Lind, L.; Peters, S.A.; den Ruijter, H.M.; Palmer, M.K.; Grobbee, D.E.; Crouse, J.R., 3rd; O'Leary, D.H.; Evans, G.W.; Raichlen, J.S.; Bots, M.L.; et al. Manual or semi-automated edge detection of the maximal far wall common carotid intima-media thickness: A direct comparison. *J. Intern. Med.* **2012**, *271*, 247–256.
58. Maloberti, A.; Meani, P.; Varrenti, M.; Giupponi, L.; Stucchi, M.; Vallerio, P.; Giannattasio, C. Structural and Functional Abnormalities of Carotid Artery and Their Relation with EVA Phenomenon. *High Blood Press Cardiovasc. Prev.* **2015**, *22*, 373–379. [CrossRef] [PubMed]
59. Touboul, P.J.; Grobbee, D.E.; Den, R.H. Assessment of subclinical atherosclerosis by carotid intima media thickness: Technical issues. *Eur. J. Prev. Cardiol.* **2012**, *19*, 18–24. [CrossRef] [PubMed]
60. 2021 ESC Guidelines on cardiovascular disease prevention in clinical practice: Developed by the Task Force for cardiovascular disease prevention in clinical practice with representatives of the European Society of Cardiology and 12 medical societies With the special contribution of the European Association of Preventive Cardiology (EAPC). *Eur. Heart J.* **2021**, *42*, 3227–3337.
61. Rosławiecka, A.; Kabłak-Ziembicka, A.; Rzeźnik, D.; Pieniążek, P.; Badacz, R.; Trystuła, M.; Przewłocki, T. Determinants of long-term outcome in patients after percutaneous stent-assisted intervention for renal artery steno-occlusive atherosclerotic disease. *Pol. Arch. Intern. Med.* **2019**, *129*, 747–760. [CrossRef]
62. Song, P.; Fang, Z.; Wang, H.; Cai, Y.; Rahimi, K.; Zhu, Y.; Fowkes, F.G.R.; Fowkes, F.J.I.; Rudan, I. Global and regional prevalence, burden, and risk factors for carotid atherosclerosis: A systematic review, meta-analysis, and modelling study. *Lancet Glob. Health* **2020**, *8*, e721–e729. [CrossRef]
63. Puz, P.; Lasek-Bal, A.; Warsz-Wianecka, A.; Kazmierski, M. Prevalence of atherosclerotic stenosis of the carotid and cerebral arteries in patients with stable or unstable coronary artery disease. *Pol. Arch. Intern. Med.* **2020**, *130*, 412–419. [CrossRef]
64. Razzouk, L.; Rockman, C.B.; Patel, M.R.; Guo, Y.; Adelman, M.A.; Riles, T.S.; Berger, J.S. Co-existence of vascular disease in different arterial beds: Peripheral artery disease and carotid artery stenosis—Data from Life Line Screening. *Atherosclerosis* **2015**, *241*, 687–691. [CrossRef] [PubMed]
65. Sirimarco, G.; Amarenco, P.; Labreuche, J.; Touboul, P.J.; Alberts, M.; Goto, S.; Rother, J.; Mas, J.L.; Bhatt, D.L.; Steg, P.G.; et al. Carotid atherosclerosis and risk of subsequent coronary event in outpatients with atherothrombosis. *Stroke* **2013**, *44*, 373–379. [CrossRef] [PubMed]

66. Kabłak-Ziembicka, A.; Przewłocki, T.; Tracz, W.; Pieniążek, P.; Musiałek, P.; Stopa, I.; Zalewski, J.; Zmudka, K. Diagnostic value of carotid intima-media thickness in indicating multi-level atherosclerosis. *Atherosclerosis* **2007**, *193*, 395–400. [CrossRef] [PubMed]
67. Bytyçi, I.; Shenouda, R.; Wester, P.; Henein, M.Y. Carotid Atherosclerosis in Predicting Coronary Artery Disease: A Systematic Review and Meta-Analysis. *Arterioscler. Thromb. Vasc. Biol.* **2021**, *41*, e224–e237. [CrossRef]
68. Stępień, E.; Kabłak-Ziembicka, A.; Musiałek, P.; Tylko, G.; Przewłocki, T. Fibrinogen and carotid intima media thickness determine fibrin density in different atherosclerosis extents. *Int. J. Cardiol.* **2012**, *157*, 411–413. [CrossRef]
69. Bots, M.L.; Witteman, J.C.; Grobbee, D.E. Carotid intima-media wall thickness in elderly women with and without atherosclerosis of the abdominal aorta. *Atherosclerosis* **1993**, *102*, 99–105. [CrossRef]
70. Kabłak-Ziembicka, A.; Przewłocki, T.; Tracz, W.; Podolec, P.; Stopa, I.; Kostkiewicz, M.; Sadowski, J.; Mura, A.; Kopeć, G. Prognostic value of carotid intima-media thickness in detection of coronary atherosclerosis in patients with calcified aortic valve stenosis. *J. Ultrasound Med.* **2005**, *24*, 461–467. [CrossRef]
71. Allan, P.L.; Mowbray, P.I.; Lee, A.J.; Fowkes, F.G. Relationship between carotid intima-media thickness and symptomatic and asymptomatic peripheral arterial disease. The Edinburgh Artery Study. *Stroke* **1997**, *28*, 348–353. [CrossRef]
72. Cohen, G.I.; Aboufakher, R.; Bess, R.; Frank, J.; Othman, M.; Doan, D.; Mesiha, N.; Rosman, H.S.; Szpunar, S. Relationship between carotid disease on ultrasound and disease on CT angiography. *JACC Cardiovasc. Imaging* **2013**, *6*, 1160–1167. [CrossRef]
73. Kabłak-Ziembicka, A.; Przewłocki, T.; Tracz, W.; Pieniążek, P.; Musiałek, P.; Sokołowski, A.; Drwila, R.; Rzeźnik, D. Carotid intima-media thickness in pre- and postmenopausal women with suspected coronary artery disease. *Heart Vessels* **2008**, *23*, 295–300. [CrossRef]
74. Ogata, T.; Yasaka, M.; Yamagishi, M.; Seguchi, O.; Nagatsuka, K.; Minematsu, K. Atherosclerosis found on carotid ultrasonography is associated with atherosclerosis on coronary intravascular ultrasonography. *J. Ultrasound Med.* **2005**, *24*, 469–674. [CrossRef] [PubMed]
75. Ikeda, N.; Kogame, N.; Iijima, R.; Nakamura, M.; Sugi, K. Carotid artery intima-media thickness and plaque score can predict the SYNTAX score. *Eur. Heart J.* **2012**, *33*, 113–119. [CrossRef] [PubMed]
76. Kabłak-Ziembicka, A.; Tracz, W.; Przewłocki, T.; Pieniążek, P.; Sokołowski, A.; Konieczynska, M. Association of increased carotid intima-media thickness with the extent of coronary artery disease. *Heart* **2004**, *90*, 1286–1290. [CrossRef] [PubMed]
77. Bots, M.L.; Hofman, A.; Grobbee, D.E. Common carotid intima-media thickness and lower extremity arterial atherosclerosis. The Rotterdam Study. *Arterioscler. Thromb.* **1994**, *14*, 1885–1891. [CrossRef] [PubMed]
78. Rohani, M.; Jogestrand, T.; Ekberg, M.; van der Linden, J.; Källner, G.; Jussila, R.; Agewall, S. Interrelation between the extent of atherosclerosis in the thoracic aorta, carotid intima-media thickness and the extent of coronary artery disease. *Atherosclerosis* **2005**, *179*, 311–316. [CrossRef]
79. Adams, M.R.; Nakagomi, A.; Keech, A.; Robinson, J.; McCredie, R.; Bailey, B.P.; Freedman, S.B.; Celermajer, D.S. Carotid intima-media thickness is only weakly correlated with the extent and severity of coronary artery disease. *Circulation* **1995**, *92*, 2127–2134. [CrossRef]
80. Azarkish, K.; Mahmoudi, K.; Mohammadifar, M.; Ghajarzadeh, M. Mean right and left carotid intima-media thickness measures in cases with/without coronary artery disease. *Acta Med. Iran.* **2014**, *52*, 884–888.
81. Liu, D.; Du, C.; Shao, W.; Ma, G. Diagnostic Role of Carotid Intima-Media Thickness for Coronary Artery Disease: A Meta-Analysis. *Biomed. Res. Int.* **2020**, *2020*, 9879463. [CrossRef]
82. Ząbczyk, M.; Natorska, J.; Undas, A. Fibrin Clot Properties in Atherosclerotic Vascular Disease: From Pathophysiology to Clinical Outcomes. *J. Clin. Med.* **2021**, *10*, 2999. [CrossRef] [PubMed]
83. Raitakari, O.T.; Juonala, M.; Kähönen, M.; Taittonen, L.; Laitinen, T.; Mäki-Torkko, N.; Järvisalo, M.J.; Uhari, M.; Jokinen, E.; Rönnemaa, T.; et al. Cardiovascular risk factors in childhood and carotid artery intima-media thickness in adulthood: The Cardiovascular Risk in Young Finns Study. *JAMA* **2003**, *290*, 2277–2283. [CrossRef]
84. Jaminon, A.; Reesink, K.; Kroon, A.; Schurgers, L. The Role of Vascular Smooth Muscle Cells in Arterial Remodeling: Focus on Calcification-Related Processes. *Int. J. Mol. Sci.* **2019**, *20*, 5694. [CrossRef]
85. Ji, X.; Leng, X.-Y.; Dong, Y.; Ma, Y.-H.; Xu, W.; Cao, X.-P.; Hou, X.-H.; Qiang Dong, Q.; Lan Tan, L.; Yu, J.-T. Modifiable risk factors for carotid atherosclerosis: A meta-analysis and systematic review. *Ann. Transl. Med.* **2019**, *7*, 632. [CrossRef]
86. Kuo, F.; Gardener, H.; Dong, C.; Cabral, D.; Della-Morte, D.; Blanton, S.H.; Elkind, M.S.V.; Sacco, R.L.; Rundek, T. Traditional Cardiovascular Risk Factors Explain the Minority of the Variability in Carotid Plaque. *Stroke* **2012**, *43*, 1755–1760. [CrossRef]
87. Zyriax, B.C.; Dransfeld, K.; Windler, E. Carotid intima–media thickness and cardiovascular risk factors in healthy volunteers. *Ultrasound J.* **2021**, *13*, 17. [CrossRef]
88. Hou, Q.; Li, S.; Gao, Y.; Tian, H. Relations of lipid parameters, other variables with carotid intima-media thickness and plaque in the general Chinese adults: An observational study. *Lipids Health Dis.* **2018**, *17*, 107. [CrossRef] [PubMed]
89. Iannuzzi, A.; Rubba, P.; Gentile, M.; Mallardo, V.; Calcaterra, I.; Bresciani, A.; Covetti, G.; Cuomo, G.; Merone, P.; Di Lorenzo, A.; et al. Carotid Atherosclerosis, Ultrasound and Lipoproteins. *Biomedicines* **2021**, *9*, 521. [CrossRef]
90. Stamler, J.; Daviglus, M.L.; Garside, D.B.; Dyer, A.R.; Greenland, P.; Neaton, J.D. Relationship of baseline serum cholesterol levels in 3 large cohorts of younger men to long-term coronary, cardiovascular, and all-cause mortality and to longevity. *JAMA* **2000**, *284*, 311–318. [CrossRef]

91. Kabłak-Ziembicka, A.; Przewłocki, T.; Kostkiewicz, M.; Pieniazek, P.; Mura, A.; Podolec, P.; Tracz, W. Relationship between carotid intima-media thickness, atherosclerosis risk factors and angiography findings in patients with coronary artery disease. *Przegl. Lek.* **2003**, *60*, 612–616. [PubMed]
92. Martinez, E.; Martorell, J.; Riambau, V. Review of serum biomarkers in carotid atherosclerosis. *J. Vasc. Surg.* **2020**, *71*, 329–341. [CrossRef]
93. Ravani, A.; Werba, J.P.; Frigerio, B.; Sansaro, D.; Amato, M.; Tremoli, E.; Baldassarre, D. Assessment and relevance of carotid intima-media thickness (C-IMT) in primary and secondary cardiovascular prevention. *Curr. Pharm. Des.* **2015**, *21*, 1164–1171. [CrossRef] [PubMed]
94. D'Agostino, R.B.; Vasan, R.S.; Pencina, M.J.; Wolf, P.A.; Cobain, M.; Massaro, J.M.; Kannel, W.B. General cardiovascular risk profile for use in primary care: The Framingham Heart Study. *Circulation* **2008**, *117*, 743–753. [CrossRef]
95. Eleid, M.F.; Lester, S.J.; Wiedenbeck, T.L.; Patel, S.D.; Appleton, C.P.; Nelson, M.R.; Humphries, J.; Hurst, R.T. Carotid ultrasound identifies high risk subclinical atherosclerosis in adults with low Framingham risk scores. *J. Am. Soc. Echocardiogr.* **2010**, *23*, 802–808. [CrossRef]
96. Nambi, V.; Chambless, L.; Folsom, A.R.; He, M.; Hu, Y.; Mosley, T.; Volcik, K.; Boerwinkle, E.; Ballantyne, C.M. Carotid intima-media thickness and presence or absence of plaque improves prediction of coronary heart disease risk: The ARIC (Atherosclerosis Risk In Communities) study. *J. Am. Coll. Cardiol.* **2010**, *55*, 1600–1607. [CrossRef] [PubMed]
97. Conroy, R.M.; Pyörälä, K.; Fitzgerald, A.P.; Sans, S.; Menotti, A.; De Backer, G.; De Bacquer, D.; Ducimetière, P.; Jousilahti, P.; Keil, U.; et al. Estimation of ten-year risk of fatal cardiovascular disease in Europe: The SCORE project. *Eur. Heart J.* **2003**, *24*, 987–1003. [CrossRef]
98. Assmann, G.; Schulte, H.; Cullen, P.; Seedorf, U. Assessing risk of myocardial infarction and stroke: New data from the Prospective Cardiovascular Munster (PROCAM) study. *Eur. J. Clin. Investig.* **2007**, *37*, 925–932. [CrossRef] [PubMed]
99. Amato, M.; Veglia, F.; de Faire, U.; Giral, P.; Rauramaa, R.; Smit, A.J.; Kurl, S.; Ravani, A.; Frigerio, B.; Sansaro, D.; et al. Carotid plaque-thickness and common carotid IMT show additive value in cardiovascular risk prediction and reclassification. *Atherosclerosis* **2017**, *263*, 412–419. [CrossRef] [PubMed]
100. Mitu, O.; Crisan, A.; Redwood, S.; Cazacu-Davidescu, I.-E.; Mitu, I.; Costache, I.-I.; Onofrei, V.; Miftode, R.-S.; Costache, A.-D.; Haba, C.M.S.; et al. The Relationship between Cardiovascular Risk Scores and Several Markers of Subclinical Atherosclerosis in an Asymptomatic Population. *J. Clin. Med.* **2021**, *10*, 955. [CrossRef] [PubMed]
101. Tunstall-Pedoe, H. Cardiovascular Risk and Risk Scores: ASSIGN, Framingham, QRISK and others: How to choose. *Heart* **2011**, *97*, 442–444. [CrossRef] [PubMed]
102. Gaibazzi, N.; Rigo, F.; Facchetti, R.; Carerj, S.; Giannattasio, C.; Moreo, A.; Mureddu, G.F.; Salvetti, M.; Grolla, E.; Faden, G.; et al. Differential incremental value of ultrasound carotid intima-media thickness, carotid plaque, and cardiac calcium to predict angiographic coronary artery disease across Framingham risk score strata in the APRES multicentre study. *Eur. Heart J. Cardiovasc. Imaging* **2016**, *17*, 991–1000. [CrossRef] [PubMed]
103. Baran, J.; Kleczyński, P.; Niewiara, Ł.; Podolec, J.; Badacz, R.; Gackowski, A.; Pieniążek, P.; Legutko, J.; Żmudka, K.; Przewłocki, T.; et al. Importance of Increased Arterial Resistance in Risk Prediction in Patients with Cardiovascular Risk Factors and Degenerative Aortic Stenosis. *J. Clin. Med.* **2021**, *10*, 2109. [CrossRef]
104. Murakamia, S.; Otsuka, K.; Hotta, N.; Yamanakaa, G.; Kuboa, Y.; Matsuokaa, O.; Yamanakaa, T.; Shinagawaa, M.; Nunodaa, S.; Nishimuraa, Y.; et al. Common carotid intima-media thickness is predictive of all-cause and cardiovascular mortality in elderly community-dwelling people: Longitudinal Investigation for the Longevity and Aging in Hokkaido County (LILAC) study. *Biomed. Pharmacother.* **2005**, *59* (Suppl. 1), S49–S53. [CrossRef]
105. Suzuki, T.; Wang, W.; Wilsdon, A.; Butler, K.R.; Adabag, S.; Griswold, M.E.; Nambi, V.; Rosamond, W.; Sotoodehnia, N.; Mosley, T.H. Carotid Intima-Media Thickness and the Risk of Sudden Cardiac Death: The ARIC Study and the CHS. *J. Am. Heart Assoc.* **2020**, *9*, e016981. [CrossRef] [PubMed]
106. Ali, Y.S.; Rembold, K.E.; Weaver, B.; Wills, M.B.; Tatar, S.; Ayers, C.R.; Rembold, C.M. Prediction of major adverse cardiovascular events by age-normalized carotid intimal medial thickness. *Atherosclerosis* **2006**, *187*, 186–190. [CrossRef] [PubMed]
107. Johnsen, S.H.; Mathiesen, E.B.; Joakimsen, O.; Stensland, E.; Wilsgaard, T.; Løchen, M.L.; Njølstad, I.; Arnesen, E. Carotid atherosclerosis is a stronger predictor of myocardial infarction in women than in men: A 6-year follow-up study of 6226 persons: The Tromso Study. *Stroke* **2007**, *38*, 2873–2880. [CrossRef] [PubMed]
108. Mathiesen, E.B.; Johnsen, S.H.; Wilsgaard, T.; Bønaa, K.H.; Løchen, M.L.; Njølstad, I. Carotid plaque area and intima-media thickness in prediction of first-ever ischemic stroke: A 10-year follow-up of 6584 men and women: The Tromso Study. *Stroke* **2011**, *42*, 972–978. [CrossRef] [PubMed]
109. Romanens, M.; Adams, A.; Sudano, I.; Bojara, W.; Balint, S.; Warmuth, W.; Szucs, T.D. Prediction of cardiovascular events with traditional risk equations and total plaque area of carotid atherosclerosis: The Arteris Cardiovascular Outcome (ARCO) cohort study. *Prev. Med.* **2021**, *147*, 106525. [CrossRef]
110. Rundek, T.; Gardener, H.; Della-Morte, D.; Dong, C.; Cabral, D.; Tiozzo, E.; Roberts, E.; Crisby, M.; Cheung, K.; Demmer, R.; et al. The relationship between carotid intima-media thickness and carotid plaque in the Northern Manhattan Study. *Atherosclerosis* **2015**, *241*, 364–370. [CrossRef] [PubMed]

111. Baber, U.; Mehran, R.; Sartori, S.; Schoos, M.M.; Sillesen, H.; Muntendam, P.; Garcia, M.J.; Gregson, J.; Pocock, S.; Falk, E.; et al. Prevalence, impact, and predictive value of detecting subclinical coronary and carotid atherosclerosis in asymptomatic adults: The BioImage study. *J. Am. Coll. Cardiol.* **2015**, *65*, 1065–1074. [CrossRef]
112. Xie, W.; Liang, L.; Zhao, L.; Shi, P.; Yang, Y.; Xie, G.; Huo, Y.; Wu, Y. Combination of carotid intima-media thickness and plaque for better predicting risk of ischaemic cardiovascular events. *Heart* **2011**, *97*, 1326–1331. [CrossRef] [PubMed]
113. Störk, S.; Feelders, R.A.; van den Beld, A.W.; Steyerberg, E.W.; Savelkoul, H.F.; Lamberts, S.W.; Grobbee, D.E.; Bots, M.L. Prediction of mortality risk in the eldery. *Am. J. Med.* **2006**, *119*, 519–525. [CrossRef]
114. Gepner, A.D.; Young, R.; Delaney, J.A.; Budoff, M.J.; Polak, J.F.; Blaha, M.J.; Post, W.M.; Michos, E.D.; Kaufman, J.; Stein, J.H. Comparison of Carotid Plaque Score and Coronary Artery Calcium Score for Predicting Cardiovascular Disease Events: The Multi-Ethnic Study of Atherosclerosis. *J. Am. Heart Assoc.* **2017**, *6*, e005179. [CrossRef]
115. Prati, P.; Tosetto, A.; Casaroli, M.; Bignamini, A.; Canciani, L.; Bornstein, N.; Prati, G.; Touboul, P.J. Carotid plaque morphology improves stroke risk prediction: Usefulness of a new ultrasonographic score. *Cerebrovasc. Dis.* **2011**, *31*, 300–304. [CrossRef] [PubMed]
116. Henein, M.J.; Faggiano, P.; Vancheri, P. Limited accuracy of carotid progression of intima-media thickness in predicting clinical cardiovascular outcome. *Pol. Arch. Intern. Med.* **2019**, *129*, 1–3. [CrossRef]
117. Cao, J.J.; Arnold, A.M.; Manolio, T.A.; Polak, J.F.; Psaty, B.M.; Hirsch, C.H.; Kuller, L.H.; Cushman, M. Association of carotid artery intima-media thickness, plaques, and C-reactive protein with cardiovascular disease and all-cause mortality: The Cardiovascular Health Study. *Circulation* **2007**, *116*, 32–38. [CrossRef]
118. Baldassarre, D.; Hamsten, A.; Veglia, F.; de Faire, U.; Humphries, S.E.; Smit, A.J.; Giral, P.; Kurl, S.; Rauramaa, R.; Mannarino, E.; et al. Measurements of carotid intima-media thickness and of inter-adventitia common carotid diameter improve prediction of cardiovascular events: Results of the IMPROVE (Carotid Intima Media Thickness [IMT] and IMT-Progression as Predictors of Vascular Events in a High Risk European Population) study. *J. Am. Coll. Cardiol.* **2012**, *60*, 1489–1499.
119. Paraskevas, K.I.; Sillesen, H.H.; Rundek, T.; Mathiesen, E.B.; Spence, J.D. Carotid Intima–Media Thickness Versus Carotid Plaque Burden for Predicting Cardiovascular Risk. *Angiology* **2020**, *71*, 108–111. [CrossRef]
120. Yang, C.H.; Guo, C.Y.; Li, C.-I.; Liu, C.-S.; Lin, C.-H.; Liu, C.-H.; Wang, M.-C.; Yang, S.-Y.; Li, T.-C.; Lin, C.-C. Subclinical Atherosclerosis Markers of Carotid Intima-Media Thickness, Carotid Plaques, Carotid Stenosis, and Mortality in Community-Dwelling Adults. *Int. J. Environ. Res. Public Health* **2020**, *17*, 4745. [CrossRef] [PubMed]
121. Sangiorgi, G.; Bedogni, F.; Sganzerla, P.; Binetti, G.; Inglese, L.; Musialek, P.; Esposito, G.; Cremonesi, A.; Biasi, G.; Jakala, J.; et al. The Virtual histology In CaroTids Observational RegistrY (VICTORY) study: A European prospective registry to assess the feasibility and safety of intravascular ultrasound and virtual histology during carotid interventions. *Int. J. Cardiol.* **2013**, *168*, 2089–2093. [CrossRef]
122. Tada, H.; Nakagawa, T.; Okada, H.; Nakahashi, T.; Mori, M.; Sakata, K.; Nohara, A.; Takamura, M.; Kawashiri, M. Clinical Impact of Carotid Plaque Score rather than Carotid Intima–Media Thickness on Recurrence of Atherosclerotic Cardiovascular Disease Events. *J. Atheroscler. Thromb.* **2020**, *27*, 38–46. [CrossRef]
123. Tadokoro, Y.; Sakaguchi, M.; Yamagami, H.; Okazaki, S.; Furukado, S.; Matsumoto, M.; Miwa, K.; Yagita, Y.; Mochizuki, H.; Kitagawa, K. Echogenicity of medium-to-large carotid plaques predicts future vascular events. *Cerebrovasc. Dis.* **2014**, *38*, 354–361. [CrossRef] [PubMed]
124. Singh, A.S.; Atam, V.; Jain, N.; Yathish, B.E.; Patil, M.R.; Das, L. Association of carotid plaque echogenicity with recurrence of ischemic stroke. *N. Am. J. Med. Sci.* **2013**, *5*, 371–376. [CrossRef]
125. Brinjikji, W.; Rabinstein, A.A.; Lanzino, G.; Murad, M.H.; Williamson, E.E.; DeMarco, J.K.; Huston, J. Ultrasound Characteristics of Symptomatic Carotid Plaques: A Systematic Review and Meta-Analysis. *Cerebrovasc. Dis.* **2015**, *40*, 165–174. [CrossRef]
126. Musiałek, P.; Pieniążek, P.; Tracz, W.; Tekieli, L.; Przewłocki, T.; Kabłak-Ziembicka, A.; Motyl, R.; Moczulski, Z.; Stepniewski, J.; Trystula, M.; et al. Safety of embolic protection device-assisted and unprotected intravascular ultrasound in evaluating carotid artery atherosclerotic lesions. *Med. Sci. Monit.* **2012**, *18*, MT7–MT18. [CrossRef] [PubMed]
127. Badacz, R.; Przewłocki, T.; Gacoń, J.; Stępień, E.; Enguita, F.J.; Karch, I.; Żmudka, K.; Kabłak-Ziembicka, A. Circulating miRNAs levels differ with respect to carotid plaque characteristics and symptom occurrence in patients with carotid artery stenosis and provide information on future cardiovascular events. *Adv. Interv. Cardiol.* **2018**, *14*, 75–84. [CrossRef] [PubMed]
128. Spence, J.D. The importance of distinguishing between diffuse carotid intima medial thickening and focal plaque. *Can. J. Cardiol.* **2008**, *24*, 61C–64C. [CrossRef]
129. Wannarong, T.; Parraga, G.; Buchanan, D.; Fenster, A.; House, A.A.; Hackam, D.G.; Spence, J.D. Progression of Carotid Plaque Volume Predicts Cardiovascular Events. *Stroke* **2013**, *44*, 1859–1865. [CrossRef] [PubMed]
130. Gacoń, J.; Przewłocki, T.; Podolec, J.; Badacz, R.; Pieniążek, P.; Ryniewicz, W.; Żmudka, K.; Kabłak-Ziembicka, A. The role of serial carotid intima-media thickness assessment as a surrogate marker of atherosclerosis control in patients with recent myocardial infarction. *Adv. Interv. Cardiol.* **2019**, *15*, 74–80. [CrossRef] [PubMed]
131. Libby, P.; Buring, J.E.; Badimon, L.; Hansson, G.K.; Deanfield, J.; Bittencourt, M.S.; Tokgözoğlu, L.; Lewis, E.F. Atherosclerosis. *Nat. Rev. Dis. Primers* **2019**, *5*, 56. [CrossRef]
132. Willeit, P.; Tschiderer, L.; Allara, E.; Reuber, K.; Seekircher, L.; Gao, L.; Liao, X.; Lonn, E.; Gerstein, H.C.; Yusuf, S.; et al. Carotid Intima-Media Thickness Progression as Surrogate Marker for Cardiovascular Risk: Meta-Analysis of 119 Clinical Trials Involving 100 667 Patients. *Circulation* **2020**, *142*, 621–642. [CrossRef] [PubMed]

133. Hirano, M.; Nakamura, T.; Kitta, Y.; Takishima, I.; Deyama, J.; Kobayashi, T.; Fujioka, D.; Saito, Y.; Watanabe, K.; Watanabe, Y.; et al. Short-term progression of maximum intima-media thickness of carotid plaque is associated with future coronary events in patients with coronary artery disease. *Atherosclerosis* **2011**, *215*, 507–512. [CrossRef] [PubMed]
134. Gacoń, J.; Przewłocki, T.; Podolec, J.; Badacz, R.; Pieniążek, P.; Mleczko, S.; Ryniewicz, W.; Żmudka, K.; Kabłak-Ziembicka, A. Prospective study on the prognostic value of repeated carotid intima-media thickness assessment in patients with coronary and extra coronary steno-occlusive arterial disease. *Pol. Arch. Intern. Med.* **2019**, *129*, 808–817. [CrossRef]
135. Huang, L.C.; Lin, R.T.; Chen, C.F.; Chen, C.H.; Juo, S.H.; Lin, H.F. Predictors of carotid intima-media thickness and plaque progression in a Chinese population. *J. Atheroscler. Thromb.* **2016**, *23*, 940–949. [CrossRef]
136. Brinjikji, W.; Lehman, V.T.; Kallmes, D.F.; Rabinstein, A.A.; Lanzino, G.; Murad, M.H.; Mulvagh, S.; Klaas, J.; Graff-Radford, J.; DeMarco, K.J.; et al. The effects of statin therapy on carotid plaque composition and volume: A systematic review and meta-analysis. *J. Neuroradiol.* **2017**, *44*, 234–240. [CrossRef] [PubMed]
137. Society of Atherosclerosis Imaging and Prevention Developed in collaboration with the International Atherosclerosis Society. Appropriate use criteria for carotid intima media thickness testing. *Atherosclerosis* **2011**, *214*, 43–46. [CrossRef] [PubMed]
138. Lorenz, M.W.; Polak, J.F.; Kavousi, M.; Mathiesen, E.B.; Völzke, H.; Tuomainen, T.P.; Sander, D.; Plichart, M.; Catapano, A.L.; Robertson, C.M.; et al. Carotid intima-media thickness progression to predict cardiovascular events in the general population (the PROG-IMT collaborative project): A meta-analysis of individual participant data. *Lancet* **2012**, *379*, 2053–2062. [CrossRef]
139. Wu, Y.; Lu, X.; Zhang, L.; Cheng, X.; Yuan, L.; Xie, M.; Lv, Q. Correlation between carotid intima-media roughness and cardiovascular risk factors. *Exp. Ther. Med.* **2019**, *18*, 49–56. [CrossRef] [PubMed]
140. Greenland, P.; Alpert, J.S.; Beller, G.A.; Benjamin, E.J.; Budoff, M.J.; Fayad, Z.A.; Foster, E.; Hlatky, M.A.; Hodgson, J.M.; Kushner, F.G.; et al. 2010 ACCF/AHA Guideline for assessment of cardiovascular risk in asymptomatic adults: A report of the American College of Cardiology Foundation/American Heart Association task force on practice guidelines developed in collaboration with the American Society of Echocardiography, American Society of Nuclear Cardiology, Society of Atherosclerosis Imaging and Prevention, Society for Cardiovascular Angiography and Interventions, Society of Cardiovascular Computed Tomography, and Society for Cardiovascular Magnetic Resonance. *J. Am. Coll. Cardiol.* **2010**, *56*, e50–e103.

Article

# Small Differences in Vitamin D Levels between Male Cardiac Patients in Different Stages of Coronary Artery Disease

Ewelina A. Dziedzic [1,*], William B. Grant [2], Izabela Sowińska [3], Marek Dąbrowski [4] and Piotr Jankowski [5,6]

1. Medical Faculty, Lazarski University in Warsaw, 02-662 Warsaw, Poland
2. Sunlight, Nutrition, and Health Research Center, P.O. Box 641603, San Francisco, CA 94164-1603, USA; wbgrant@infionline.net
3. Medical Faculty, Medical University of Warsaw, 02-091 Warsaw, Poland; sowinska.izabela@gmail.com
4. Department of Cardiology, Bielanski Hospital, 01-809 Warsaw, Poland; mardab@wp.pl
5. Department of Internal Medicine and Geriatric Cardiology, Centre of Postgraduate Medical Education, 01-813 Warsaw, Poland; piotrjankowski@interia.pl
6. Institute of Cardiology, Jagiellonian University Medical College, 31-008 Krakow, Poland
* Correspondence: ewelinadziedzic82@gmail.com; Tel.: +48-792207779

**Abstract:** Cardiovascular diseases are the main cause of mortality in males older than 65 years of age. The prevalent vitamin D deficiency in the worldwide population may have multiple effects on the cardiovascular system. This study sought to determine the association between serum levels of 25-hydroxyvitamin D (25(OH)D) and the stage of coronary artery disease (CAD) in Polish male subjects. Additionally, subjects with a history of myocardial infarction (MI) were analyzed for potential differences in 25(OH)D levels in comparison with those diagnosed with stable CAD. The study was conducted prospectively in a group of 669 male patients subjected to coronarography examination. CAD stage was defined using the Coronary Artery Surgery Study Score. Patients without significant coronary lesions had significantly higher 25(OH)D levels than patients with single-, double-, or triple-vessel disease (median, 17 vs. 15 ng/mL; $p < 0.01$). Significantly lower levels of 25(OH)D were apparent when MI was identified as the cause of the then-current hospitalization in comparison with stable CAD, as well as in patients with a history of MI; all of these cases had lower levels of 25(OH)D in comparison with patients with no such history. Male patients with single-, double-, or triple-vessel CAD, acute coronary syndrome, or a history of MI presented lower serum 25(OH)D.

**Keywords:** vitamin D; coronary artery disease; myocardial infarction; males; Coronary Artery Surgery Study Score

## 1. Introduction

The aging of the worldwide population is being observed in recent decades. Consequently, the subpopulation of male individuals older than 65 years in Poland has gradually increased [1–4]. In this group of patients, cardiovascular diseases account for more than half of all deaths [5]. Despite the observed improvement concerning mortality rates, a large difference between the average male and female lifespans persisted (73 and 81 years, respectively) [5]. Elderly men should be considered a unique group of patients liable to major cardiovascular events. Considering exceedingly high rates of the risk of death, cardiovascular diseases (CVDs) continue to prompt the need for the relentless investigation of their risk factors and new therapies [6]. As a result of advancements in treatment, including non-pharmacological prevention, the risk of death from CVDs has dropped by 20% over the last few decades [7]. Despite these improvements, CVD remains responsible for about 18 billion deaths per year, the majority of which are a consequence of myocardial infarction or stroke [8]. Appropriate physical activity and dietary interventions both reduce the cardiovascular risk [9,10] and affect the level of 25-hydroxyvitamin D. Notably, calcitriol deficiency is identified as one of the new cardiovascular disease risk factors and has been proven to be prevalent in human populations worldwide [11–13].

The discovery of the biological mechanisms underlying vitamin D effects justifies studies of the association between its deficiency and the risk of cardiovascular diseases. The 1,25-dihydroxyvitamin D (calcitriol) receptor is present in numerous cells of the cardiovascular system [14]. Studies conducted on an animal model have shown an adverse effect of vitamin D deficiency on the functions of endothelial cells, vascular smooth muscle, and cardiomyocytes [14]. Due to the presence of the enzyme 1-α hydroxylase, these cells are capable of autocrine calcitriol synthesis [15,16]. This hormone is a negative regulator of the axis of the renin–angiotensin–aldosterone system, the increased activity of which leads to the development of arterial hypertension and myocardial hypertrophy [17–19]. The relationship between calcitriol deficiency and individual stages of plaque formation and destabilization, as well as documented risk factors for coronary artery disease, has been documented [13,20].

To date, the results of studies do not offer an explicit agreement on how vitamin D affects the cardiovascular system [21]. However, some reports suggest that 25(OH)D levels below the reference range may increase the risk of CVD [21], whereas optimum levels may exert a protective effect on both musculoskeletal and cardiovascular systems [21–23]. The main objective of this study was to assess the potential association between serum 25(OH)D levels and the stage of coronary artery disease (CAD) in Polish males.

## 2. Materials and Methods

### 2.1. Population

This study is part of a research project focused on the relationship between the level of vitamin D and the severity of coronary artery atherosclerosis in Polish cardiac patients. Results of the analysis of this association among 637 patients are presented in previously published articles, in which details of the study population and measurements (diabetes diagnosis, acute coronary syndrome (ACS) diagnosis, interview questionnaire, body mass index (BMI), concentration of total cholesterol (TC) and/or triglycerides (TG), systolic and diastolic blood pressure, coronary angiography, and total 25(OH)D in participant serum and plasma) were described [24–26]. Abnormal serum levels of phosphate, calcium and parathyroid hormone (PTH) treatments, or supplementation containing vitamin D or calcium served as exclusion criteria. Patients with stages III-V chronic kidney disease, active malignancy, and elevated inflammatory markers or fever were also excluded from the study. New patients were continuously examined, and final pooled data of Polish patients hospitalized in the Cardiology Department who underwent diagnostic catheter angiography for the evaluation of coronary artery disease in the years 2013 to 2017 were presented in the most previous study [27]. This study presents data for male patients.

The serum level of 25(OH)D was determined with the Vitamin D total assay by Roche Diagnostics, certified by VDSP. The Roche Diagnostics Vitamin D total assay is a competitive electrochemiluminescence protein-binding assay intended for the quantitative determination of the total 25-OH vitamin D in human serum and plasma. The assay utilizes a vitamin-D-binding protein (VDBP) as the capture protein, which binds to both 25-OH D3 and 25-OH D2 [28].

The status of vitamin D levels was classified according to the Endocrine Society Clinical Practice Guidelines for Vitamin D Deficiency [29]: 25(OH)D level <10 ng/mL was considered as a severe deficiency; $\geq$10 to <20 ng/mL as a moderate deficiency; $\geq$20 to <30 ng/mL as a mild deficiency; $\geq$30 ng/mL as optimal.

Coronary atherosclerosis was assessed by Coronary Artery Surgery Study Score (CASSS) according to the following rules [30]. Stenosis $\geq$50% of the left main coronary artery (LMCA) was scored at 2 points. Stenosis >70% in any of the large epicardial coronary arteries (anterior descending branch, LAD; circumflex branch, LCx; right coronary artery, RCA) was scored at 1 point. The sum of all points equaled the score, which may indicate, respectively a one-, two-, or three-vessel CAD [30].

The study project was approved by the University Bioethical Committee (KB/124/2014) and followed the rules and principles of the Helsinki Declaration.

## 2.2. Statistics

The Shapiro–Wilk test was used to evaluate the normal distribution of data. The Poisson regression analysis was used to assess the relationship between 25(OH)D levels and selected variables. To compare the results of continuous variables between the two groups, the Mann–Whitney test or $t$-test was used. For comparisons of three or more independent groups, the Kruskal–Wallis test or one-way analysis of variance were used, depending on the presence of a Gaussian distribution (Shapiro–Wilk normality test). Pearson's chi-squared test or Fisher's exact test was used to determine differences between prevalence in selected groups. Statistical analyses were performed with a significance level of 5% ($p$ value < 0.05). The statistical analysis was carried out with STATISTICA 12.5 software.

## 3. Results

### 3.1. Characteristics of the Study Group

The study was conducted on 1345 patients admitted to the Department of Cardiology in the Bielanski Hospital in Warsaw (Poland) for coronarographic examination as a result of suspected CAD as identified in an outpatient setting. Final statistical analysis was carried out in 1043 patients (669 males, 374 females). The data of 302 subjects were excluded, as they met the study exclusion criteria (for details, see [27]).

### 3.2. Comparisons between Female and Male Subpopulations

Statistically significant differences were observed between females and males with regard to age, total cholesterol, high-density lipoprotein (HDL) cholesterol, and low-density lipoprotein (LDL) cholesterol levels. Statistically significant disproportions were observed between the female and male subpopulations with regard to smoking status, history of myocardial infarction, and the number of arteries presenting with significant stenosis (Table 1).

**Table 1.** Results between female and male subpopulations.

| Variable | Females | Males | p |
|---|---|---|---|
| N | 374 | 669 | N/A |
| Age (years) | 70 ± 11 | 65 ± 11 | <0.001 |
| Body mass index (kg/m$^2$) | 28 ± 5 | 28 ± 5 | 0.75 |
| Body mass index class (1/2/3) [†] | 100/120/131 | 156/274/197 | <0.05 |
| Diabetes (No/Yes/Prediabetes) | 242/120/12 | 418/225/26 | 0.72 |
| Total cholesterol (mg/Dl) | 189 ± 49 | 172 ± 46 | <0.001 |
| High-density lipoprotein (mg/dL) | 55 ± 16 | 46 ± 14 | <0.001 |
| Low-density lipoprotein (mg/dL) | 108 ± 44 | 100 ± 41 | <0.01 |
| Triglycerides (mg/dL) | 129 ± 57 | 130 ± 74 | 0.82 |
| Hyperlipidemia (No/Yes) | 131/218 | 265/348 | 0.08 |
| Hypertension (No/Yes) | 57/317 | 124/545 | 0.18 |
| Smoking (No/Yes/Ex) | 272/72/30 | 371/221/77 | <0.001 |
| History of myocardial infarction (No/Yes) | 254/120 | 389/280 | <0.01 |
| Cause of hospitalization (0/1) [‡] | 232/141 | 389/277 | 0.23 |
| Coronary Artery Surgery Study Score (0/1/2/3) | 142/96/74/62 | 126/180/208/155 | <0.001 |

Table 1. Cont.

| Variable | Females | Males | p |
|---|---|---|---|
| Level of 25-hydroxyvitamin D (ng/mL (range)) | 14 (4–55) | 16 (4–48) | 0.07 |
| 25(OH)D level (1/2/3/4) ** | 101/168/76/29 | 128/357/149/35 | <0.01 |
| Season (October–April/May–September) | 291/83 | 494/175 | 0.16 |

25(OH)D = 25-hydroxyvitamin D; BMI, body mass index; CASSS, Coronary Artery Surgery Study Score; HDL, high-density lipoprotein; LDL, low-density lipoprotein. † BMI class 1, <25; class 2, 25–30; class 3, >30; ‡ 0, stable coronary artery disease; 1, myocardial infarction; ** 1: <10 ng/mL severe deficiency, 2: ≥10 to <20 ng/mL moderate deficiency, 3: ≥20 to <30 ng/mL mild deficiency, 4: ≥30 ng/mL optimal.

Statistically significant differences were observed between females and males with regard to age, total cholesterol, high-density lipoprotein (HDL) cholesterol, and low-density lipoprotein (LDL) cholesterol levels. Statistically significant disproportions were observed between the female and male subpopulations with regard to smoking status, history of myocardial infarction, and the number of arteries presenting with significant stenosis.

### 3.3. Analysis of Male Subpopulation, Correlation between 25(OH)D Levels or Other Parameters, and the CASSS Stage of Coronary Artery Disease in Male Subpopulation

Among male patients divided into individual CASSS severity groups (Table 2), analysis of variance revealed statistically significant differences in age, total cholesterol levels, HDL cholesterol levels, and LDL cholesterol levels.

Table 2. Characteristics of the examined group divided according to degree of coronary atherosclerosis (the Coronary Artery Surgery Study Score (CASSS)) into four subgroups.

| Variable | CASSS 0 | CASSS 1 | CASSS 2 | CASSS 3 | p |
|---|---|---|---|---|---|
| N | 126 | 180 | 208 | 155 | |
| Age (years) | 64 ± 11 | 64 ± 12 | 64 ± 10 | 68 ± 10 | <0.001 |
| Body mass index (kg/m$^2$) | 29 ± 6 | 28 ± 5 | 28 ± 5 | 28 ± 5 | 0.07 |
| Body mass index class (1/2/3) † | 30/45/47 | 38/71/53 | 49/93/55 | 39/65/42 | 0.50 |
| Diabetes (No/Yes/Prediabetes) | 88/34/4 | 122/52/6 | 123/73/12 | 85/66/4 | <0.05 |
| Total cholesterol (mg/dL) | 180 ± 45 | 176 ± 44 | 171 ± 49 | 163 ± 45 | <0.05 |
| High-density lipoprotein (mg/dL) | 52 ± 18 | 46 ± 13 | 46 ± 13 | 43 ± 12 | <0.001 |
| Low-density lipoprotein (mg/dL) | 104 ± 38 | 105 ± 40 | 100 ± 43 | 92 ± 39 | <0.05 |
| Triglycerides (mg/dL) | 124 ± 68 | 127 ± 66 | 130 ± 68 | 137 ± 93 | 0.54 |
| Hyperlipidemia (No/Yes) | 43/66 | 61/107 | 90/103 | 71/71 | 0.07 |
| Hypertension (No/Yes) | 34/92 | 36/144 | 29/179 | 25/130 | <0.05 |
| Smoking (No/Yes/Ex) | 88/26/12 | 90/74/16 | 104/72/32 | 89/49/17 | <0.01 |
| History of myocardial infarction (No/Yes) | 115/11 | 112/68 | 96/112 | 66/89 | <0.001 |
| Cause of hospitalization (0/1) ‡ | 113/13 | 86/93 | 115/91 | 75/80 | <0.001 |
| Level of 25-hydroksyvitamin D (ng/mL (range)) | 17 (5–47) | 15 (4–48) | 15 (4–37) | 15 (4–43) | 0.05 |
| 25(OH)D level (1/2/3/4) ** | 19/64/35/8 | 36/102/32/10 | 35/124/41/8 | 38/67/41/9 | 0.08 |
| Season (October–April/May–September) | 96/30 | 129/51 | 157/51 | 112/43 | 0.73 |

25(OH)D = 25-hydroxyvitamin D; BMI, body mass index; CASSS, Coronary Artery Surgery Study Score; HDL, high-density lipoprotein; LDL, low-density lipoprotein. † BMI class 1: <25; class 2: 25–30; class: 3 >30; ‡ 0, stable coronary artery disease; 1, myocardial infarction; ** 1: <10 ng/mL severe deficiency, 2: ≥10 to <20 ng/mL moderate deficiency, 3: ≥20 to <30 ng/mL mild deficiency, 4: ≥30 ng/mL optimal.

Post hoc analyses in unequal subgroup populations revealed that CASSS 3 patients were significantly older than patients in all other CASSS groups ($p < 0.01$ for all comparisons). Individual subgroups of patients with different CASSS scores were characterized by statistically significant differences in the prevalence of diabetes, hypertension, smoking, history of myocardial infarction, or the cause of the then ongoing hospitalization.

No significant differences were observed in 25(OH)D levels, BMI values, or triglyceride levels between patients across all CASSS groups. Neither could significant differences be observed in the prevalence of hyperlipidemia or the season of examination between individual CASSS groups.

Poisson distribution and multiple regression analysis were used to identify factors that significantly determined the CASSS in the male population. Factors/determinants in the analysis included serum 25(OH)D levels, age, BMI, smoking status, hypertension, concomitant diabetes, hyperlipidemia, history of myocardial infarction, cause of the then-current hospitalization, and season during the examination. Factors significantly determining the CASSS value included age ($p < 0.05$), cause of ongoing hospitalization ($p < 0.001$), smoking status ($p < 0.05$), and history of myocardial infarction ($p < 0.001$).

### 3.4. Male Patients without Significant Arterial Stenosis (CASSS 0) in Comparison with Patients with Significant Arterial Stenosis (CASSS 1–3)

The group of patients without significant changes within the coronary arteries (CASSS 0) presented with higher 25(OH)D levels than patients with single-, double-, or triple-vessel disease (CASSS 1, 2, or 3, respectively). Considering the above, we carried out further analyses with the study population divided into two subgroups: the CASSS 0 subgroup and the CASSS 1–3 subgroup (Table 3).

**Table 3.** Characteristics of the examined group divided according to degree of coronary atherosclerosis (CASSS) into two subgroups.

| Variable | CASSS 0 | CASSS 1–3 | p |
|---|---|---|---|
| N | 126 | 543 | |
| Age (years] | 64 ± 11 | 65 ± 11 | 0.78 |
| Body mass index (kg/m$^2$) | 29 ± 5 | 28 ± 5 | <0.01 |
| Body mass index class (1/2/3) [†] | 30/45/47 | 126/229/150 | 0.13 |
| Diabetes (No/Yes/Prediabetes) | 88/34/4 | 330/191/22 | 0.17 |
| Total cholesterol (mg/dL) | 180 ± 45 | 170 ± 46 | <0.05 |
| High-density lipoprotein (mg/dL) | 52 ± 18 | 45 ± 13 | <0.001 |
| Low-density lipoprotein (mg/dL) | 104 ± 38 | 99 ± 41 | 0.28 |
| Triglycerides (mg/dL) | 124 ± 68 | 131 ± 75 | 0.38 |
| Hyperlipidemia (No/Yes) | 43/66 | 222/282 | 0.38 |
| Hypertension (No/Yes) | 34/92 | 90/453 | <0.01 |
| Smoking (No/Yes/Ex) | 88/26/12 | 283/195/65 | <0.01 |
| History of myocardial infarction (No/Yes) | 115/11 | 274/269 | <0.001 |
| Cause of hospitalization (0/1) [‡] | 113/13 | 276/264 | <0.001 |
| Level of 25-hydroxyvitamin D (ng/mL (range)) | 17 (5–47) | 15 (4–48) | <0.01 |
| 25(OH)D level (1/2/3/4) ** | 19/64/35/8 | 109/293/114/27 | 0.26 |
| Season (October–April/May–September) | 96/30 | 398/145 | 0.51 |

[†] BMI class 1 < 25; class 2 25–30; class 3 > 30; [‡] 0, stable coronary artery disease; 1, myocardial infarction; ** 1: <10 ng/mL severe deficiency, 2: ≥10 to <20 ng/mL moderate deficiency, 3: ≥20 to <30 ng/mL mild deficiency, 4: ≥30 ng/mL optimal.

Statistically significant differences were observed between male patients with and without significant coronary stenosis with regard to serum 25(OH)D, BMI values, total cholesterol levels, and HDL cholesterol levels.

Statistically significant disproportions were observed between subgroups with regard to arterial hypertension status, smoking status, history of myocardial infarction, and cause of the then ongoing hospitalization.

Only 13 patients from the CASSS 0 subgroup were hospitalized for myocardial infarction; the remaining 113 subjects were hospitalized as a result of stable CAD. In addition, 11 patients in the CASSS 0 subgroup had a history of myocardial infarction. About half of the patients from the CASSS 1–3 subgroup were hospitalized for myocardial infarction; about half also had a history of myocardial infarction.

Factors significantly determining the CASSS value in the entire male subpopulation included age ($p < 0.05$), cause of the then-current hospitalization ($p < 0.001$), smoking status ($p < 0.05$), and history of myocardial infarction ($p < 0.001$). Among the CASSS 1–3 subgroup of male patients, larger percentages of patients had arterial hypertension, were smokers, had a history of myocardial infarction, and reported to the department because of an acute coronary syndrome rather than stable CAD.

*3.5. Determinants of Serum 25(OH)D Levels in Male Cardiac Patients*

In the presented study group, significant determinants of serum 25(OH)D levels included the season of the year ($p < 0.001$) and hyperlipidemia ($p < 0.01$). Lower serum 25(OH)D levels were presented independently by patients with hyperlipidemia and those examined between October and April.

*3.6. Identifying the Group with the Lowest 25(OH)D Levels among Male Cardiac Patients*

Factors significantly determining the CASSS value included age ($p < 0.05$), cause of the then-ongoing hospitalization ($p < 0.001$), smoking status ($p < 0.05$), and history of myocardial infarction ($p < 0.001$). The lowest serum 25(OH)D levels were measured in elderly male cardiac patients hospitalized for an acute coronary syndrome, presenting with a history of myocardial infarction, positive smoking status, and diagnosis of hyperlipidemia, as well as undergoing examination between October and April.

### 4. Discussion

Cardiovascular diseases are ranked as the main cause of death in male patients aged over 65 years old, remaining the second in younger individuals [8]. Mortality rates due to CVD for males are higher than those for females [31]. To date, numerous studies suggested a correlation between low 25(OH)D levels and increased risk of death from cardiovascular causes was suggested [32,33]. The aim of our research was to assess the association between vitamin D serum levels the severity of CAD.

The findings of this research are consistent with the results of previous studies examining the association between serum 25(OH)D levels and CVD [12]. However, only a few studies thus far were conducted in male subpopulations only; most were carried out in mixed-sex populations [34–38]. In our study, male patients without significant coronary lesions (CASSS 0) presented with statistically higher serum vitamin D levels than patients with significant stenosis of coronary arteries (CASSS 1–3); however, the nominal difference was negligible. We showed that calcitriol serum levels were significantly lower in patients with a history of MI. Elderly patients with hyperlipidemia, actively smoking, hospitalized for an ACS, with a history of MI, were a subgroup presenting with the lowest 25(OH)D serum levels.

The impact of serum vitamin D level on the established cardiovascular risk factors (i.e., development of type 2 diabetes, metabolic syndrome) was repeatedly proven in the literature [39,40].

Both nuclear vitamin D receptor (VDR) and the enzyme 25-hydroxyvitamin D3-1α-hydroxylase have been identified in various cells of the cardiovascular system, indicating a direct involvement of this hormone group in the initiation and progression of CVD [41]. Importantly, in patients with heart failure, atrial fibrillation, or coronary artery disease vitamin D deficiency was associated with a worse prognosis [42–44]. Moreover, hypovitaminosis D was proven to affect the established cardiovascular risk factors such as arterial hypertension [45], type 2 diabetes [44], or dyslipidemia [44]. Calcitriol inhibits the renin-angiotensin–aldosterone system (RAAS) and the secretion of natriuretic peptides, thus having a hypotensive effect [46]. Activation of the VDR receptor has a protective effect on the excess of angiotensin II by inhibiting fibrosis and exerting anti-inflammatory and antiproliferative effects [47]. Mediated by cells of the immune system, calcitriol modulates the secretion of miR-106b-5p and inhibits the secretion of renin by the glomerular apparatus [48]. The impact of vitamin D on various stages of atherosclerosis is currently being a subject of some studies [13]. Previous studies demonstrated that vitamin D affects atherosclerotic plaque formation in numerous ways, including reducing the inflammatory response, inhibiting the NF-κB pathway [49], and suppressing the post-infarction scar formation [50]. Proper serum 25(OH)D level was proven to reduce the activity of the metalloproteinases, which degrade the fibrous cap of the atherosclerotic plaque [51]. In addition, vitamin D also inhibits the activity of vascular endothelial growth factors, preventing the formation of new vessels within an already formed plaque, thus contributing to its better stability [52]. After plaque rupture, vitamin D exerts an antithrombotic effect by increasing the production of thrombomodulin and reducing the expression of platelet tissue factors. Hence, it inhibits the adhesion of platelets to vascular endothelial cells [53]. This process may be a way of vitamin D contributing to the prevention of ACS.

A study based on an analysis of more than 1000 Polish patients confirmed the already reported low vitamin D levels in the Polish population [54,55], as well as the higher 25(OH)D levels in males than in females [26]. On the other hand, Verdoia emphasizes the importance of higher 25(OH)D levels noted in men, compared with women [56]. The results of that study provided a stimulus to expand the research and reassess how 25(OH)D levels affect the stage of CAD and incidence of MI in the entirely male cohort. The results of the above-mentioned studies stimulated us to evaluate the impact of 25(OH)D levels on the stage of coronary artery disease and the incidence of MI in an all-male cohort. The influence of vitamin D deficiency on episodes of MI in men is supported by several cohort studies [57,58]. Patients with 25(OH)D levels of ≤15 ng/mL were proven to have a more than 1.5-fold increase in the risk of adverse cardiovascular events (i.e., MI, angina pectoris, stroke, TIA, and heart failure) [57] and a twofold increase in the risk of ACS [58]. Moreover, low vitamin D levels and a history of MI were associated with a significant increase in the risk of further major adverse cardiovascular events (MACE), including reoccurrence of MI [37]. In addition, serum 25 (OH) D levels above 7.3 ng/mL were associated with a 40% reduction in the risk of non-fatal MACE in patients with ACS.

To date, several studies examining vitamin D supplementation in patients with CVD have been conducted. Although none of the large cohort studies showed a favorable cardiovascular outcome, individual experiments have proven that six-month calcitriol supplementation significantly reduced the inflammation of coronary arteries [59] and declined SYNTAX score (67). However, poor bioavailability and large intervals between consecutive doses of cholecalciferol should be underlined as potentially resolvable issues [59]. Another possible mechanism by which vitamin D may affect the degree of progression of coronary disease is its effect on the metabolism of sex hormones. In the MESA study, lower 25(OH)D levels were found to be associated with lower sex-hormone-binding globulin concentrations and higher levels of free testosterone, which are important in the course of coronary artery disease [60].

Our research suffers from several limitations. The study group consisted of residents of only central Poland, most residing in urban areas. Expanding the study group to include residents of other provinces would facilitate the translation of the results to the entire Polish population. CAD staging was classified based on the results of coronary angiography using the CASSS. The classification of the severity of atherosclerosis based on the SYNTAX might change our results.

The results of the observational studies carried out so far have shown that the endocrine system of vitamin D, in addition to its documented effect on the skeletal system, exerts a wide spectrum of extra-skeletal activity [61,62]. In these studies, low vitamin D levels were found to be associated with an increased risk of cardiovascular diseases, including hypertension, congestive heart failure, as well as adverse cardiovascular events (MACE, heart attacks, and strokes). In a meta-analysis involving nearly 850,000 people, low serum 25(OH)D levels were associated with a 1.42 times higher risk of developing MACE, compared with patients with higher levels of vitamin D [63]. On the other hand, the results of randomized clinical trials (VITAL, ViDa, D2d), which included over 30,000 participants, showed that supplementation with vitamin D does not prevent cardiovascular events or the progression of type 2 diabetes [64–66]. It should be emphasized that the initial serum level of 25 (OH) D in the respondents of the above-mentioned studies fluctuated above 50 nmol/L, and post hoc analysis suggested some extra-skeletal benefits in the vitamin D deficiency group. The causal association between calcitriol and cardiovascular mortality continues to be the subject of much debate. New information was provided by the recently presented results of the non-linear MR analysis carried out at UK Biobank [67]. The authors of the cited study presented the association between the genetically predicted serum 25 (OH) D levels and the risk of cardiovascular diseases to be L shaped. This research seems to confirm the results of observational and interventional studies and determines a specific range of vitamin D levels within which vitamin D supplementation may have a beneficial effect in short- and long-term observations. At the same time, it explains why supplementing people rich in vitamin D does not generate overall health benefits, and correction of a severe deficiency of this hormone may be necessary. At present, the opinions of scientists around the world unanimously recommend the correction of vitamin D (25 (OH) D serum deficiency <30 nmol/L), and most scientific societies recommend a target level of >50 nmol/L as optimal for bone health. In our opinion, vitamin D deficiency may also be an easily modifiable risk factor of the acute coronary syndrome in men, which should undoubtedly be the subject of further research. Perhaps, well-designed and conducted social campaigns in the field of proper exposure to solar radiation, food fortification, or pharmacological supplementation of vitamin D could considerably contribute to the prevention of CAD and its complications.

## 5. Conclusions

In conclusion, we demonstrated that male patients with a history of ACS and MI presented reduced serum calcitriol levels. Patients with advanced CAD presented with significantly lower levels of 25(OH)D than those without significant atherosclerotic lesions; however, the difference should be considered as clinically negligible. Further studies should be undertaken in specific subgroups, to assess the potential beneficial effects of vitamin D supplementation in this group of patients.

**Author Contributions:** Conceptualization, E.A.D.; methodology, E.A.D.; formal analysis, E.A.D.; investigation, E.A.D.; resources, E.A.D.; data curation, E.A.D.; writing—original draft preparation, E.A.D., W.B.G., I.S., M.D. and P.J.; writing—review and editing, E.A.D., W.B.G., I.S., M.D. and P.J.; funding acquisition, E.A.D. All authors have read and agreed to the published version of the manuscript.

**Funding:** This research was partly supported by a statutory grant to the Cardiology Clinic of Physiotherapy Division from the Second Faculty of Medicine, Medical University of Warsaw, Poland Grant Number 2F5/PM2/16. The APC was funded by the Medical University of Warsaw.

**Institutional Review Board Statement:** The study was conducted according to the guidelines of the Declaration of Helsinki and approved by the Bioethical Committee of Medical University (KB/124/2014).

**Informed Consent Statement:** Informed consent was obtained from all subjects involved in the study.

**Data Availability Statement:** Data can be provided by the authors upon reasonable request.

**Conflicts of Interest:** William B. Grant receives funding from Bio-Tech Pharmacal, Inc. (Fayetteville, AR, USA). Other authors declare no conflict of interest.

## References

1. Crimmins, E.; Beltrán-Sánchez, H. Mortality and morbidity trends: Is there compression of morbidity? *J. Gerontol. B Psychol. Sci. Soc. Sci.* **2011**, *66*, 75–86. [CrossRef]
2. Kibele, E.U.; Jasilionis, D.; Shkolnikov, V.M. Widening socioeconomic differences in mortality among men aged 65 years and older in Germany. *J. Epidemiol. Community Health* **2013**, *67*, 453–457. [CrossRef]
3. Krumholz, H.M.; Nuti, S.V.; Downing, N.S.; Normand, S.L.; Wang, Y. Mortality, hospitalizations, and expenditures for the medicare population aged 65 years or older, 1999–2013. *JAMA* **2015**, *314*, 355–365. [CrossRef]
4. Leszko, M.; Zając-Lamparska, L.; Trempala, J. Aging in Poland. *Gerontologist* **2015**, *55*, 707–715. [CrossRef]
5. Maniecka-Bryła, I.; Bryła, M.; Bryła, P.; Pikala, M. The burden of premature mortality in Poland analysed with the use of standard expected years of life lost. *BMC Public Health* **2015**, *15*, 1–8. [CrossRef]
6. Liu, K.; Daviglus, M.L.; Loria, C.M.; Colangelo, L.A.; Spring, B.; Moller, A.C.; Lloyd-Jones, D.M. Healthy lifestyle through young adulthood and the presence of low cardiovascular disease risk profile in middle age: The Coronary Artery Risk Development in Young Adults (CARDIA) study. *Circulation* **2012**, *125*, 996–1004. [CrossRef]
7. Lozano, R.; Naghavi, M.; Foreman, K.; Lim, S.; Shibuya, K.; Aboyans, V.; Abraham, J.; Adair, T.; Aggarwal, R.; Ahn, S.Y.; et al. Global and regional mortality from 235 causes of death for 20 age groups in 1990 and 2010: A systematic analysis for the Global Burden of Disease Study 2010. *Lancet* **2012**, *380*, 2095–2128. [CrossRef]
8. Roth, G.A.; Mensah, G.A.; Johnson, C.O.; Addolorato, G.; Ammirati, E.; Baddour, L.M.; Barengo, N.C.; Beaton, A.Z.; Benjamin, E.J.; Benziger, C.P.; et al. Global Burden of Cardiovascular Diseases and Risk Factors, 1990–2019: Update from the GBD 2019 Study. *J. Am. Coll. Cardiol.* **2020**, *76*, 2982–3021. [CrossRef]
9. Suzuki, T.; Kohro, T.; Hayashi, D.; Yamazaki, T.; Nagai, R. Frequency and impact of lifestyle modification in patients with coronary artery disease: The Japanese Coronary Artery Disease (JCAD) study. *Am. Heart J.* **2012**, *163*, 268–273. [CrossRef]
10. Dehghan, M.; Mente, A.; Teo, K.K.; Gao, P.; Sleight, P.; Dagenais, G.; Avezum, A.; Probstfield, J.L.; Dans, T.; Yusuf, S.; et al. Relationship between healthy diet and risk of cardiovascular disease among patients on drug therapies for secondary prevention: A prospective cohort study of 31 546 high risk individuals from 40 countries. *Circulation* **2012**, *126*, 2705–2712. [CrossRef]
11. Holick, M.F. Vitamin D deficiency. *NEJM* **2007**, *357*, 266–281. [CrossRef]
12. Michos, E.D.; Cainzos-Achirica, M.; Heravi, A.S.; Appel, L.J. Vitamin D, Calcium Supplements, and Implications for Cardiovascular Health: JACC Focus Seminar. *J. Am. Coll. Cardiol.* **2021**, *77*, 437–449. [CrossRef]
13. Kassi, E.; Adamopoulos, C.; Basdra, E.K.; Papavassiliou, A.G. Role of vitamin D in atherosclerosis. *Circulation* **2013**, *128*, 2517–2531. [CrossRef]
14. Al Mheid, I.; Quyyumi, A.A. Vitamin D and Cardiovascular Disease: Controversy Unresolved. *J. Am. Coll. Cardiol.* **2017**, *70*, 89–100. [CrossRef]
15. Somjen, D.; Weisman, Y.; Kohen, F.; Gayer, B.; Limor, R.; Sharon, O.; Jaccard, N.; Knoll, E.; Stern, N. 25-hydroxyvitamin D3-1alpha-hydroxylase is expressed in human vascular smooth muscle cells and is upregulated by parathyroid hormone and estrogenic compounds. *Circulation* **2005**, *111*, 1666–1671. [CrossRef]
16. Zehnder, D.; Bland, R.; Chana, R.S.; Wheeler, D.C.; Howie, A.J.; Williams, M.C.; Stewart, P.M.; Hewison, M. Synthesis of 1,25-dihydroxyvitamin D(3) by human endothelial cells is regulated by inflammatory cytokines: A novel autocrine determinant of vascular cell adhesion. *J. Am. Soc. Nephrol.* **2002**, *13*, 621–629.
17. Li, Y.C. 1,25-Dihydroxyvitamin D(3) is a negative endocrine regulator of the renin-angiotensin system. *J. Clin. Investig.* **2002**, *110*, 229–238. [CrossRef]
18. Zhou, C.; Lu, F.; Cao, K.; Xu, D.; Goltzman, D.; Miao, D. Calcium-independent and 1,25(OH)2D3-dependent regulation of the renin-angiotensin system in 1alpha-hydroxylase knockout mice. *Kidney Int.* **2008**, *74*, 170–179. [CrossRef]
19. Chen, S.; Law, C.S.; Grigsby, C.L.; Olsen, K.; Hong, T.T.; Zhang, Y.; Yeghiazarians, Y.; Gardner, D.G. Cardiomyocyte-specific deletion of the vitamin D receptor gene results in cardiac hypertrophy. *Circulation* **2011**, *124*, 1838–1847. [CrossRef]
20. Izzo, M.; Carrizzo, A.; Izzo, C.; Cappello, E.; Cecere, D.; Ciccarelli, M.; Iannece, P.; Damato, A.; Vecchione, C.; Pompeo, F. Vitamin D: Not Just Bone Metabolism but a Key Player in Cardiovascular Diseases. *Life* **2021**, *11*, 452. [CrossRef]
21. Spiro, A.; Buttriss, J.L. Vitamin D: An overview of vitamin D status and intake in Europe. *Nutr. Bull.* **2014**, *39*, 322–350. [CrossRef]
22. Lee, J.H.; Gadi, R.; Spertus, J.A.; Tang, F.; O'Keefe, J.H. Prevalence of vitamin d deficiency in patients with acute myocardial infarction. *Am. J. Cardiol.* **2011**, *107*, 1636–1638. [CrossRef]
23. Pludowski, P.; Holick, M.F.; Pilz, S.; Wagner, C.L.; Hollis, B.W.; Grant, W.B.; Shoenfeld, Y.; Lerchbaum, E.; Llewellyn, D.J.; Kienreich, K.; et al. Vitamin D effects on musculoskeletal health, immunity, autoimmunity, cardiovascular disease, cancer, fertility, pregnancy, dementia and mortality-a review of recent evidence. *Autoimmun. Rev.* **2013**, *12*, 976–989. [CrossRef]
24. Dziedzic, E.A.; Gąsior, J.S.; Pawłowski, M.; Dąbrowski, M. Association of Vitamin D Deficiency and Degree of Coronary Artery Disease in Cardiac Patients with Type 2 Diabetes. *J. Diabetes Res.* **2017**, *2017*, 3929075. [CrossRef]
25. Dziedzic, E.A.; Gąsior, J.S.; Pawłowski, M.; Wodejko-Kucharska, B.; Saniewski, T.; Marcisz, A.; Dąbrowski, M.J. Vitamin D level is associated with severity of coronary artery atherosclerosis and incidence of acute coronary syndromes in non-diabetic cardiac patients. *Arch. Med. Sci.* **2019**, *15*, 359–368. [CrossRef]
26. Dziedzic, E.A.; Przychodzeń, S.; Dąbrowski, M. The effects of vitamin D on severity of coronary artery atherosclerosis and lipid profile of cardiac patients. *Arch. Med. Sci.* **2016**, *12*, 1199–1206. [CrossRef]

27. Dziedzic, E.A.; Gasior, J.S.; Saniewski, T.; Dąbrowski, M. Vitamin D deficiency among Polish patients with angiographically confirmed coronary heart disease. *Pol. Tow. Lek.* **2021**, *49*, 278–282.
28. Cobas E411 Vitamin D Total Reagent Insert (07464215190V2.0), Roche Diagnostics. Available online: http://labogids.sintmaria.be/sites/default/files/files/vit._d_total_ii_2017-11_v2.pdf (accessed on 29 December 2021).
29. Płudowski, P.; Karczmarewicz, E.; Bayer, M.; Carter, G.; Chlebna-Sokół, D.; Czech-Kowalska, J.; Dębski, R.; Decsi, T.; Dobrzańska, A.; Franek, E.; et al. Practical guidelines for the supplementation of vitamin D and the treatment of deficits in Central Europe—Recommended vitamin D intakes in the general population and groups at risk of vitamin D deficiency. *Endokrynol. Pol.* **2013**, *64*, 319–327. [CrossRef]
30. Ringqvist, I.; Fisher, L.D.; Mock, M.; Davis, K.B.; Wedel, H.; Chaitman, B.R.; Passamani, E.; Russell, R.O., Jr.; Alderman, E.L.; Kouchoukas, N.T.; et al. Prognostic value of angiographic indices of coronary artery disease from the Coronary Artery Surgery Study (CASS). *J. Clin. Investig.* **1983**, *71*, 1854–1866. [CrossRef]
31. Gao, Z.; Chen, Z.; Sun, A.; Deng, X. Gender differences in cardiovascular disease. *Med. Nov. Technol. Devices* **2019**, *4*, 100025. [CrossRef]
32. Szulc, P.; Claustrat, B.; Delmas, P.D. Serum concentrations of 17beta-E2 and 25-hydroxycholecalciferol (25OHD) in relation to all-cause mortality in older men—the MINOS study. *Clin. Endocrinol. (Oxf.)* **2009**, *71*, 594–602. [CrossRef]
33. Johansson, H.; Odén, A.; Kanis, J.; McCloskey, E.; Lorentzon, M.; Ljunggren, Ö.; Karlsson, M.K.; Thorsby, P.M.; Tivesten, Å.; Barrett-Connor, E.; et al. Low serum vitamin D is associated with increased mortality in elderly men: MrOS Sweden. *Osteoporos. Int.* **2012**, *23*, 991–999. [CrossRef]
34. Scragg, R.; Jackson, R.; Holdaway, I.M.; Lim, T.; Beaglehole, R. Myocardial-infarction is inversely associated with plasma 25-hydroxyvitamin-D3 levels—a community based study. *Int. J. Epidemiol.* **1990**, *19*, 559–563. [CrossRef]
35. Ng, L.L.; Sandhu, J.K.; Squire, I.B.; Davies, J.E.; Jones, D.J. Vitamin D and prognosis in acute myocardial infarction. *Int. J. Cardiol.* **2013**, *168*, 2341–2346. [CrossRef]
36. De Metrio, M.; Milazzo, V.; Rubino, M.; Cabiati, A.; Moltrasio, M.; Marana, I.; Campodonico, J.; Cosentino, N.; Veglia, F.; Bonomi, A.; et al. Vitamin D plasma levels and in-hospital and 1-year outcomes in acute coronary syndromes: A prospective study. *Medicine* **2015**, *94*, e857. [CrossRef]
37. Aleksova, A.; Belfiore, R.; Carriere, C.; Kassem, S.; La Carrubba, S.; Barbati, G.; Sinagra, G. Vitamin D deficiency in patients with acute myocardial infarction: An italian single-center study. *Int. J. Vitam. Nutr. Res.* **2015**, *85*, 23–30. [CrossRef]
38. Correia, L.C.; Sodré, F.; Garcia, G.; Sabino, M.; Brito, M.; Kalil, F.; Barreto, B.; Lima, J.C.; Noya-Rabelo, M.M. Relation of severe deficiency of vitamin D to cardiovascular mortality during acute coronary syndromes. *Am. J. Cardiol.* **2013**, *111*, 324–327. [CrossRef]
39. Gagnon, C.; Lu, Z.X.; Magliano, D.J.; Dunstan, D.W.; Shaw, J.E.; Zimmet, P.Z.; Sikaris, K.; Ebeling, P.R.; Daly, R.M. Low serum 25-hydroxyvitamin D is associated with increased risk of the development of the metabolic syndrome at five years: Results from a national, population-based prospective study (The Australian Diabetes, Obesity and Lifestyle Study: AusDiab). *J. Clin. Endocrinol. Metab.* **2012**, *97*, 1953–1961. [CrossRef]
40. Pittas, A.G.; Lau, J.; Hu, F.B.; Dawson-Hughes, B. The role of vitamin D and calcium in type 2 diabetes. A systematic review and meta-analysis. *J. Clin. Endocrinol. Metab.* **2007**, *92*, 2017–2029. [CrossRef]
41. Cosentino, N.; Campodonico, J.; Milazzo, V.; De Metrio, M.; Brambilla, M.; Camera, M.; Marenzi, G. Vitamin D and Cardiovascular Disease: Current Evidence and Future Perspectives. *Nutrients* **2021**, *13*, 3603. [CrossRef]
42. Mensah, G.A.; Wei, G.S.; Sorlie, P.D.; Fine, L.J.; Rosenberg, Y.; Kaufmann, P.G.; Mussolino, M.E.; Hsu, L.L.; Addou, E.; Engelgau, M.M.; et al. Decline in Cardiovascular Mortality: Possible Causes and Implications. *Circ. Res.* **2017**, *120*, 366–380. [CrossRef] [PubMed]
43. Norman, P.E.; Powell, J.T. Vitamin D and cardiovascular disease. *Circ. Res.* **2014**, *114*, 379–393. [CrossRef]
44. Zittermann, A. Vitamin D Status, Supplementation and Cardiovascular Disease. *Anticancer Res.* **2018**, *38*, 1179–1186.
45. Karadeniz, Y.; Özpamuk-Karadeniz, F.; Ahbab, S.; Ataoğlu, E.; Can, G. Vitamin D Deficiency Is a Potential Risk for Blood Pressure Elevation and the Development of Hypertension. *Medicina* **2021**, *57*, 1297. [CrossRef]
46. Pilz, S.; Tomaschitz, A. Role of vitamin D in arterial hypertension. *Expert Rev. Cardiovasc. Ther.* **2010**, *8*, 1599–1608. [CrossRef]
47. Cui, C.; Xu, P.; Li, G.; Qiao, Y.; Han, W.; Geng, C.; Liao, D.; Yang, M.; Chen, D.; Jiang, P. Vitamin D receptor activation regulates microglia polarization and oxidative stress in spontaneously hypertensive rats and angiotensin II-exposed microglial cells: Role of renin-angiotensin system. *Redox Biol.* **2019**, *26*, 101295. [CrossRef]
48. Oh, J.; Matkovich, S.J.; Riek, A.E.; Bindom, S.M.; Shao, J.S.; Head, R.D.; Barve, R.A.; Sands, M.S.; Carmeliet, G.; Osei-Owusu, P.; et al. Macrophage secretion of miR-106b-5p causes renin-dependent hypertension. *Nat. Commun.* **2020**, *11*, 4798. [CrossRef]
49. Chen, S.; Swier, V.J.; Boosani, C.S.; Radwan, M.M.; Agrawal, D.K. Vitamin D deficiency accelerates coronary artery disease progression in swine. *Arterioscler. Thromb. Vasc. Biol.* **2016**, *36*, 1651–1659. [CrossRef]
50. Ahmad, M.I.; Chevli, P.A.; Li, Y.; Soliman, E.Z. Vitamin D deficiency and electrocardiographic subclinical myocardial injury: Results from national health and nutrition examination survey-iii. *Clin. Cardiol.* **2018**, *41*, 1468–1473. [CrossRef]
51. Bahar-Shany, K.; Ravid, A.; Koren, R. Upregulation of MMP-9 production by TNFalpha in keratinocytes and its attenuation by vitamin D. *J. Cell. Physiol.* **2010**, *222*, 729–737.
52. Mantell, D.J.; Owens, P.E.; Bundred, N.J.; Mawer, E.B.; Canfield, A.E. 1 Alpha,25-dihydroxyvitamin D (3) inhibits angiogenesis in vitro and in vivo. *Circ. Res.* **2000**, *87*, 214–220. [CrossRef] [PubMed]

53. Koyama, T.; Shibakura, M.; Ohsawa, M.; Kamiyama, R.; Hirosawa, S. Anticoagulant effects of 1alpha,25dihydroxyvitamin D3 on human myelogenous leukemia cells and monocytes. *Blood* **1998**, *92*, 160–167. [CrossRef] [PubMed]
54. Płudowski, P.; Ducki, C.; Konstantynowicz, J.; Jaworski, M. Vitamin D status in Poland. *Pol. Arch. Med. Wewn* **2016**, *126*, 530–539. [CrossRef] [PubMed]
55. Pludowski, P.; Grant, W.B.; Bhattoa, H.P.; Bayer, M.; Povoroznyuk, V.; Rudenka, E.; Ramanau, H.; Varbiro, S.; Rudenka, A.; Karczmarewicz, E.; et al. Vitamin D status in Central Europe. *Int. J. Endocrinol.* **2014**, *2014*, 589587. [CrossRef]
56. Verdoia, M.; Schaffer, A.; Barbieri, L.; Di Giovine, G.; Marino, P.; Suryapranata, H.; De Luca, G.; Novara Atherosclerosis Study Group (NAS). Impact of gender difference on vitamin D status and its relationship with the extent of coronary artery disease. *Nutr. Metab. Cardiovasc. Dis.* **2015**, *25*, 464–470. [CrossRef]
57. Wang, T.J.; Pencina, M.J.; Booth, S.L.; Jacques, P.F.; Ingelsson, E.; Lanier, K.; Benjamin, E.J.; D'Agostino, R.B.; Wolf, M.; Vasan, R.S. Vitamin D deficiency and risk of cardiovascular disease. *Circulation* **2008**, *117*, 503–511. [CrossRef]
58. Giovannucci, E.; Liu, Y.; Hollis, B.W.; Rimm, E.B. 25-hydroxyvitamin d and risk of myocardial infarction in men: A prospective study. *Arch. Intern Med.* **2008**, *168*, 1174–1180. [CrossRef]
59. Dalle Carbonare, L.; Valenti, M.T.; Del Forno, F.; Caneva, E.; Pietrobelli, A. Vitamin D: Daily vs. Monthly use in children and elderly—what is going on? *Nutrients* **2017**, *9*, 652. [CrossRef]
60. Zhao, D.; Ouyang, P.; de Boer, I.H.; Lutsey, P.L.; Farag, Y.M.; Guallar, E.; Siscovick, D.S.; Post, W.S.; Kalyani, R.R.; Billups, K.L.; et al. Serum vitamin D and sex hormones levels in men and women: The Multi-Ethnic Study of Atherosclerosis (MESA). *Maturitas* **2017**, *96*, 95–102. [CrossRef]
61. Bouillon, R.; Marcocci, C.; Carmeliet, G.; Bikle, D.; White, J.H.; Dawson-Hughes, B.; Lips, P.; Munns, C.F.; Lazaretti-Castro, M.; Giustina, A.; et al. Skeletal and Extraskeletal Actions of Vitamin D: Current Evidence and Outstanding Questions. *Endocr. Rev.* **2019**, *40*, 1109–1151. [CrossRef]
62. Bouillon, R.; Manousaki, D.; Rosen, C.; Trajanoska, K.; Rivadeneira, F.; Richards, J.B. The health effects of vitamin D supplementation: Evidence from human studies. *Nat. Rev. Endocrinol.* **2022**, *18*, 96–110. [CrossRef]
63. Manson, J.E.; Cook, N.R.; Lee, I.M.; Christen, W.; Bassuk, S.S.; Mora, S.; Gibson, H.; Gordon, D.; Copeland, T.; D'Agostino, D.; et al. Vitamin D Supplements and Prevention of Cancer and Cardiovascular Disease. *N. Engl. J. Med.* **2019**, *380*, 33–44. [CrossRef]
64. Scragg, R.; Khaw, K.T.; Toop, L.; Sluyter, J.; Lawes, C.M.M.; Waayer, D.; Giovannucci, E.; Camargo, C.A., Jr. Monthly High-Dose Vitamin D Supplementation and Cancer Risk: A Post Hoc Analysis of the Vitamin D Assessment Randomized Clinical Trial. *JAMA Oncol.* **2018**, *4*, e182178. [CrossRef]
65. Pittas, A.G.; Dawson-Hughes, B.; Sheehan, P.; Ware, J.H.; Knowler, W.C.; Aroda, V.R.; Brodsky, I.; Ceglia, L.; Chadha, C.; Chatterjee, R.; et al. Vitamin D supplementation and prevention of type 2 diabetes. *N. Engl. J. Med.* **2019**, *381*, 520–530. [CrossRef]
66. Barbarawi, M.; Kheiri, B.; Zayed, Y.; Barbarawi, O.; Dhillon, H.; Swaid, B.; Yelangi, A.; Sundus, S.; Bachuwa, G.; Alkotob, M.L.; et al. Vitamin D Supplementation and Cardiovascular Disease Risks in More Than 83,000 Individuals in 21 Randomized Clinical Trials: A Meta-analysis. *JAMA Cardiol.* **2019**, *4*, 765–776. [CrossRef]
67. Zhou, A.; Selvanayagam, J.B.; Hyppönen, E. Non-linear Mendelian randomization analyses support a role for vitamin D deficiency in cardiovascular disease risk. *Eur. Heart J.* **2021**, *11*, 809. [CrossRef]

MDPI
St. Alban-Anlage 66
4052 Basel
Switzerland
Tel. +41 61 683 77 34
Fax +41 61 302 89 18
www.mdpi.com

*Journal of Clinical Medicine* Editorial Office
E-mail: jcm@mdpi.com
www.mdpi.com/journal/jcm

www.ingramcontent.com/pod-product-compliance
Lightning Source LLC
LaVergne TN
LVHW070611100526
838202LV00012B/621